RECENT ADVANCES IN DRUG ADDICTION RESEARCH AND CLINICAL APPLICATIONS

Edited by **William M. Meil**
and **Christina L. Ruby**

Recent Advances in Drug Addiction Research and Clinical Applications
http://dx.doi.org/10.5772/61445
Edited by William M. Meil and Christina L. Ruby

Contributors

Patrizia Zeppegno, Carla Gramaglia, Ada Lombardi, Annalisa Rossi, Alessandro Feggi, Janet Neisewander, Ryan Bastle, Selena Bartlett, Omkar Patkar, Arnauld Belmer, Anton J.M. Loonen, Arnt F.A. Schellekens, Svetlana A. Ivanova, Elisabet Jerlhag, John Mills, Melanie Marie Pina, Amy Williams, Jennifer Willford, Conner Smith, Tyler Kuhn, Brady Weber

Published by InTech

Janeza Trdine 9, 51000 Rijeka, Croatia

Publishing Process Manager Dajana Pemac
Technical Editor SPi Global
Cover InTech Design team

First published July, 2016
Printed in Croatia

Additional hard copies can be obtained from orders@intechopen.com

Recent Advances in Drug Addiction Research and Clinical Applications, Edited by William M. Meil and Christina L. Ruby
p. cm.
Print ISBN 978-953-51-2491-7
Online ISBN 978-953-51-2492-4

For EU product safety concerns:
IN TECH d.o.o., Prolaz Marije Krucifikse Kozulić 3, 51000 Rijeka, Croatia,
info@intechopen.com or visit our website at intechopen.com.

Meet the editors

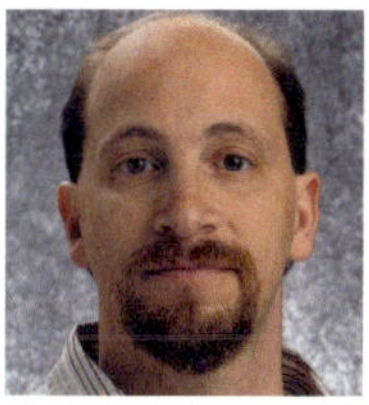

Dr. William M. Meil is a full-time professor in the Psychology Department at the Indiana University of Pennsylvania. He previously was a postdoctoral fellow at The Northeastern Ohio Universities Colleges of Medicine and Pharmacy in Rootstown, Ohio. He was awarded an MA degree in Psychology from The University of Hartford in West Hartford, Connecticut, and PhD in Psychology from Washington State University in Pullman, Washington. His research has spanned human and laboratory animal studies investigating the neurobiological basis of substance abuse and addiction. The current focus of his research is the examination of ecologically valid measures of executive function as predictors of substance abuse and recovery from addiction. He is the author of many peer-reviewed book chapters and journal articles.

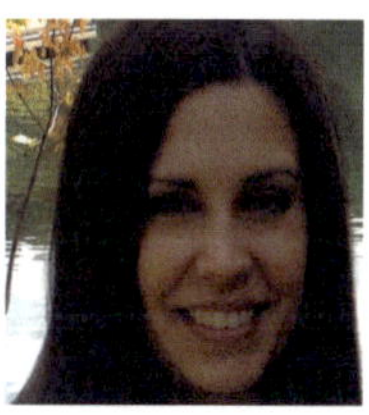

Dr. Christina L. Ruby is an assistant professor of Biology at Indiana University of Pennsylvania. Prior to her current appointment, she held a postdoctoral fellowship at Mayo Clinic College of Medicine in Rochester, Minnesota. She earned her PhD in Physiology from Kent State University in Kent, Ohio. Christina has over 10 years of research experience studying the neurobiology of alcohol addiction. She has authored numerous peer-reviewed original research articles, reviews, and book chapters, some of which has been highlighted in the popular press. She has also provided several manuscript reviews for journals.

Contents

Preface

Drug addiction represents a major public health concern. This statement has been echoed at the beginning of many of our papers and presentations over the last 20 years, and we imagine this has been the same for the majority of our colleagues. Indeed, substance use disorders have taken and continue to take a major toll on individuals, families, clinicians, and society at large. However, beyond this beginning statement, the majority of this book does not resemble one that might have been written 20 years ago. Technological advances and the findings that have followed from their application have allowed our understanding of drug addiction to progress. Moreover, we are seeing an emphasis on translating our growing knowledge to advances into clinical practice. This book includes eight chapters that not only review the past and present status of various topics related to drug addiction, but also illustrate how our increasing understanding of the neurobiological basis of drug addiction is laying the foundation for future clinical approaches that will benefit those suffering from addictive disorders.

This book opens with a discussion of the neurocircuitry underlying addictive behavior through the lens of evolution. From this unique perspective, Chapter 1 describes the roles of the lateral and medial habenula in modulating the activity of the monoaminergic reward pathways (classically the primary focus of addiction research) and the stress/anxiety pathways (increasingly recognized as central to addiction). The authors present an anatomical model in which the lateral habenula gates reward-seeking depending on the valence of the expected reward, and the medial habenula activates misery-fleeing behavior and dysphoria that accompany drug craving. Consequently, the authors postulate that the habenula has a dual-role in transition to addiction and relapse during abstinence. Chapter 2 continues with epigenetic mechanisms in addiction, a relatively nascent, but intriguing field of study. Epigenetic modifications, such as DNA methylation, histone modification, and non-coding RNAs, induce long-lasting, even intergenerational, changes in gene expression and are thus poised to contribute uniquely to the relapsing nature of addiction. Although studies to date have focused primarily on alcohol and cocaine, evidence that epigenetic modifications mediate many of the persistent molecular changes in the brain occurring with repeated drug exposure, or life experiences that confer risk for addiction (such as stress), is compelling.

Chapter 3 summarizes the commonly used rodent models of alcohol intake and seeking behavior and discusses how they have combined with recent methodological advances to reveal neurobiological substrate regulating aspects of alcohol use disorders. The authors present the strengths and limitations of drinking paradigms as well as operant self-administration and place conditioning, which reflect the importance of environmental cues in relapse. Chapter 3 then describes the classical and modern techniques used to elucidate the molecular mechanisms and neural structures that mediate alcohol-related behavior. Finally, the authors discuss some key findings in the alcohol research field made possible by these approaches. Chapter 4 further develops the well-established role of dopaminergic signaling in alcohol drinking and reward. It reviews the efficacy and tolerability of pharmacological treatments targeting dopamine transmission and suggests that newer agents that stabilize or indirectly modulate the mesolimbic dopamine system may be superior therapies, reflecting the paradigm shift from potent selective pharmaceuticals to more moderate approaches that target drug reward with fewer side effects. Chapter 5 further illustrates how our understanding of addiction now extends well beyond the mesolimbic dopamine system. This chapter highlights how dysregulation of serotonin and noradrenaline within the basolateral amygdala results in stress-induced negative emotional states upon alcohol withdrawal and subsequent craving and vulnerability to relapse. The potential of several putative pharmacotherapies for alcohol use disorders that target these transmitter systems are addressed.

Despite being endorsed by the majority of psychological and medical organizations, the medical or disease model of drug addiction remains overshadowed by the view that drug addiction represents a moral failing among wide swaths of the population. The continued controversy surrounding these theoretical perspectives can be seen across Chapter 6, which provides an overview of major approaches to treating substance use disorders, outlining their origins and core features. Moreover, this chapter provides the reader with a platform to consider advances in clinical practices, the importance of evidence-based approaches to treating addiction, and considers how drug courts may represent a potential reconciliation of the medical and moral approaches to addressing substance use disorders. The value of appreciating the dynamic nature of factors related to the development of drug addiction is well illustrated in Chapter 7, which compares two cohorts of dual diagnosis patients admitted to an acute psychiatry ward 10 years apart. This chapter highlights that while our current knowledge of substance use disorders can be informed by past research, we cannot solely rely on our previous understanding as a variety of changing demographic, societal, and pharmacological influences can shape the nature of problems faced by addicts and healthcare professionals alike. Chapter 8 reviews recent neuroimaging studies examining the effects of prenatal exposure across of a variety of addictive drugs on brain structure, function, developmental trajectory, and behavior. While emphasizing the challenges associated with research examining the effects of prenatal drug exposure this chapter also raises the possibilities that biomarkers will emerge that might ultimately inform prevention and intervention programs.

Perhaps believing we will one day be saying that drug addiction is no longer a major public health concern is both optimistic and unrealistic? It is our hope that in coming decades we will see many of the ideas and translational approaches articulated here come to fruition and the next wave of technological advances will build upon our cumulative understanding of addictive processes and reduce the suffering of those directly and indirectly impacted by substance use disorders.

William M. Meil Ph.D.
Professor of Psychology
Indiana University of Pennsylvania

Christina L. Ruby Ph.D.
Assistant Professor of Biology
Indiana University of Pennsylvania

Chapter 1

Circuits Regulating Pleasure and Happiness: A Focus on Addiction, Beyond the Ventral Striatum

Anton J.M. Loonen, Arnt F.A. Schellekens and
Svetlana A. Ivanova

Additional information is available at the end of the chapter

http://dx.doi.org/10.5772/62707

Abstract

A recently developed anatomical model describes how the intensity of reward-seeking and misery-fleeing behaviours is regulated. The first type of behaviours is regulated within an extrapyramidal cortical–subcortical circuit containing as first relay stations, the caudate nucleus, putamen and core of the accumbens nucleus. The second type of behaviours is controlled by a limbic cortical–subcortical circuit with as first stations, the centromedial amygdala, extended amygdala, bed nucleus of the stria terminalis and shell of the accumbens nucleus. We hypothesize that sudden cessation of hyperactivity of the first circuit results in feelings of pleasure and of the second circuit in feelings of happiness. The insular cortex has probably an essential role in the perception of these and other emotions. Motivation to show these behaviours is regulated by monoaminergic neurons projecting to the accumbens from the midbrain: dopaminergic ventral tegmental nuclei, adrenergic locus coeruleus and serotonergic upper raphe nuclei. The activity of these monoaminergic nuclei is in turn regulated through a ventral pathway by the prefrontal cortex and through a dorsal pathway by the medial and lateral habenula. The habenula has this role since the first vertebrate human ancestors with a brain comparable to that of modern lampreys. The lateral habenula promotes or inhibits reward-seeking behaviours depending upon the gained reward being larger or smaller than expected. It is suggested that the ventral pathway is essential for maintaining addiction based on the observation of specific cues, while the dorsal pathway is essential for becoming addicted and relapsing during periods of abstinence.

Keywords: addiction, mood, habenula, basal ganglia, amygdala, insula

1. Introduction

The dominant view on the neuro-pathology of addiction is that of deficient control processes resulting from impaired prefrontal cortex function and increased saliency of drug-related cues over normal rewarding stimuli [1]. The latter results from altered reward processing in the ventral striatum [1]. An important starting point in this respect has been the work of Koob [2, 3], who integrated knowledge from different fields of science in order to describe a scheme for the neuro-circuitry of addiction. An important component of the work of Koob [4] is the characterization of anti-reward or negative reinforcement in particularly in the more advanced stages of addiction. In his work, he assigns a major role to the activation of the brain stress systems, the amygdala, in particular, in addiction. In line with Koob's work, we propose additional neuro-circuitry to be involved in addiction. In this review, we apply a neuro-evolutionary approach to addiction, in order to identify potential additional subcortical structures that might have relevance for addiction.

Two basic principles of animal life are essential for survival of the individual and as a species. Firstly, the animal should be motivated to obtain food, warmth, sexual gratification and comfort. Secondly, the animal should be motivated to escape from predators, cold, sexual competitors and misery. As the human species currently exists, even our oldest ocean-dwelling ancestors living over 540 million years ago must have been capable to react to the environment to feed, evade predators, defend territory and reproduce. Thus, their primitive nervous systems must have regulated the necessary behaviours and incorporated the most essential structures of all today's freely moving Animalia. However, since then the human brain passed through a long evolutionary pathway during which particularly the forebrain showed major changes. The earliest vertebrate's brain almost completely lacked the human neocortex and the dorsal parts of the basal ganglia [5, 6]. These newer parts of the brain are believed to determine human behaviour to a high extent and consequently receive most attention in research of processes explaining the genesis of mental disorders. This contrasts the involvement in psychiatric disorders of those behavioural processes described above as also being displayed by the most primitive vertebrates. We want to suggest that these actions are still regulated in humans by brain structures derived from the primitive forebrain of the earliest vertebrates. Therefore, we describe the anatomy of the forebrain of the earliest human vertebrate ancestors [6]. From a comparison of the striatum of lampreys to that of anuran amphibians and younger vertebrates, it can be concluded that the striatum of lampreys is the forerunner of the human centromedial (i.e. nuclear) amygdala. In anuran amphibians (frogs and toads), the lamprey's striatum is retrieved as central and medial amygdaloid nuclei, while a dorsal striatum for the first time appears in its direct vicinity [6, 7]. The lampreys forebrain also contains a structure of which the connections are very well conserved in more recent human ancestors: the habenula. The habenula constitutes—together with the stria medullaris and pineal gland—the epithalamus and consists of medial and lateral parts [8]. The habenula has received much attention because of it asymmetry in certain vertebrate species [9] and its role in mediating biorhythms [10]. The habenula regulates the intensity of reward-seeking and misery-fleeing behaviour probably in all our vertebrate ancestors. In lampreys, the activity of the lateral habenula is in turn regulated by a specific structure: the habenula-projecting globus

http://dx.doi.org/10.5772/62707

pallidus. It is tempting to speculate that this structure has a similar role in humans, but a clear anatomical human equivalent with the same function has not yet been identified. Based upon the evolution of the basal ganglia in vertebrates and the mechanism of the emotional response, we postulate the existence of two systems regulating the intensity of the aforementioned behaviours [11]. These two circuits include the extrapyramidal and limbic basal ganglia, which are collaborating in a reciprocal (i.e. Yin-and-Yang) fashion. The two basal ganglia systems are linked together by the core and shell parts of the nucleus accumbens (NAcb), which regulates motivation to show reward-seeking and misery-fleeing behaviour, respectively. Hijacking of the reward-seeking mechanism by certain substances such as alcohol or illicit drugs is considered the essential mechanism behind addiction.

In this chapter, we will describe the evolution of the vertebrate forebrain and the functioning of the described regulatory circuits in somewhat more detail. Thereafter, the putative role of the habenula in initiating addiction and causing relapse after abstinence is depicted. The described model also explains the mood and anxiety symptoms that accompany the addictive process. We will start with a brief description of the mechanism of the emotional process [11, 12].

2. Model for emotional regulation

A suitable model for the regulation of the emotional response can be derived from the paper of Terence and Mark Sewards [13]. According to their model, the control centre for emotional response types such as *sexual desire*, *hunger*, *thirst*, *fear*, *nurturance* and *sleep-need* drives and *power-dominance* drives is the hypothalamus. The output of the hypothalamus proceeds along three channels. The first route projects via the thalamus to the cortex, including a pathway that contributes to the perception of emotion and one for the initiation and planning of cognitive and motor responses (drives). The second output pathway is a projection at least partly via the periaqueductal grey (PAG) to several brainstem nuclei, including nuclei that regulate the autonomic components of the emotional response (e.g. increased circulation and respiration). The PAG also activates the serotonergic raphe nuclei, the adrenergic locus coeruleus complex and the dopaminergic ventral tegmental area. From these nuclei, projections pass back to the hypothalamus (e.g. regulating hypophysiotropic hormones) and through the medial forebrain bundle to the forebrain (activating the frontal cortex). The PAG also constitutes an important input structure generating signals to the emotional forebrain. Apart from hormone release mediated through various brainstem nuclei, a third direct hypothalamic projection system regulates the endocrine component of the emotional response (also by releasing hypophysiotropic hormones), enabling adaptation of the milieu interne, or correction of a possible misbalance. The hypothalamus also exerts a receptor function for various substances in the circulating blood.

This model corresponds to a significant extent with the model of Liotti and Panksepp [14]. However, they follow a different approach, describing seven emotional systems for *seeking*, *rage*, *fear*, *panic* (separation distress and social bonding), *care* (nursing and empathy), *lust* (sexual love) and *play* (joy and curiosity), which are not all regulated by the autonomic hypothalamus. Within the context of this article, the first three systems of Liotti and Panksepp deserve a more detailed description.

The appetitive motivation-*seeking* system stimulates the organism to acquire the many things needed for survival. This motivation is coupled to a reward feeling that can—but not necessarily does—result from these activities. The nature of the specific rewards is of a lesser importance; the system works equally well for seeking food, water, warmth, and illicit drugs, as well as for social goals such as sexual gratification, maternal engagement and playful entertainment. The system promotes interest, curiosity and desire for engagement with necessary daily life activities. The process of reward pursuing consists of at least three psychological components: learning to value (attentive salience), incentive salience or 'wanting' and experiencing pleasure resulting in 'liking'. The first component is believed to be addressed by the amygdala. The amygdala can 'learn' by conditioning to appreciate sensory appetitive information within the context of external and internal circumstances and to initiate a proper response. Incentive salience is regulated by mesocorticolimbic mechanisms, with a central role for the NAcb. Later, in this chapter, we will describe that the insula plays an essential role in perceiving pleasure.

The amygdala additionally takes a central position with respect to valuing aversive stimuli, playing a critical role in anxiety and aggression. The anger-promoting rage system is associated with irritation and frustration. In this system, the emotional circuit is stimulated by projections

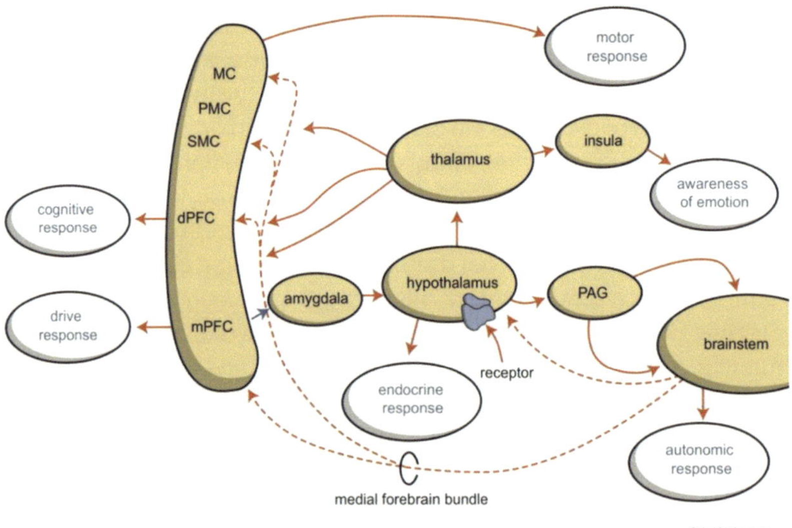

Figure 1. Simplified model for the regulation of emotional response. The hypothalamus is considered to be the principle controller and the amygdala the initiator of emotional response. In this depiction, the amygdala represents all limbic structures involved in emotional response. The amygdala is inhibited by the mPFC (blue arrow). MC = motor cortex, PAG = periaqueductal grey substance, dPFC = dorsolateral prefrontal cortex, mPFC = medial prefrontal cortex, PMC = premotor cortex, SMC = supplementary motor cortex.

between the medial amygdala and the medial hypothalamus via the stria terminalis. Neurons also project reciprocally between specific parts of the PAG in the mesencephalon and the medial hypothalamus. The fear system is organized in a fashion parallel to the rage system, in which both the amygdala and the PAG project to the medial hypothalamus. Activity within this system can lead to freezing or flight behaviour. Sustained fear (anxiety) is also mediated by the amygdala but follows a slightly different anatomical route and links the fear and stress systems.

Taken together, the regulation of the described forms of emotional output can be summarized and simplified into the scheme in **Figure 1**. The hypothalamus can be considered one of the principle control centres for emotional (non-behavioural) output (especially gratification, fear and aggression-driven). The hypothalamus regulates three components of this response: a thalamic one, a brainstem one and a pituitaric one. As explained above, the hypothalamus itself receives a stimulating input function from the amygdala, among other regions. The amygdala is responsible for the initiation of a suitable response type. In this process of initiating the emotional response, the amygdala is inhibited by the medial prefrontal cortex. This scheme describes the process of response selection, but another mechanism is regulating the level of motivation to exhibit the selected response type.

3. Perception of feelings of pleasure and happiness

According to Terence and Mark Sewards [13], the cortical representations of their emotional response types are located on the medial prefrontal and anterior cingulate areas. However, these cortical areas represent the fields initiating the corresponding drives for finding relief and are unlikely directly involved in the perception of feelings of thirst, hunger, sleepiness, somatic pain, etcetera, as these anterior cerebral areas are generally implicated in generating output. A better candidate for the perception of feelings of pleasure (reward) and happiness (euphoria) would be the insular cortex (**Figure 2**) as the posterior part of the insula contains areas for gustation, thermo-sensation, pain, somato-sensation, and viscera-sensation [15]. Indeed, the insular cortex has been demonstrated to be involved in processing emotions, such as anger, fear, happiness, sadness or disgust, and has been shown to display treatment-responsive changes of activity in different mood disorders [16]. However, the exact position of the insular cortex with respect to the perception of the discussed feelings remains unclear. The insular cortex, being located in the centre of the cerebral hemisphere, is reciprocally connected with almost every other input and output structure of the emotional response system. It could also be suggested that the insula's most important role is the integration and adjustment of the activities of such other brain structures without being primarily involved in the perception of emotional feelings itself.

However, yet another possibility comes into mind, which can be considered a revival of the late nineteenth century hypothesis developed independently by the US American William James (1842–1910) and the Dane Carl Lange (1834–1900) [17]. Their theories on the origin and nature of emotions states that once we become aware of the physiological bodily changes induced by, for example, danger, we feel the corresponding emotion of fear [18, 19]. So, the

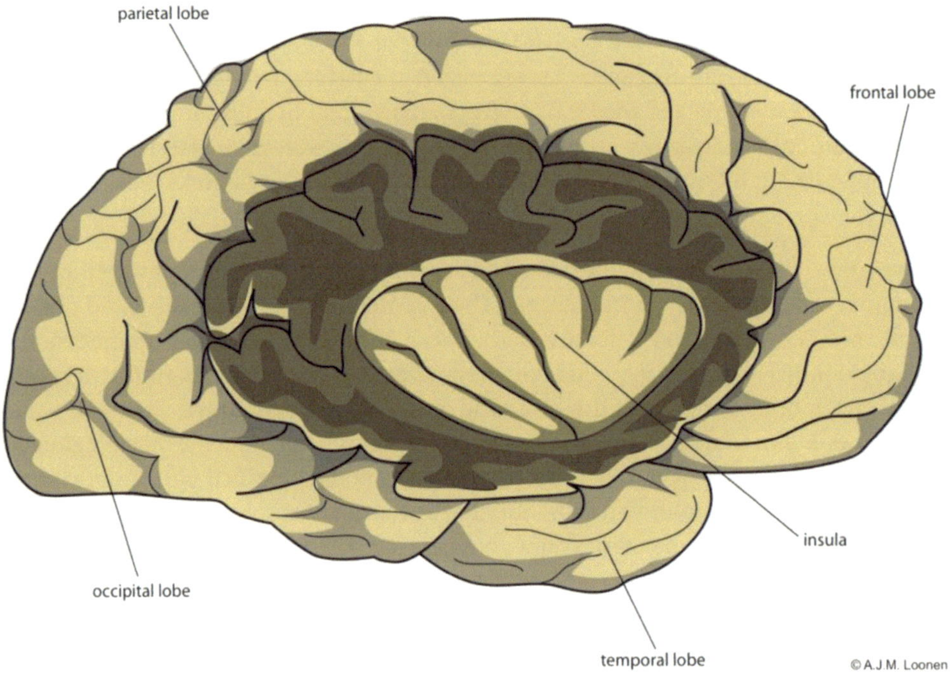

Figure 2. Position of the insular cortex. The human insular cortex forms a distinct, but entirely hidden cerebral lobe, situated in the depth of the Sylvian fissure. It is a phylogenetically ancient part of the cerebral hemisphere and entirely overgrown by adjacent regions of the hemispheres and the temporal lobe (cf. [15]).

basic premise of this theory is that the perception of interoceptive stimuli instigates the experience of an emotional feeling as well as its phenomenal consciousness. This could easily be expanded with the perception of other changes including environmental factors, which then would induce exteroceptive stimuli [19]. The anteriorly directed processing stream within the insula would make the anterior insula perfectly suitable to fulfil the requirements for the neuronal representative of such functions [20]. The upper part of the anterior insula is strongly and reciprocally connected with the anterior cingulate cortex, and the lower part is functionally linked to the adjacent caudal orbitofrontal cortex, which makes the anterior insula involved in food-related stimuli and the urge to take drugs as well [15].

The orbitofrontal cortex is the neuronal structure, which is most intricately involved in motivating for reward bringing behaviours [21, 22]. Perhaps the insula is involved in experiencing pleasure, but in our opinion, this is unlike to occur directly as sensing these positive feelings. As a matter of fact, the orbitofrontal cortex induces motivation to go for the possibility to obtain food, sex or drugs, which results in an unpleasant urge to exhibit this behaviour, called 'craving' [2–4]. This craving feeling results from hyperactivity of the motivational cortical–striatal–thalamic–cortical (CSTC) reentry circuit, running from the orbitofrontal cortex, through the core part of the NAcb, ventral pallidum and thalamus back to the orbitofrontal cortex [23]. It has been suggested that the NAcb itself is responsible for sensing pleasure, but this is unlike to be true. Probably, the nucleus accumbens core (NAcbC) has a classical role of adapting the activity when reward is expected based upon information about other significant factors [24]. We want to hypothesize that the experience of pleasure is more likely related with the sudden ceasing of the urge to obtain the delightful objects once they are acquired.

Evidence for this last proposal can be derived from investigating neuro-activation during a very pleasurable activity; that is having sex. The activity pattern during sexual activity has been extensively studied [24, 25]. In women, first the medial amygdala and insula become activated, among other structures; then, the cingulate cortex is added to this activation; and then, at orgasm itself, the NAcb, paraventricular nucleus of the hypothalamus (secretes oxytocin) and hippocampus become active [25]. Specific experiments by Georgiadis and colleagues [26, 27] have shown that during orgasm, which is the moment that true pleasure is perceived, the activation of brain structures is very much the same in men and women. What is particularly interesting is that they found a profound deactivation in the anterior part of the orbitofrontal cortex (and also in the temporal lobe). Georgiades and colleagues [27] interpret the decreased activity of the orbitofrontal cortex and the temporal lobe to reflect the occurrence of satiety. But this idea may be too limited. In our opinion, they also make a case that the relief that accompanies the disappearance of the urge to reach orgasm is indeed the most important representation of pleasure itself. The reaction within the orbitofrontal cortex may be due to the loss of anticipating achieving the important goal (because it has been reached). The profound deactivation of the motivational reentry circuit would result in abrupt ceasing of craving, what in itself could result in pleasure. This would also indicate that without craving also pleasure cannot occur.

A prefrontal structure that has consistently been implicated in negative mood states (i.e. dysphoria) is the subgenual part of the anterior cingulate cortex (Brodmann's areas 25 and the caudal portions of Brodmann's areas 32 and 24). Anatomical studies have shown that the volume of the infralimbic sgACC is reduced in certain depressed groups [28]. Moreover, the activity of the sgACC is affected following successful treatment with SSRIs, electroconvulsive therapy, transcranial magnetic stimulation (rTMS), ablative surgery and deep brain stimulation [29]. Moreover, this sgACC has been found to be metabolically overactive in depressed states and reacts to the treatment with a decrease of its activity [30].

As shown in **Figure 3**, the infralimbic subgenual part of the anterior cingulate cortex is one of the structures, which feeds the shell part of the NAcb [31]. Hyperactivity of this structure might well result in hyperactivity within a putative emotional reentry circuit, which starts and ends within the anterior cingulate cortex. The subgenual cingulate gyrus sends efferents to all subcortical structures of our limbic basal ganglia and receives afferents from several hypothalamic and thalamic nuclei [32]. This hyperactivation of the subgenual cingulate gyrus might in turn results in increased stimulation of the anterior insula [32], which might lead to experiencing feelings of dysphoria. Abrupt termination of this hyperactivity might result in happiness in the same manner as ending craving would result in pleasure.

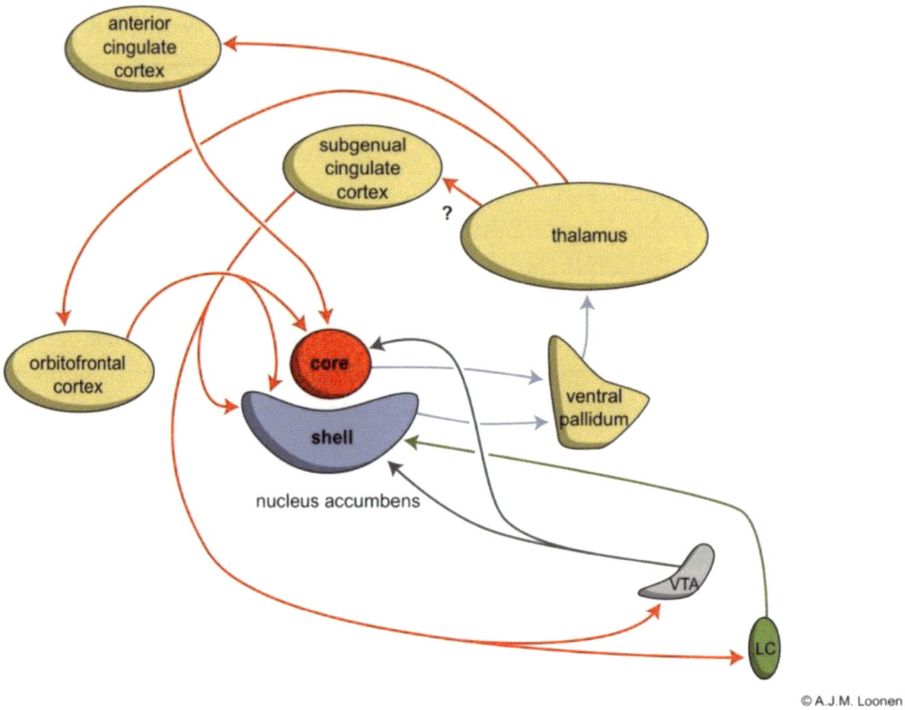

Figure 3. Stimulation of the core and shell of the nucleus accumbens. (Adapted from Ref. [31], reproduced with permission of the author). VTA = ventral tegmental area; LC = locus coeruleus. Red = glutamatergic, blue = GABAergic, grey = dopaminergic and green = adrenergic.

In conclusion, we want to hypothesize that two parallel cortical–subcortical reentry circuits regulate motivation to exert reward-bringing and misery-escaping behaviours, respectively. These circuits are involved in causing pleasure and happiness. Hyperactivity of the NAcb core-containing CSTC circuit induces craving and its abrupt ending is experienced as pleasure. Hyperactivity of the NAcb shell-containing CSTC circuit induces dysphoria and abrupt termination of the activity within this circuit would induce happiness.

4. Two complementary regulating circuits

In a previous paper, we have proposed to distinguish two separate circuits regulating skilled (cognitively controlled) and intuitive (emotionally controlled) behaviour: extrapyramidal and limbic circuits [11].

The 'extrapyramidal' circuit is often mainly associated with motor activity but also regulates other behavioural responses. The first relay station of this cortical–subcortical circuit is formed by the striatum, which consists of three parts that correspond to three parallel divisions of the extrapyramidal system: the caudate nucleus (cognitive system), putamen (motor system) and ventral striatum (emotional/motivational system) [23, 33–35]. This last part is formed by the NAcb, which consists of a core (NAcbC) and a shell (NAcbS). The core belongs to the extrapyramidal basal ganglia and is primarily involved in motivating the organism to exhibit skilled behaviour. The shell belongs to the limbic basal ganglia and is primarily involved in facilitating intuitive (emotional) behaviour [23, 35].

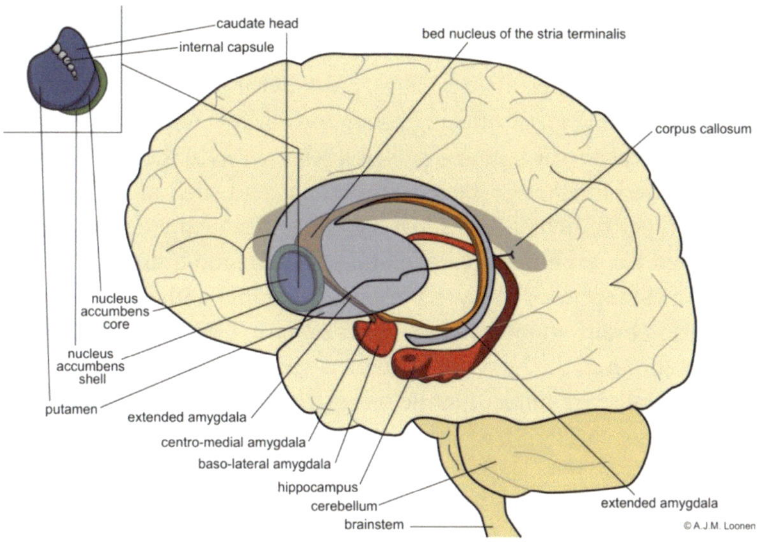

Figure 4. Position of the limbic basal ganglia (centromedial amygdala, extended amygdala, bed nucleus of the stria terminalis and nucleus accumbens shell) relative to the extrapyramidal basal ganglia (caudate nucleus, putamen, nucleus accumbens core) and hippocampus. The figure only shows the first relay stations of the extrapyramidal (light and dark blue) and limbic (orange and green) cortical–subcortical circuits.

The 'limbic' circuit is for a significant extent covered by the amygdala. The amygdala consists of a heterogeneous group of nuclei and cortical regions and is divided into cortical (basolateral) and ganglionic (centromedial) sections [36–38]. The various nuclei differ in the number and type of brain areas to which they are connected. Apart from extensive connectivity with a variety of cortical areas [37], the various parts of the complex are mutually massively connected with each other [37, 38]. Nevertheless, it is possible to consider the centromedial (ganglionic) part as an output channel to the diencephalon and brain stem, while the basolateral (cortical) part is more easily regarded as an input channel for cortical information. Moreover, the amygdaloid complex has widespread connectivity with many subcortical regions [37], including the dorsal and ventral striatum, the bed nucleus of the stria terminalis, and the basal forebrain nuclei. The centromedial amygdala is continuous with the extended amygdala, which is in turn continuous through the bed nucleus of the stria terminalis with the shell part of the NAcb [23, 39]. This extended amygdala takes a position to the allocortex (olfactory cortex and hippocampus) that is similar to that which the neocortex takes to the striatum [39]. This idea can be extended to distinguishing limbic and extrapyramidal basal ganglia. The centromedial amygdala, proper extended amygdala, bed nucleus of the stria terminalis, and the shell of the NAcb form the limbic basal ganglia, with a function for the limbic cortex that reflects that of the extrapyramidal basal ganglia for the rest of the neocortex (**Figure 4**).

5. The evolution of the forebrain in vertebrates

We have developed an anatomical model how the intensity of reward-seeking and misery-fleeing behaviours is regulated. We propose that the first type of reward-seeking behaviours is controlled within a converging extrapyramidal neocortical–subcortical–frontocortical circuit containing as first stations, the caudate nucleus, putamen and core of the accumbens nucleus (NAcbC). The second type of misery-fleeing behaviours is then regulated by a limbic cortical–subcortical–frontocortical circuit containing as first relay stations, the centromedial amygdala, extended amygdala, bed nucleus of the stria terminalis and shell of the accumbens nucleus (NAcbS). As these types of behaviours must also have been exhibited by our most ancient ancestors, we studied the evolutionary development of the forebrain [6]. We found out that the earliest vertebrates, supposed to have a brain comparable with the modern lamprey, had an olfactory bulb, forebrain, diencephalon, brain stem and spinal cord, but not yet a true cerebellum. The forebrain of the lamprey contains a striatum with a modern extrapyramidal system, which is activated by dopaminergic mesostriatal fibres coming from the nucleus of the tuberculum posterior (NTP) [5], which is comparable with human ventral tegmental area

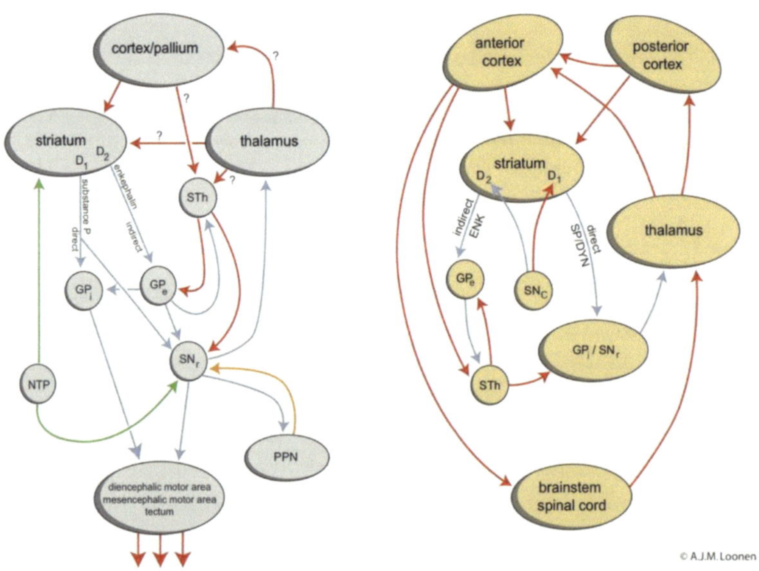

Figure 5. Simplified representation of the extrapyramidal system of lampreys (left) and humans (right). In lampreys, the internal and external parts of the globus pallidus are intermingled within the dorsal pallidum but functionally segregated. For further explanations, consult Refs. [33, 40, 41]. GPe = globus pallidus externa; GPi = globus pallidus interna; NTP = nucleus tuberculi posterior; PPN = pedunculopontine nucleus; SNr = substantia nigra pars reticulata; STh = subthalamic nucleus. Left figure: red = glutamatergic, blue = GABAergic, green = dopaminergic, orange = cholinergic; Right figure: red = excitatory, blue = inhibitory.

(VTA). An extrapyramidal circuit has not yet been developed and the extrapyramidal output ganglia directly activate motor control centres of the brainstem (**Figure 5**). In addition, the dorsal thalamus is very small and the forerunner of the neocortex has hardly developed.

It has been suggested that during evolution of vertebrates, the development of the cerebral cortex resulted in the successive addition of concise modules to the extrapyramidal basal ganglia, each regulating a newly acquired function of the species (**Figure 6**) [5]. What happened on the limbic side is not entirely clear. The amygdaloid complex was moved laterally to the pole of the temporal lobe. The centromedial amygdaloid nuclei can be considered to be a remaining part of the lampreys striatum, but whether the extended amygdala and the bed nucleus of the stria terminalis also evolved from this structure is uncertain. Amphibians already have a bed nucleus of the stria terminalis, which is closely associated with the central and medial nuclear amygdala [42]. The nucleus accumbens can be considered to be the interface between motor and limbic basal ganglia [35]. So, our theory is to a certain extent supported by these evolutionary considerations. We suggest that the core of the accumbens nucleus regulates the motivation to exhibit reward-driven (approach) behaviour and the shell of the accumbens nucleus regulates the motivation to exhibit misery-driven (avoidance) behaviour.

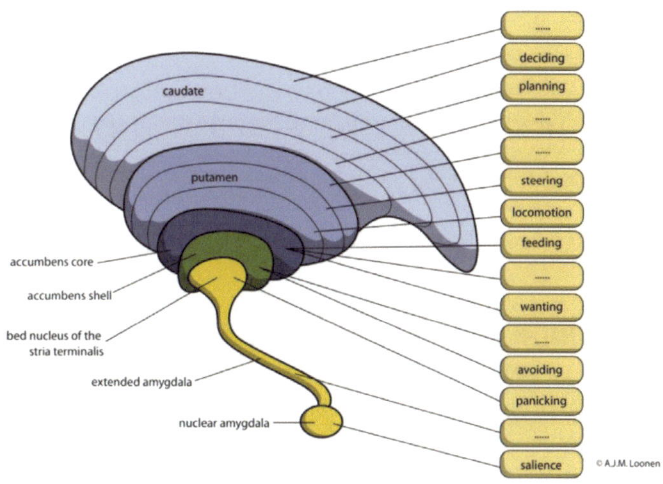

Figure 6. Modular expansion of the basal ganglia during evolution of vertebrates (adapted from [5]). The figure only shows the first relay stations of the extrapyramidal (light and dark blue) and limbic (yellow and green) cortical–subcortical circuits.

But how is this motivation to show these two types of behaviours adapted to the changing demands of environment? At this point, again, considering the forebrain of lampreys can shed some light on this matter. Within the lamprey's forebrain, a specific nuclear structure has been identified within the subhippocampal region, called the habenula-projecting globus pallidus (GPh) [6]. This nucleus receives inhibitory control from the striatum and excitatory input from both thalamus and pallium. It activates the lateral habenula, and from there, glutamatergic fibres run directly to the dopaminergic NTP (excitatory) or indirectly via the GABAergic rostromedial tegmental nucleus (inhibitory). These dopaminergic fibres of the NTP regulate the activity of the striatum. So, in lampreys, the activity of the dopaminergic NTP is under the control of an evaluative system with input from the striatum and pallium in order to decide whether the locomotor activity should be increased or not (**Figure 7**). These structures increase activity during reward situations and decrease activity when an expected reward does not occur. A cholinergic circuitry from the medial habenula to the interpeduncular nucleus and periaqueductal grey regulates the fear/flight response.

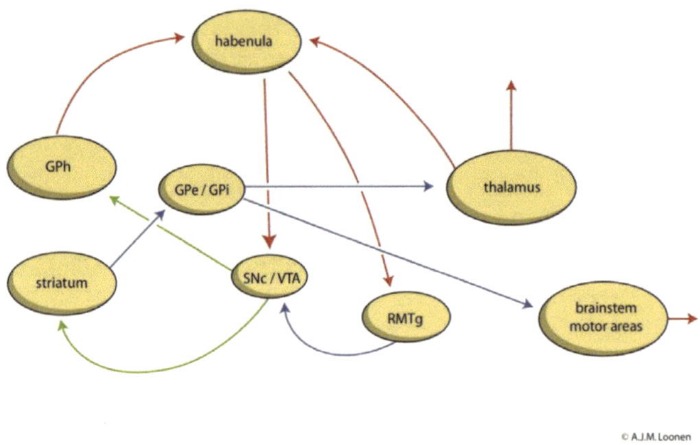

Figure 7. Circuitry of habenula-projecting globus pallidus of lampreys. Red = glutamatergic, blue = GABAergic, green = dopaminergic.

6. The habenula

The habenula in the epithalamus has recently received much attention for possibly playing a role in depression and addiction [43–47]. This is strongly related to the influence of the habenula on the activity of monoaminergic control centres of the brainstem [46, 47]. The habenula is subdivided into two nuclei: the medial habenula and lateral habenula. In lampreys, a direct pathway runs from the homologue of the lateral habenula to the nucleus of the tuberculum posterior (NTP; considered to be a homologue of the SNc/VTA), next to a pathway to a homologue of the GABAergic rostromedial tegmental nucleus (RMTg; which inhibits the NTP) [5, 48]. Other efferents of the lateral habenula run to (diencephalic) histaminergic and serotonergic areas. In lampreys, a projection system from the homologue of the medial habenula to the interpeduncular nucleus was also identified. These habenular output structures are well conserved across species. All the vertebrates examined possess the same efferent pathway, called fasciculus retroflexus, running to the ventral midbrain [9, 46, 47]. In mammals, the medial habenula projects, almost exclusively, to the cholinergic interpeduncular nucleus [49], whereas the lateral habenula projects to a variety of nuclei including the rostromedial tegmental nucleus (RMTg), raphe nuclei, substantia nigra, ventral tegmental area, and the nucleus incertus [9]. Moreover, the medial habenula has direct output to the lateral habenula and may regulate the latter's activity [46, 47] (**Figure 8**).

However, the input to the epithalamus appears to be less well conserved during evolution. In lampreys, the input of the homologue of the medial habenula comes from the medial olfactory bulb, the parapineal organ, the pretectum and the striatum [48]. The input of the lateral habenula comes from subhippocampal lobe (habenula-projecting globus pallidus; GPh) and the lateral hypothalamus, but not from the diagonal band of Broca. Mammals do not have a distinct GPh. It has been suggested that its homologue in primates is localized in the border of the globus pallidus interna (GPb) [5, 50]. Whether the function of the lampreys' GPh is retained within this GPb, is far from certain. The mammalian habenula receives input via the stria medullaris from the posterior septum, as well as from the medial septum, the nucleus of the diagonal band and midbrain structures [47, 49]. Major input to the medial habenula arises from septal nuclei, which in turn receive the majority of their input from the hippocampus [48]. Afferents of the lateral habenula come from the hippocampus, ventral pallidum, lateral hypothalamus, globus pallidus and other basal ganglia structures [46]. It is hypothesized that during evolution from lampreys to mammals, the originally direct sensory innervation of the habenula has been replaced by inputs from the so-called limbic system (i.e. the septum and diagonal band of Broca) [48]. We prefer to say that this is not a replacement, but a maintainment as the human limbic system is considered to be a derivative of the lamprey's forebrain.

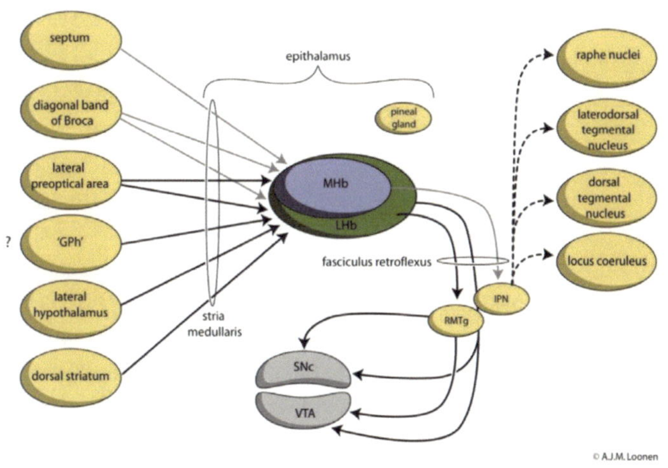

Figure 8. Connectivity through the epithalamus. GPh = habenula-projecting globus pallidus, IPN = interpeduncular nucleus, RMTg = rostromedial tegmental nucleus, SNc = substantia nigra, pars compacta, VTA = ventral tegmental nucleus (adapted from Ref. [47]).

In our opinion, the amygdala plays an essential role in value-based selection of behaviour (salience attribution) and this idea is supported by the history of the amygdaloid complex in our ancestors. When the habenula-projecting globus pallidus still exists and functions in humans, this structure should receive input from the amygdala and hippocampus and give glutamatergic output to the lateral habenula. The amygdala and hippocampus would then regulate both the activity of the medial habenula (misery-fleeing behaviour) via septal nuclei as well as the activity of the lateral habenula (reward-seeking behaviour) via the homologue of the GPh. The amygdala and hippocampus should then be in an essential position for response selection of behaviour.

7. Idea for a possible role of habenula in addiction

In order to be considered to have a substance addiction, the individual must start to abuse a drug, he/she should maintain this abuse and/or he/she should relapse to abuse after a period of abstinence. Several lines of evidence suggest that indeed patients go through different stages of substance use, from intoxication, through repeated cycles of withdrawal and increasing tolerance to an end stage of addiction and relapse [3, 4]. It has also been shown that during this process, the motivation to use substances develops from 'liking' to 'wanting/needing' [3, 4]. In line with these findings, the neurobiological changes develop from more ventral striatal, reward-related, circuits to more dorsal striatal circuits involved in habit formation and stress [3, 4]. Moreover, addicted patients no longer use substances because it is nice (positive reinforcement), but because it reduces a negative affective state, related to increased activity of the brain stress systems, including the amygdala and hypothalamus-pituitary axis (negative reinforcement). This theory describes a development of addiction in three stages: *binge/intoxication*, *withdrawal/negative affect* and *preoccupation/anticipation* [3, 4].

Our proposal of staging is slightly different in order to let it correspond better to the described primitive subcortical regulation of behaviour. Abuse is probably largely maintained by the pathological process of craving for drugs, which is activated by the observation of certain phenomena (cues), the getting involved in social and emotional circumstances or executing specific habits which all are related to the individuals' personal circumstances of drug abuse. We want to suggest that this mechanism (i.e. activation of craving by cues) explains the usage of the illicit drug by the individual on a regular basis. It has been described that the craving process is activated by stimulation of the dopaminergic input to the NAcb from the VTA. This VTA is in turn activated by glutamatergic fibres from the prefrontal cortex by a ventral connection, which are reacting upon analysis of the circumstances that predict the availability of the illicit drug [51]. The glutamatergic synapses with mesencephalic dopaminergic neurons carry nicotinic cholinergic receptors, which allow long term potentiation of this excitatory synaptic transmission [51].

The above mechanism explains how addiction is maintained, but not how it is initiated. We want to hypothesize that in this second process, the habenula is involved (for a description of the role of the habenula in addiction see Refs. [46, 47]). The lateral habenula stimulates or inhibits the VTA depending upon the result of the behaviour. It stimulates the behaviour when the result is more rewarding than expected [52, 53] and inhibits it when the behaviour has more or less disappointing results [54]. The lateral habenula also encodes reward probability, reward magnitude and the upcoming availability of information about reward [54, 55]. So, when an individual uses an illicit drug and the results are very rewarding (biological, psychological or social) the habenula disinhibits the VTA to continue and expand this behaviour. The same is true concerning the rapid reactivation of craving for example tobacco, cocaine or GHB in the case of relapse after a period of abstinence. The lateral habenula could then signal vividly that the individual likes these effects very much. So it could be interesting to study the activity of the pathways during a phase of active drug abuse and after re-usage after a period of abstinence. This could also shed some light on the pharmacological mechanisms to prevent relapse.

Besides craving for the positive effects of substances, craving for addictive substances is also often accompanied by dysphoria and anxiety. This process has been described as the 'dark side of addiction' and has been associated with the development of a powerful negative reinforcement process [4]. This dysphoria is particularly true during relatively long-lasting periods of abstinence when even a clear depression can develop. Koob [4] has introduced the term 'anti-reward' to describe the background of this phenomenon. This is unfortunate, because it suggests a fictitious relationship with the reward-seeking system. However, this dysphoria could very well result from a dysfunction of another pathway connecting amygdaloid complex and hippocampus through the epithalamus with the midbrain. The misery-fleeing (fear/flight) response could be regulated via septal nuclei and medial habenula with the interpeduncular nucleus. Through this pathway, the medial habenula regulates the activity of the adrenergic locus coeruleus and the serotonergic dorsal raphe nucleus [47]. This could result in the activation of the misery-fleeing mechanism, causing dysphoria. The reward-seeking response could be regulated by a parallel pathway via a homologue of GPh and lateral habenula with the ventral tegmental area [56]. Hypoactivity of the reward-driven reentry circuit with as first station NAcbC would result in anhedonia and lack of energy, two main symptoms of depression.

8. Conclusions

Studying the evolution of the vertebrate's forebrain offers interesting clues about the mechanism of addiction. In lampreys, motor activity is regulated by a striatum, which can be considered to be the forerunner of the nuclear amygdala. The lamprey's striatum contains a quite modern extrapyramidal system (**Figure 5**). The activity of this striatum is regulated by dopaminergic fibres coming from the forerunner of the VTA in the midbrain. The activity of the VTA is in turn regulated by the habenula, with a connectivity that is very well conserved during the evolution into finally humans. During this evolution, the basal ganglia developed in a modular fashion with the addition of new layers on the dorsal side of the basal ganglia once new functions developed (**Figure 6**). The evolution of the ventral part of the basal ganglia is less certain, but these structures also became connected with parts of the (limbic) neocortex via the diencephalon. Therefore, it is possible to distinguish extrapyramidal and limbic CSTC circuits, which regulate the magnitude of reward-seeking and misery-fleeing behaviours. Motivation to express these two behaviours is regulated by the NAcbC and NAcbS, respectively. In turn, the VTA determines the activity of NAcb, and the locus coeruleus only of the NAcbS (**Figure 3**). Directly and indirectly, the upper raphe nuclei also determine the activity of both parts of the NAcb [57]. As part of a dorsal pathway, the lateral habenula controls the activity of the VTA and the medial habenula the activity of locus coeruleus and raphe nuclei. The activity of both lateral and medial habenula is controlled by the amygdala and hippocampus. Via a ventral route, the prefrontal cortex also influences the activity of the VTA. We hypothesize that this ventral route is involved in maintaining substance abuse, while the dorsal route is primarily involved in initiating addiction and causing relapse into dependence after using illicit drugs after a period of abstinence.

Author details

Anton J.M. Loonen[1,2*], Arnt F.A. Schellekens[3,4] and Svetlana A. Ivanova[5,6]

*Address all correspondence to: a.j.m.loonen@rug.nl

1 Department of Pharmacy, University of Groningen, Groningen, The Netherlands

2 Mental Health Institute (GGZ) Westelijk Noord-Brabant, Halsteren, The Netherlands

3 Department of Psychiatry, Radboud University Medical Centre, Nijmegen, The Netherlands

4 Centre for Neuroscience, Donders Institute for Brain Cognition and Behaviour, Nijmegen, The Netherlands

5 Mental Health Research Institute, Tomsk, Russian Federation

6 National Research Tomsk Polytechnic University, Tomsk, Russian Federation

References

[1] Tang YY, Posner MI, Rothbart MK, Volkow ND. Circuitry of self-control and its role in reducing addiction. Trends Cogn Sci. 2015;19(8):43944. doi:10.1016/j.tics.2015.06.007

[2] Koob GF, Le Moal M. Drug abuse: hedonic homeostatic dysregulation. Science. 1997;278(5335):52–58. Stable URL: http://www.jstor.org/stable/2894498

[3] Koob GF, Volkow ND. Neurocircuitry of addiction. Neuropsychopharmacology. 2010;35(1):217–238. doi:10.1038/npp.2009.110

[4] Koob GF, Buck CL, Cohen A, Edwards S, Park PE, Schlosburg JE, Schmeichel B, Vendruscolo LF, Wade CL, Whitfield TW Jr, George O. Addiction as a stress surfeit disorder. Neuropharmacology. 2014;76 (Pt B):370–382. doi:10.1016/j.neuropharm.2013.05.024

[5] Robertson B, Kardamakis A, Capantini Pérez-Fernández J, Suryanarayana SM, Wallén P, Stephenson-Jones M, Grillner S. The lamprey blueprint of the mammalian nervous system. Prog Brain Res. 2014;212:337–349. doi: 10.1016/B978-0-444-63488-7.00016-1

[6] Loonen AJM, Ivanova SA. Circuits regulating pleasure and happiness: the evolution of reward-seeking and missery-fleeing behavioral mechanisms in vertebrates. Front Neurosci. 2015;9:394. doi: 10.3389/fnins.2015.00394

[7] Moreno N, González A. The common organization of the amygdaloid complex in tetrapods: new concepts based on developmental, hodological and neurochemical data in anuran amphibians. Prog Neurobiol. 2006;78(2):61–90. doi: 10.1016/j.pneurobio.2005.12.005

[8] Benarroch EE. Habenula: recently recognized functions and potential clinical relevance. Neurology. 2015;85(11):992–1000. doi: 10.1212/WNL.0000000000001937

[9] Aizawa H. Habenula and the asymmetric development of the vertebrate brain. Anat Sci Int. 2013;88(1):1–9. doi: 10.1007/s12565-012-0158-6

[10] Salaberry NL, Mendoza J. Insights into the role of the habenular circadian clock in addiction. Front Psychiatry. 2015;6:179. doi: 10.3389/fpsyt.2015.00179

[11] Loonen AJM, Ivanova SA. Circuits regulating pleasure and happiness in major depression. Med Hypotheses. 2016;87(1):14–21. doi: 10.1016/j.mehy.2015.12.013

[12] Bruinsma F, Loonen A. Neurobiologie van cognitieve en emotionele motivatie. [Neurobiology of cognitive and emotional motivation] Neuropraxis. 2006;10(3):77–88. doi: 10.1007/BF03079087

[13] Sewards TV, Sewards MA. Representations of motivational drives in mesial cortex, medial thalamus, hypothalamus and midbrain. Brain Res Bull. 2003;61(1):25–49. doi: 10.1016/S0361-9230(03)00069-8

[14] Liotti M, Panksepp J. Imaging human emotions and affective feelings: implications for biological psychiatry. In: Panksepp J, editor. Textbook of biological psychiatry. Hoboken, NJ: Wiley-Liss; 2004. pp. 33–74. doi: 10.1002/0471468975.ch2

[15] Nieuwenhuys R. The insular cortex: a review. Prog Brain Res. 2012;195:123–163. doi: 10.1016/B978-0-444-53860-4.00007-6

[16] Nagai M, Kishi K, Kato S. Insular cortex and neuropsychiatric disorders: a review of recent literature. Eur Psychiatry. 2007;22(6):387–394. doi: 10.1016/j.eurpsy.2007.02.006

[17] Schioldann J. 'On periodical depressions and their pathogenesis' by Carl Lange (1886). Hist Psychiatry. 2011;22(1):108–130. doi: 10.1177/0957154X10396807

[18] Craig AD. Human feelings: why are some more aware than others? Trends Cogn Sci. 2004 Jun;8(6):239–241. doi: 10.1016/j.tics.2004.04.004

[19] Northoff G. From emotions to consciousness—a neuro-phenomenal and neuro-relational approach. Front Psychol. 2012;3:303. doi: 10.3389/fpsyg.2012.00303

[20] Craig AD. How do you feel—now? The anterior insula and human awareness. Nat Rev Neurosci. 2009;10(1):59–70. doi: 10.1038/nrn2555

[21] Starkstein SE, Kremer J. The disinhibition syndrome and frontal-subcortical circuits. In: Lichter DF, Cummings JL, editors. Frontal-subcortical circuits in psychiatric and neurological disorders. New York, NY: Guilford Press; 2001. pp. 163–176. ISBN: 9781572306233.ch7

[22] Zald DH, Rauch SL, editors. The orbitofrontal cortex. Oxford: Oxford University Press, 2006. doi: 10.1093/acprof:oso/9780198565741.001.0001

[23] Heimer L. A new anatomical framework for neuropsychiatric disorders and drug abuse. Am J Psychiatry. 2003;160(10):1726–1739. doi: 10.1176/appi.ajp.160.10.1726

[24] Georgiadis JR, Kringelbach ML. The human sexual response cycle: brain imaging evidence linking sex to other pleasures. Prog Neurobiol. 2012;98(1):49–81. doi: 10.1016/j.pneurobio.2012.05.004

[25] Bianchi-Demicheli F, Ortigue S. Toward an understanding of the cerebral substrates of woman's orgasm. Neuropsychologia. 2007;45(12):2645–2659. doi: 10.1016/j.neuropsychologia.2007.04.016

[26] Georgiadis JR, Kortekaas R, Kuipers R, Nieuwenburg A, Pruim J, Reinders AA, Holstege G. Regional cerebral blood flow changes associated with clitorally induced orgasm in healthy women. Eur J Neurosci. 2006;24(11):3305–3316. doi: 10.1111/j.1460-9568.2006.05206.x

[27] Georgiadis JR, Reinders AA, Paans AM, Renken R, Kortekaas R. Men versus women on sexual brain function: prominent differences during tactile genital stimulation, but not during orgasm. Hum Brain Mapp. 2009;30(10):3089–3101. doi: 10.1002/hbm.20733

[28] Soares JC, Mann JJ. The functional neuroanatomy of mood disorders. J Psychiatr Res. 1997;31(4):393–432. doi: 10.1016/S0022-3956(97)00016-2

[29] Mayberg HS. Modulating dysfunctional limbic-cortical circuits in depression: towards development of brain-based algorithms for diagnosis and optimised treatment. Br Med Bull. 2003;65(1):193–207. doi: 10.1093/bmb/65.1.193

[30] Seminowicz DA, Mayberg HS, McIntosh AR, Goldapple K, Kennedy S, Segal Z, Rafi-Tari S. Limbic-frontal circuitry in major depression: a path modeling metanalysis. Neuroimage. 2004;22(1):409–418. doi: 10.1016/j.neuroimage.2004.01.015

[31] Dalley JW, Mar AC, Economidou D, Robbins TW. Neurobehavioral mechanisms of impulsivity: fronto-striatal systems and functional neurochemistry. Pharmacol Biochem Behav. 2008;90(2):250–260. doi: 10.1016/j.pbb.2007.12.021

[32] Hamani C, Mayberg H, Stone S, Laxton A, Haber S, Lozano AM. The subcallosal cingulate gyrus in the context of major depression. Biol Psychiatry. 2011;69(4):301–308. doi: 10.1016/j.biopsych.2010.09.034

[33] Loonen AJ, Ivanova SA. New insights into the mechanism of drug-induced dyskinesia. CNS Spectr. 2013;18(1):15–20. doi: 10.1017/S1092852912000752

[34] Alexander GE, DeLong MR, Strick PL. Parallel organization of functionally segregated circuits linking basal ganglia and cortex. Annu Rev Neurosci. 1986;9:357–381. doi: 10.1146/annurev.ne.09.030186.002041

[35] Groenewegen HJ, Trimble M. The ventral striatum as an interface between the limbic and motor systems. CNS Spectr. 2007;12(12):887–892. doi: 10.1017/S1092852900015650

[36] Balleine BW, Killcross S. Parallel incentive processing: an integrated view of amygdala function. Trends Neurosci. 2006;29(5):272–279. doi: 10.1016/j.tins.2006.03.002

[37] Freese JL, Amaral DG. Neuroanatomy of the primate amygdala. In: Whalen PJ, Phelps AE, editors. The human amygdala. New York, NY: Guildford Press; 2009. pp. 3–42. ISBN: 9781606230336.ch1

[38] Pitkänen A. Connectivity of the rat amygdaloid complex. In: Aggleton JP, editor. The Amygdala. A functional analysis. Oxford, UK: Oxford University Press; 2000: pp. 31–115. ISBN: 9780198505013.ch2

[39] Elias WJ, Ray DK, Jane JA. Lennart Heimer: concepts of the ventral striatum and extended amygdala. Neurosurg Focus. 2008;25(1):E8. doi: 10.3171/FOC/2008/25/7/E8

[40] Stephenson-Jones M, Samuelsson E, Ericsson J, Robertson B, Grillner S. Evolutionary conservation of the basal ganglia as a common vertebrate mechanism for action selection. Curr Biol. 2011;21(13):1081–1091. doi: 10.1016/j.cub.2011.05.001

[41] Stephenson-Jones M, Ericsson J, Robertson B, Grillner S. Evolution of the basal ganglia: dual-output pathways conserved throughout vertebrate phylogeny. J Comp Neurol. 2012;520(13):2957–2973. doi: 10.1002/cne.23087

[42] Moreno N, Morona R, López JM, Domínguez L, Joven A, Bandín S, González A. Characterization of the bed nucleus of the stria terminalis in the forebrain of anuran amphibians. J Comp Neurol. 2012;520(2):330–363. doi: 10.1002/cne.22694

[43] Belzung C, Willner P, Philippot P. Depression: from psychopathology to pathophysiology. Curr Opin Neurobiol. 2014;30C:24–30. doi: 10.1016/j.conb.2014.08.013

[44] Savitz JB, Nugent AC, Bogers W, Roiser JP, Bain EE, Neumeister A, Zarate CAJr, Manji HK, Cannon DM, Marrett S, Henn F, Charney DS, Drevets WC. Habenula volume in bipolar disorder and major depressive disorder: a high-resolution magnetic resonance imaging study. Biol Psychiatry. 2011;69(4):336–343. doi: 10.1016/j.biopsych.2010.09.027

[45] Schneider TM, Beynon C, Sartorius A, Unterberg AW, Kiening KL. Deep brain stimulation of the lateral habenular complex in treatment-resistant depression: traps

and pitfalls of trajectory choice. Neurosurgery. 2013;72(2 Suppl Operative):ons184–193. doi: 10.1227/NEU.0b013e318277a5aa

[46] Velasquez KM, Molfese DL, Salas R. The role of the habenula in drug addiction. Front Hum Neurosci. 2014;8:174. doi: 10.3389/fnhum.2014.00174

[47] Antolin-Fontes B, Ables JL, Görlich A, Ibañes-Tallon I. The habenulo-interpeduncular pathway in nicotine aversion and withdrawal. Neuropharmacology. 2015;96(Pt B):213–222. doi: 10.1016/j.neuropharm.2014.11.019.

[48] Stephenson-Jones M, Floros O, Robertson B, Grillner S. Evolutionary conservation of the habenular nuclei and their circuitry controlling the dopamine and 5-hydroxytryptophan (5-HT) systems. Proc Natl Acad Sci USA. 2012;109(3):E164–E173. doi: 10.1073/pnas.1119348109.

[49] Viswanath H, Carter AQ, Baldwin PR, Molfese DL, Salas R. The medial habenula: still neglected. Front Hum Neurosci. 2014;7:931. doi: 10.3389/fnhum.2013.00931

[50] Grillner S, Robertson B. The basal ganglia downstream control of brainstem motor centres-an evolutionarily conserved strategy. Curr Opin Neurobiol. 2015;33:47–52. doi: 10.1016/j.conb.2015.01.019

[51] Wu J, Gao M, Shen JX, Shi WX, Oster AM, Gutkin BS. Cortical control of VTA function and influence on nicotine reward. Biochem Pharmacol. 2013;86(8):1173–1180. doi: 10.1016/j.bcp.2013.07.013

[52] Matsumoto M, Hikosaka O. Lateral habenula as a source of negative reward signals in dopamine neurons. Nature. 2007;447(7148):1111–1115. doi: 10.1038/nature05860

[53] Jhou TC, Good CH, Rowley CS, Xu SP, Wang H, Burnham NW, Hoffman AF, Lupica CR, Ikemoto S. Cocaine drives aversive conditioning via delayed activation of dopamine-responsive habenular and midbrain pathways. J Neurosci. 2013;33(17):7501–7512. doi: 10.1523/JNEUROSCI.3634-12.2013

[54] Matsumoto M, Hikosaka O. Representation of negative motivational value in the primate lateral habenula. Nat Neurosci. 2009;12(1):77–84. doi: 10.1038/nn.2233

[55] Bromberg-Martin ES, Matsumoto M, Hikosaka O. Distinct tonic and phasic anticipatory activity in lateral habenula and dopamine neurons. Neuron. 2010;67(1):144–155. doi: 10.1016/j.neuron.2010.06.016

[56] Lecca S, Meye FJ, Mameli M. The lateral habenula in addiction and depression: an anatomical, synaptic and behavioral overview. Eur J Neurosci. 2014;39(7):1170–1178. doi: 10.1111/ejn.12480

[57] Loonen AJM, Ivanova SA. Role of 5-HT2C receptors in dyskinesia. Int J Pharm Pharm Sci. 2016;8(1):5–10. http://innovareacademics.in/journals/index.php/ijpps/article/viewFile/8736/3470

Chapter 2

Epigenetics and Drug Abuse

Ryan M. Bastle and Janet L. Neisewander

Additional information is available at the end of the chapter

http://dx.doi.org/10.5772/101986

Abstract

Gene expression and inheritance are not only a function of the DNA code, but also epigenetic mechanisms that regulate DNA accessibility, transcription, and translation of the genetic code into a functional protein. Epigenetic mechanisms are invoked by life experiences, including stress and exposure to drugs of abuse, and the resulting changes in gene expression can be inherited by future generations. This chapter highlights recent research demonstrating epigenetic changes in response to drug exposure with a focus on three different mechanisms: DNA methylation, histone modification, and noncoding RNAs. We briefly describe each of these mechanisms and then provide key examples of drug-induced changes involving these mechanisms, as well as epigenetic manipulations that alter effects of drugs. We then review cutting-edge technologies, including viral-mediated gene transfer and gene editing, that are being used to manipulate epigenetic processes with temporal and cell-type specificity. We also describe and provide examples of intergenerational epigenetic modifications, a topic that has interesting implications for how addiction-related traits may be passed down across generations. Finally, we discuss how this research provides a greater understanding of drug addiction and may lead to novel molecular targets for preventions and interventions for drug abuse.

Keywords: DNA methylation, histone modification, noncoding RNA, cocaine, alcohol

1. Introduction

One of the most compelling questions in the field of drug abuse is why some individuals who experiment with drugs go on to develop substance use disorders (SUDs) while others do not. Both a family history of SUDs and stressful life events increase one's vulnerability to develop SUDs [1, 2]. Historically, these risk factors were viewed as "nature and nurture" making separate contributions to an addiction phenotype. However, recent advances in the field of epigenetics demonstrate that "nurture" changes "nature" by modifying whether or not a given gene will be expressed. Understanding how one's environment (e.g., drug-taking behavior, stress, and learning) can alter gene expression in the brain may give insight into how drug addiction develops, how it may be passed down into future generations, and perhaps, how it can be better treated.

While the DNA sequence of a gene can be modified directly (e.g., mutations, deletions, insertions, translocations, etc.) resulting in altered gene expression, epigenetics regulates gene expression by mechanisms other than changes to the DNA sequence. It has long been known that epigenetic mechanisms largely control cell differentiation by allowing some genes to be expressed and others to be silenced at various points in time during development. Indeed, even though all human cells possess the same DNA (with the exception of egg and sperm cells), what differentiates a given cell type from others (e.g., a neuron versus a liver cell) is the epigenetic mechanisms that permit or deny its genes to be transcribed and translated into cell type-specific functional proteins [3]. Beyond the hard-wire epigenetic programming of gene expression during development, epigenetic mechanisms also provide dynamic and heritable means of altering gene expression in response to environmental change. For example, either stressful life experiences or a history of chronic drug intake can invoke chemical modifications to either the DNA or the histone proteins that are involved in storing the DNA. Such epigenetic changes have an impact on how accessible the DNA is for gene transcription. Epigenetic changes can also be long lasting and passed down to future generations. In this way, not only does experience with stress and/or drugs place one's self at risk for SUDs, but also one's offspring due to heritable epigenetic modifications. Even in the more proximal time frame of an individual's lifespan, epigenetic mechanisms provide a "working memory" for gene expression changes that are involved in brain plasticity [4]. Brain plasticity changes resulting from drug exposure are thought to be the crux of the dysfunction underlying addiction [5]. An exciting implication of understanding the role of epigenetic changes in drug-induced brain plasticity is that new strategies for therapeutic interventions may be discovered.

In this chapter, we review three epigenetic mechanisms that have been found to impact drug abuse-related behaviors in animal models: (1) chemical modifications to DNA, (2) chemical modifications to histones, and (3) the induction of noncoding RNAs that regulate gene expression. We will begin with a brief explanation of how drugs modify intracellular signaling pathways that propagate to the cell nucleus, leading to epigenetic changes. We will then provide a brief description of the epigenetic mechanisms listed above, followed by examples of how drugs of abuse invoke these mechanisms and how pharmacologically targeting the epigenome can alter drug-abuse-related behavior. Next, we will cover the latest developments in genetic tools that provide precise manipulation of epigenetic enzymes, further elucidating the roles of these specific molecules. We will also review literature supporting transgenerational inheritance of epigenetic changes associated with a history of drug intake. We conclude by discussing important future directions for research investigating epigenetic mechanisms associated with drug addiction.

http://dx.doi.org/10.5772/101986

2. The link between drug action, intracellular signaling, and epigenetic changes

Both endogenous neurotransmitters and drugs interact with neuronal proteins, such as neurotransmitter receptors, proteins involved in synaptic homeostasis (e.g., neurotransmitter metabolic enzymes, transporters, etc.), and proteins involved in intracellular signaling pathways. These intracellular signaling pathways can propagate to the cell nucleus, leading to changes in gene expression [6]. Often, the first change observed in the cell nucleus following an environmental perturbation (e.g., drug use, stress, novelty, etc.) is the expression of immediate early genes (IEGs). Common IEGs encode transcription factors that increase expression of other target genes by binding to the genes' promoter region, which is a sequence in the DNA that signals the cell to initiate transcription [7, 8]. IEGs are rapidly induced and are often used as a marker of changes in neuronal signaling activity [9]. Both IEGs and target genes may undergo epigenetic modifications that regulate their expression. Thus, either natural signaling in response to environmental stimuli or drug-induced changes in signaling can invoke epigenetic mechanisms that alter gene expression. The dynamics of the epigenetic changes may be specific to the degree and phase of drug exposure, where particular epigenetic marks may only arise (or disappear) following acute or chronic drug administration, or during a period of withdrawal from drug use [10].

3. DNA epigenetic modification

A given gene is composed of a sequence of nucleotide base pairs in the DNA that are unique to that gene. For coding genes, the DNA sequence of base pairs serves as the blueprint for making a particular protein. Given that proteins are the machinery for cell structure and function, gene expression changes in a neuron can alter cell protein composition and, in turn, change the way that the neuron functions and communicates with other neurons.

There are four different nucleotide bases that compose the sequence portion of the DNA molecule, including the pyrimidines cytosine (C) and thymine (T), and the purines adenine (A) and guanine (G). Due to the structures of these nucleotides, the chemical bond responsible for base pairing can only form between C and G or A and T, respectively. Cs followed by Gs in the DNA sequence (i.e., CpGs) can be modified by a reaction in which DNA methyltransferases (DNMTs) add a methyl group (CH3) to the 5-position of the C to form 5mC. Intracellular signals may initiate newly synthesized *de novo* DNA methylation, which is mediated by DNMT subtypes DNMT3a and DNMT3b. Subtype DNMT1, on the other hand, maintains DNA methylation patterns across cell replication, such that the newly synthesized DNA has the exact methylation pattern that existed before DNA replication. In general, DNA methylation is correlated with a decrease in DNA accessibility and therefore is thought to be a mechanism of silencing gene expression. Methylated DNA can silence gene expression by interfering with the binding of transcriptional activators or by binding to proteins with a methyl-CpG-binding domain (MBD), such as methyl-CpG binding protein 2 (MECP2), that then form a complex with other proteins that together repress DNA accessibility [11].

Historically, DNA methylation was believed to be a permanent modification. However, demethylation of DNA can occur and also contributes to dynamic changes in gene expression. While passive demethylation in dividing cells may be due to malfunctioning of DNMT1, active demethylation occurs in both dividing and nondividing cells by enzymatic reactions. One reaction changes 5mC into a T, which is then recognized as a G/T mismatch. The mismatch activates a base excision repair (BER) pathway that utilizes thymine DNA glycosylase (TDG) and ultimately replaces T with a nonmethylated C [12]. Another reaction catalyzed by 10–11 translocation enzymes (TET) adds a hydroxyl (–OH) group to 5mC forming 5hmC. 5hmC itself has effects on gene expression and it can undergo further reactions that convert it back to a nonmethylated C [13]. Therefore, demethylation of DNA is generally correlated with an increase in DNA accessibility.

4. DNA methylation changes associated with drugs of abuse

Although DNA methylation is typically a stable epigenetic process, drugs of abuse have been shown to alter both DNA methylation and its associated enzymes. Much of this research has focused on DNA methylation in the nucleus accumbens (NAc), a brain region involved in reward and motivation learning [14]. A well-established marker of repeated exposure to drugs of abuse is an increase in the transcription factor ΔFosB protein in the NAc [15]. Acute or repeated cocaine administration decreases methylation at the *fosB* promoter in the NAc of rodents, which co-occurs with increases in *fosB* mRNA expression [16]. This may serve as a mechanism by which exposure to drugs of abuse produces stable increases in ΔFosB protein expression. Acute or chronic cocaine administration also increases *Dnmt3a* mRNA and MeCP2 protein expression in the NAc [16–18]. These increases are accompanied by decreases in psychostimulant reward as measured by conditioned place preference (CPP), a procedure in which an animal experiences a drug state while confined to one compartment of an apparatus and a neutral state while confined to an alternate compartment during conditioning, resulting in a shift in the animal's preference for the drug-paired compartment when given free access to both compartments. The decreased CPP effects are believed to be mediated by *Dnmt3a*- and MeCP2-induced silencing of genes that encode proteins that are needed for adaptation and functioning of NAc neurons [17, 18]. In addition, the TET enzyme that catalyzes DNA demethylation and subsequent transcriptional activation via conversion of 5mC to 5hmC [19] is decreased in the NAc in both rodents following cocaine administration and in postmortem tissue from human cocaine addicts [20]. Paradoxically, this decrease in TET is associated with increases in 5hmC expression at specific gene loci that have previously been linked to addiction [20]. Further investigation is needed to explain this complex pattern of epigenetic changes.

5. Histone modification

In order for the long strands of DNA to fit within a cell's nucleus, DNA is tightly condensed into chromatin. Chromatin is made up of nucleosomes that contain a histone protein core comprised of two copies of each of four different histone proteins, H2A, H2B, H3, and H4, as well as 147 base pairs of DNA that is wrapped around the histone core (**Figure 1**). Chromatin can either be tightly (i.e., heterochromatin) or loosely packaged (i.e., euchromatin), where the former restricts and the latter permits gene expression. Chromatin is able to undergo dynamic remodeling by chemical modification of amino acid residues of the histone core proteins. Similar to DNA methylation, histone proteins can undergo post-translational addition or removal of one of several chemical groups via enzymatic reactions. There are more than 100 different posttranslational modifications that may occur and these changes correlate with either the activation or the suppression of gene expression.

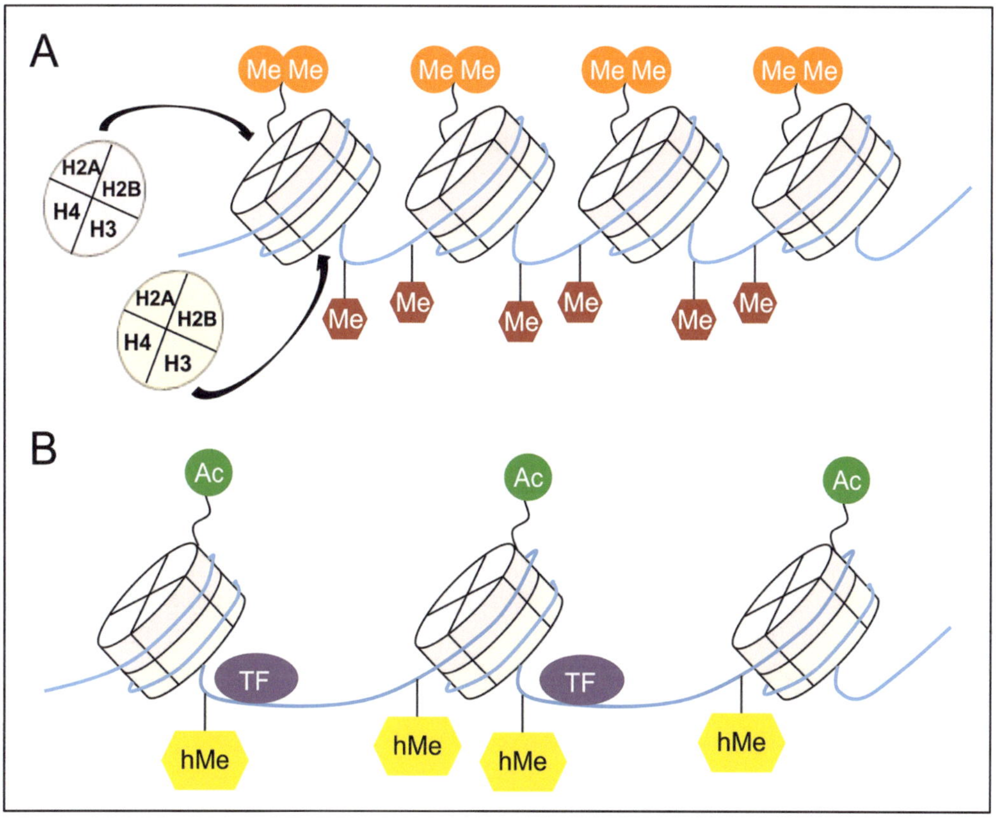

Figure 1. DNA and histone chemical modifications. DNA (blue lines) wraps around pairs of histone proteins H2A, H2B, 3, and 4 (light pink and tan) that form an octomer histone protein core. (A) Closed chromatin, due to DNA methylation (Me; red) and histone dimethylation on H3K9 (Me; orange), leads to transcriptional repression. (B) Open chromatin, due to DNA hydroxymethylation (hMe; yellow) and histone acetylation (Ac; green), allows for transcription factors (TF; purple) to recruit RNA polymerase for transcription initiation.

A powerful technique for studying post-translational histone modifications is chromatin immunoprecipitation (ChIP). ChIP utilizes antibodies that bind specifically to chemically modified histone proteins, which can then be isolated along with the associated DNA (i.e., promoter regions, gene bodies, etc.) from the rest of the tissue. Next, histones and DNA segments are denatured and levels of specific DNA sequences are measured. This technique can be used to (1) determine which gene or gene promoter may be associated with a specific histone modification, (2) correlate changes in histone modification with expression of specific genes, and (3) suggest possible mechanisms for how a gene is turned on or off following an experimental manipulation (e.g., drug administration).

6. Histone modifications associated with drugs of abuse

6.1. Acetylation

Acetyl groups are added to histone proteins, typically on a lysine residue, by histone acetyl transferases (HATs). Addition of acetyl groups leads to a more relaxed, less condensed chromatin state by negating the positive charge of the histone protein that is attracted to the negatively charged DNA (**Figure 1B**). Indeed, increases in drug-induced gene expression often positively correlate with the levels of histone acetylation.

Previous work has found widespread changes in acetylation of histone H3 and H4 subunits in the NAc following acute and repeated psychostimulant administration in rodents [21, 22], suggesting that many genes in the NAc may be primed for transcription, while others are suppressed. Acute cocaine administration induces expression of the IEGs *c-fos* and *fosB* in rodents [16, 23], and ChIP analysis revealed increases in H4 acetylation at the respective promoter regions of these genes [21]. With repeated cocaine administration, the increase in *fosB* expression is maintained and is associated with increases in H3 acetylation at the *fosB* promoter region [21]. This mechanism likely contributes to ΔFosB protein accumulation in the NAc following repeated drug exposure. Repeated cocaine administration also reduces the ability of cocaine to induce *c-fos* and this is accompanied by a reduction in H4 acetylation at the *c-fos* promoter region [21, 24]. Furthermore, chronic opiate administration decreases expression of another IEG, brain-derived neurotrophic factor (*Bdnf*), and decreases H3 acetylation at the *Bdnf* promoter in the ventral tegmental area (VTA) [25]. *Bdnf* is critical for the development and maintenance of synaptic structure and function [26, 27] and drugs of abuse exert their reinforcing effect primarily by activating mesocorticolimbic dopamine neurons that originate in the VTA and project to the NAc, prefrontal cortex (PFC), amygdala, and hippocampus [28, 29].

Additionally, alcohol withdrawal in rodents reduces expression of the IEGs activity-regulated cytoskeleton protein (*Arc*) and *Bdnf* in the amygdala along with decreases in H3 acetylation at the respective gene promoters [30]. The amygdala is involved in processing emotional memories and it plays a critical role in alcohol-related behavior and anxiety [31]. Although these examples suggest functional links between degree of acetylation and associated gene expression, histone acetylation may occur even without changes in gene expression [32]. Therefore, further work into the causal role of acetylation in drug-induced gene expression is required.

6.2. Methylation

In contrast to histone acetylation, methylation can be associated with both transcriptional activation and repression, depending on which histone residue is modified. For example, dimethylation of histone H3 Lysine 9 (i.e., H3K9me2) is commonly associated with transcriptional repression. One histone methyltransferase that catalyzes H3K9me2, G9a, is decreased in the NAc following both chronic cocaine and opiate administration [33, 34]. It should be noted that this also occurs following chronic social stress in mice that produces depressive-like behavioral phenotypes, including decreased social interaction and increased anhedonia [35]. Similarly, G9a is decreased in postmortem NAc tissue of clinically depressed patients [35]. Decreases in G9a are associated with increases in cocaine and morphine CPP [33, 34]. Interestingly, G9a opposes expression of ΔFosB [33, 34]. In turn, ΔFosB represses G9a expression, creating a feedback loop that perpetuates its own expression through disinhibition. Similarly, postmortem NAc brain tissue of human cocaine addicts exhibits decreases in G9a expression [36] and increases in ΔFosB expression [37], providing further support for a functional link between these two molecules. In addition to specific genes, compelling work using ChIP and high-throughput sequencing of the associated genome has shown that cocaine-induced downregulation of H3K9me2 expression preferentially occurs in nongenic regions of chromosomes [38], suggesting additional roles of histone methylation that may be independent of traditional effects on specific protein-coding genes.

7. Noncoding RNAs

Before the 1990s, noncoding RNA was often referred to as "junk DNA" that was thought to have little relevance to biological function. A growing body of research over the past 25 years has shown that noncoding RNAs have pivotal roles in almost every cellular process investigated. One class of noncoding RNAs that has received much attention is microRNAs (miRNAs). miRNAs are small transcripts (~22 nucleotides) that regulate gene expression post-transcriptionally. They are transcribed from DNA in a manner similar to protein-coding transcripts, where transcription factors recognize promoter sequences upstream of miRNA genes and initiate transcription (**Figure 2**). Once transcribed, the several hundred nucleotide long transcript folds and binds to itself, producing a stem-loop hairpin structure referred to as a pri-miRNA. The enzyme, Drosha, trims the pri-miRNA into a smaller form known as pre-miRNA (~70 nucleotides long). Pre-miRNA is then transported out of the nucleus into the cytoplasm, where the loop portion of the pre-miRNA is cleaved by the enzyme Dicer [39]. Now as a double-stranded RNA molecule, it is unwound and one strand joins with several proteins to form the miRNA-induced silencing complex (miRISC). The mature miRNA binds to complementary sequences in the 3′ untranslated region (UTR) of a target mRNA where miRISC causes either translational repression, deadenylation, or endonucleolytic cleavage of the target mRNA, preventing its expression [40]. Importantly, the mature miRNA needs only ~6–8 complementary nucleotides for which to base pair with the 3′ UTR of the target mRNA, and therefore, one miRNA can target several hundreds of different mRNAs in a given cell. For this reason, miRNAs have been regarded as "master regulators" of gene expression. Changes

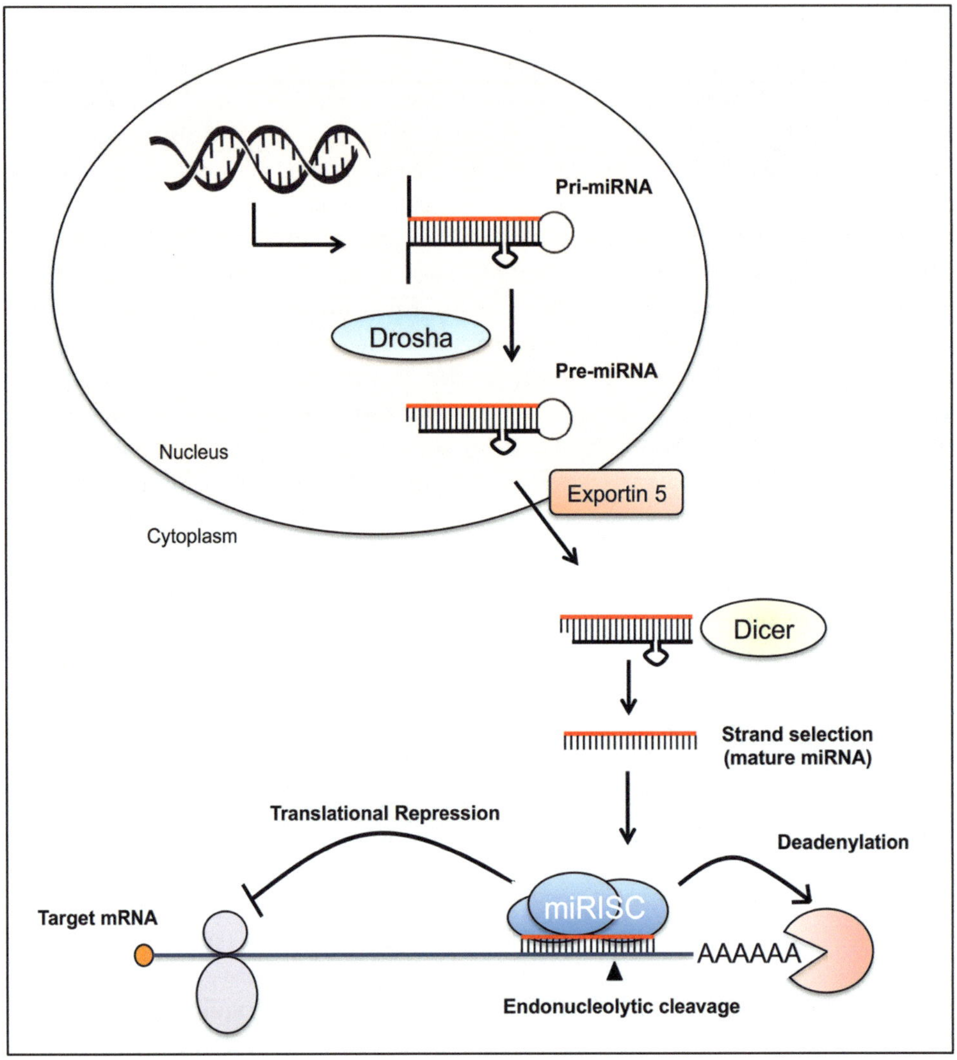

Figure 2. MicroRNA processing and function. MicroRNAs are transcribed similarly to protein-coding RNAs, except they form a stem-loop structure following transcription (i.e., pri-miRNA). The enzyme, Drosha, trims the ends of the stem (i.e., pre-miRNA) to prepare for exportation from the nucleus via Exportin 5. Once in the cytoplasm, Dicer cleaves the loop of the pre-miRNA that produces a double-stranded RNA. One strand (i.e., mature miRNA) is chosen to be incorporated into the miRNA-induced silencing complex (miRISC). Upon binding to a complementary sequence in the 3′ untranslated region of a target mRNA, either translational repression, deadenylation, or endonucleolytic cleavage may occur. All three mechanisms lead to decreases in protein product.

in miRNA expression can therefore lead to widespread changes in gene expression and alteration in several cellular signaling cascades. Other types of noncoding RNAs include: (1) PIWI-interacting RNA (piRNA), which regulates sperm development, (2) small nuclear RNA (snRNA), which regulates mRNA splicing, and (3) long noncoding RNA (lncRNA), which has widespread effects on chromatin modification and transcription [41].

8. Noncoding RNA changes associated with drugs of abuse

Given that most drug abuse research has focused on miRNAs, we will focus on this subclass. One approach to finding candidate addiction-related miRNAs is to examine miRNA expression changes within brain regions implicated in addiction following varying levels of drug exposure. Using this approach, Hollander and colleagues [42] found that rats given extended (6 h/day), but not restricted (2 h/day), access to cocaine self-administration exhibited upregulation of miR-212 in the dorsal striatum, a region involved in establishing habitual behavior [43]. Since the extended access self-administration model produces a behavioral phenotype that mimics the escalation of drug intake observed in human drug addicts, the findings suggest that upregulated miR-212 may play a role in the development of compulsive drug taking. One gene target of miR-212 is MeCP2 [44], a protein whose increased expression in the NAc is associated with reductions in amphetamine reward CPP [17]. However in the dorsal striatum, decreases in MeCP2 via miR-212 regulation are associated with decreases in compulsive-like cocaine self-administration [44]. These findings highlight the importance of examining the roles of epigenetic modulators across different drug classes, brain regions, and drug abuse models.

Another approach to identify candidate miRNAs is through bioinformatics. Databases exist that identify predicted targets of miRNAs and their distribution within the brain. We recently identified miR-495 as a lead candidate that has targets enriched in the Knowledgebase of Addiction-Related Genes database [45] and exhibits high expression in the NAc [46]. We found that cocaine self-administration decreases levels of NAc miR-495 and increases expression of several addiction-related genes. These effects suggest that cocaine dysregulates NAc miR-495, leading to disinhibition of addiction-related gene expression.

miRNAs and other noncoding RNAs have also been implicated in brain changes observed with other drugs of abuse. Alcohol-dependent rats exhibit increases in miR-206 in the medial PFC (mPFC) [47], a brain region involved in executive control of drug-seeking behavior [48]. miR-206 directly targets and suppresses BDNF expression in the mPFC [47], where increases in BDNF in this region are associated with inhibiting motivation for cocaine [49, 50]. This suggests increases in miR-206 likely contribute to the development of alcohol dependency through suppression of BDNF. Additionally, several lncRNAs exhibit expression changes in the NAc of heroin addicts postmortem [51]. These promising findings suggest that noncoding RNAs provide a treasure trove of novel targets for regulating addiction-related gene changes and behaviors.

9. Pharmacological manipulations of epigenetic mechanisms

Pharmacological agents that target specific epigenetic machinery have been used to further understand the role of epigenetic mechanisms in the effects of drugs of abuse and to explore their potential use as treatments for drug addiction. Most preclinical studies have utilized both systemic and intracranial administration of these compounds, where the former has a more human translational value, while the latter allows for greater brain region specificity.

9.1. Methyl supplementation and DNMT inhibitors.

DNA methylation can be altered pharmacologically by using methionine or DNMT inhibitors. Methionine is an amino acid commonly found in diet, where methionine metabolism yields methyl groups that serve as donors for methylating DNA. DNMT inhibitors exert the opposite effect by preventing DNMT from catalyzing DNA methylation. Daily, systemic administration of methionine has been shown to reduce both the rewarding and motivating effects of cocaine in rodents [18, 52]. In contrast, intracranial administration of a DNMT inhibitor (i.e., RG108) into the NAc increases the rewarding effects of cocaine [18]. However, this same manipulation decreases drug-seeking behavior following a prolonged abstinence period [53]. These findings suggest that the effect of DNA methylation in the NAc may depend on whether or not there has been a period of abstinence following cocaine exposure. Indeed, our lab and others have shown that dynamic changes occur during forced abstinence from cocaine in animal models, and that these changes can result in opposing effects of pharmacological challenge on cocaine abuse-related behavior depending on whether the manipulation occurs during active drug intake versus abstinence [54–56]. It should be noted that work using DNA methyl supplementation and DNMT inhibitors has primarily been done with cocaine and needs to be tested on other drug classes.

9.2. Histone deacetylase inhibitors

The removal of an acetyl group from a histone is catalyzed by histone deacetylases (HDACs). This reaction results in condensing the chromatin and repressing transcription. HDAC inhibitors prevent this reaction from occurring, thereby maintaining DNA accessibility. There are five different classes of HDACs (e.g., I, IIa, IIb, III, and IV) and each class contains multiple HDAC enzymes (e.g., HDAC1, HDAC8, SIRT1, etc.). HDAC inhibitors range in their selectivity for specific HDAC classes. Drugs that target both class I and II HDACs (e.g., Tricostatin A, sodium butyrate, and SAHA) have been found to enhance cocaine locomotor sensitization [21, 57, 58], cocaine and opiate CPP [21, 58, 59], and cocaine self-administration [60] when administered systemically prior to cocaine exposure. In contrast, administration of HDAC compounds *following* cocaine exposure attenuates cocaine CPP [61]. Similarly, these compounds appear to produce mixed effects with alcohol, with some reporting increases [62] and others reporting decreases [63, 64] in consumption. While these effects were found during active drug administration, HDAC inhibitors have also been shown to alleviate anxiety symptoms during alcohol withdrawal [30, 65]. Additionally, several studies have found that the effects of the class I/II HDAC inhibitors were specific to drug self-administration, as no effects were found with these drugs on food reinforcement [60, 63, 64]. Collectively, it appears that class I/II HDAC inhibitors can produce both increases and decreases in drug-abuse-related behavior, and that the effects may vary depending on whether testing occurs during drug exposure or withdrawal.

More consistent effects have been observed with selective HDAC inhibitors. For instance, the selective class I HDAC inhibitor, MS-275, decreases both alcohol and cocaine abuse-related behavior in rodents [63, 64, 66, 67]. Also, the highly selective HDAC3 inhibitor, RGF-P966, decreases cocaine CPP [68]. These findings suggest that the use of more selective HDAC inhibitors may improve behavioral outcomes.

10. Genetic tools for uncovering epigenetic roles in drug-abuse-related behavior

While pharmacological approaches have translational value for development of therapeutic agents, efficacy may be compromised by the widespread drug distribution if the effects of an epigenetic manipulation vary depending on the brain region of interest. Also, pharmacological manipulations used to date have widespread effects on the genome, whereas sharpening the mechanism/location targeted may improve desired outcomes. Recent preclinical research has shed light on this area with technologies that selectively manipulate genes in specific brain pathways and cell types.

10.1. Viral vectors

One approach to manipulating a certain gene within a particular brain region is the use of viral vectors. Viral vectors are constructed to be nonreplicative so that they do not produce more viral particles after infecting the cell. They enter the cell through endocytosis and insert a gene of interest (i.e., transgene) into the genome of specific neurons (**Figure 3**). There are many different modes of transfection that vary in length from days to months. In order to achieve high levels of expression in a particular cell type, within the viral vector the transgene is typically downstream from a promoter sequence that is specific to that cell. Thus, upon viral transfection, the cells own transcriptional machinery will recognize and bind to the promoter that will then activate transcription of the transgene. The direction of regulation (i.e., increase vs. decrease expression) is determined by the sequence of the transgene. For instance, an increase in gene expression is obtained by inserting the sequence of the transgene into the viral vector with a strong upstream promoter. In order to decrease gene expression, a couple of methods may be used. One involves transfecting a short-hairpin RNA (shRNA) that is processed into a mature short-interfering RNA (siRNA). siRNAs are similar to miRNAs, except that they are perfectly complementary to the target mRNA and will therefore selectively downregulate only one target gene, in contrast to the multiple targets of most miRNAs. This is referred to as a 'knockdown,' rather than a 'knockout,' as it is preventing translation of the gene rather than completing deleting it from the genome. In order to accomplish a 'knockout' using viral vectors, transgenes that express a new gene editing approach, called the CRISPR-Cas9 system, can be used. The latter uses a guide RNA that is complementary to specific sequences in the DNA (e.g., gene of interest) that directs enzymes to that site and excises the sequence from the DNA, therefore deleting it.

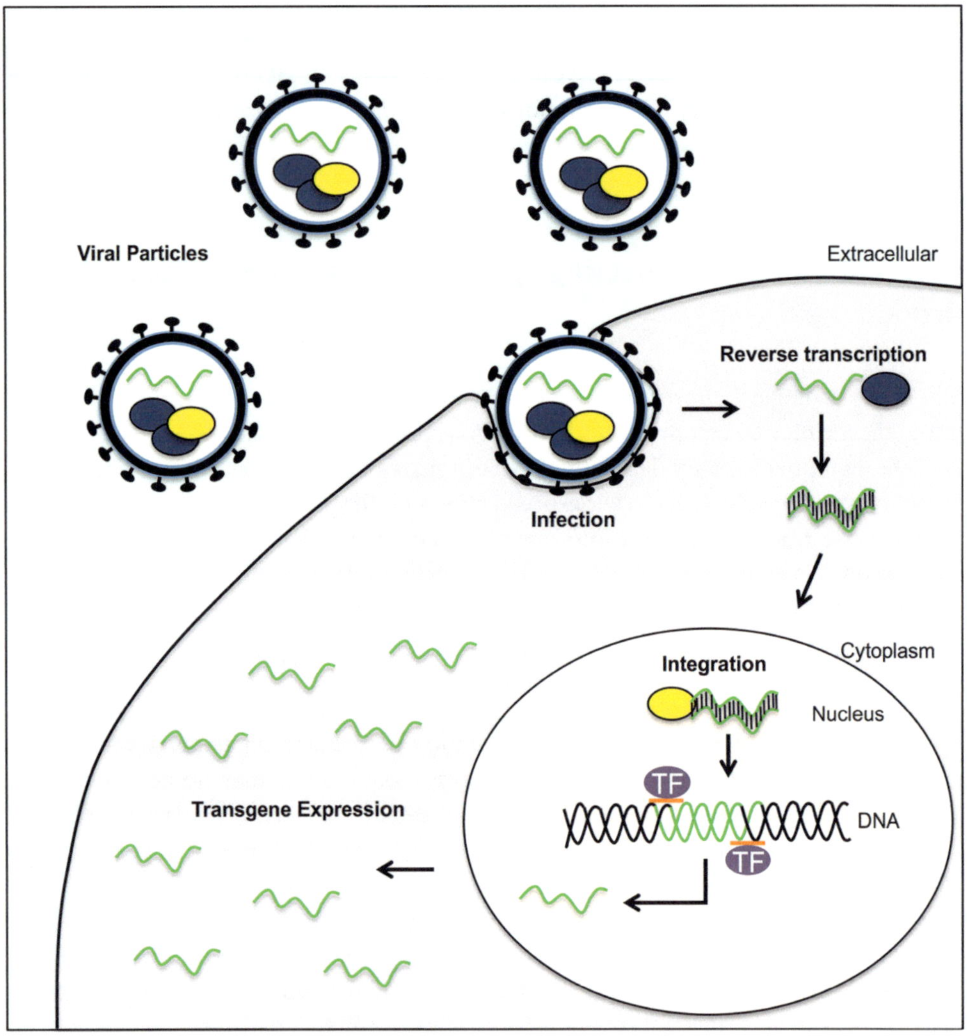

Figure 3. Viral-mediated gene transfer. Viral particles are infused into a region of interest and infect local cells through receptor-mediated endocytosis. Once viral particles are released from the vesicle inside the infected cell, viral RNA is reverse-transcribed into DNA (via reverse transcriptase; dark blue) and transported into the nucleus, where it becomes integrated into the genome (via integrase; yellow). By using a strong promoter (orange line) upstream of the transgene, the cell's transcriptional machinery produces an abundance of viral transgene expression in the cell. TF = transcription factor.

Research using viral vectors has furthered our understanding of the impact of epigenetic manipulations on drug-abuse-related behavior. As previously described, DNA methylation is thought to inhibit cocaine abuse-related behaviors in animal models [16, 18, 52]. To test whether *Dnmt3a* expression in the NAc specifically mediates these effects, LaPlant et al. [18] infused viral vectors into this region that either increased or decreased *Dnmt3a* levels. Increasing NAc *Dnmt3a* expression countered cocaine CPP in mice, while decreasing expression increased this behavior [18]. Interestingly, this same manipulation also increases depressive-

http://dx.doi.org/10.5772/101986

like behavior following repeated social stress in mice [18], suggesting the blunted rewarding effects of cocaine may be due to increases in anhedonia. This illustrates the importance of testing the role of epigenetic modulators in both drug abuse and mood disorder models.

Another exciting use of viral vectors is to express synthetically engineered transcription factors that bind to specific sequences in the DNA and regulate histone modifications at one specific gene loci. Heller and colleagues [69] recently used this approach and found that histone acetylation or methylation near the *fosB* gene locus increases or decreases cocaine reward CPP, respectively. Again, this same manipulation produces either anti- or pro-depressive behaviors, respectively, following repeated social stress [69], further demonstrating the complex role of these molecules in both reward and emotional regulation processes. Bidirectional manipulation of cocaine self-administration in rats has also been demonstrated for miR-212 levels in the dorsal striatum where viral-mediated increases prevent escalation of cocaine self-administration, whereas knockdown increases cocaine self-administration [42]. In some cases, decreasing miRNA levels may be needed to attenuate addiction-related behavior. For instance, viral-mediated increases in miR-206 expression in the prefrontal cortex create an alcohol-dependent phenotype in rats [47], and, therefore, it is possible that decreasing miR-206 levels in the PFC may be protective against alcoholism. These examples suggest that the development of new therapeutics that target epigenetic mechanisms have potential for treating addiction. Currently, there are no pharmacological agents for manipulating miRNAs, although development is in the initial stages for their delivery in drug compounds [70]. A future challenge for this avenue of research will be to develop methods of site-selective drug delivery.

10.2. Cre-Lox recombination

Another approach to manipulating gene expression is the use of Cre-Lox recombination (**Figure 4**). Cre recombinase is an enzyme that identifies sequences in the DNA called LoxP sites. When Cre recognizes these sites, it catalyzes a reaction that can either excise or invert the DNA sequence contained between the two sites, depending on which direction the LoxP sites are oriented. If the two LoxP sites are in the same direction, Cre will excise the DNA, effectively deleting a gene that is between those two sites. If the LoxP sites are in the opposite direction, Cre will then invert the two LoxP sites along with inverting the flanked DNA sequence. This latter effect allows for gene activation, where a previous nonfunctional inverted gene sequence becomes functional after Cre-Lox mediated-inversion.

Cre-lox recombination is carried out in rodents that are bred to have LoxP sites at specific locations in the DNA that flank a gene of interest (e.g., *Bdnf*$^{fl/fl}$). A viral vector expressing Cre recombinase can then be infused into a specific brain region and Cre-expressing infected cells will recognize the LoxP sites and either excise or invert the flanked gene. This will result in region- and temporal-specific manipulation of gene expression. Another approach with even greater precision involves breeding mice to express Cre in only certain cell types. This is accomplished by breeding rodents that express Cre downstream from a promoter that is specific for only one type or subtype of cells. For instance, Cre can be expressed specifically in catecholamine neurons when used downstream of a promoter for tyrosine hydroxylase (TH). TH is an enzyme involved in synthesizing catecholamines (e.g., dopamine). Only cells with

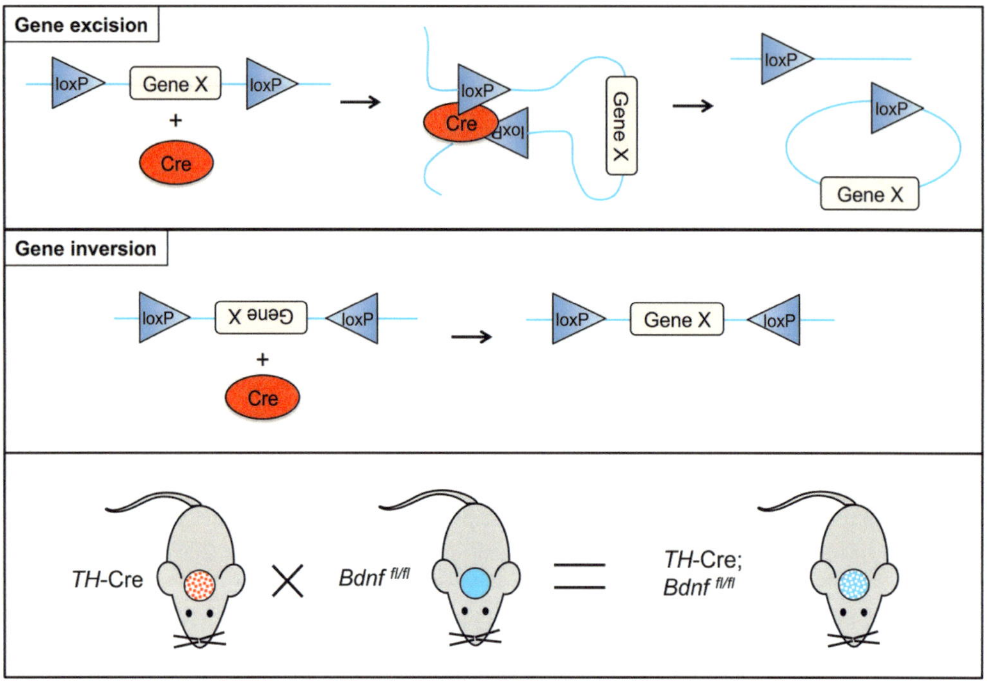

Figure 4. Cre-lox recombination. The top panel illustrates how Cre-lox recombination can result in gene excision, where Cre recombinase (red) recognizes two loxP sites in the same orientation and joins the two ends of DNA, then cleaves one end to join the other, resulting in excision of the flanked gene between the two loxP sites. The middle panel illustrates how Cre recognizes two loxP sites in opposite orientations and inverts the intervening DNA sequence (e.g., Gene X). Gene inversion can be used to turn on a gene that is initially inverted and inactive. The bottom panel depicts how crossbreeding two transgenic mice that express Cre recombinase only in tyrosine hydroxylase-expressing cells (*TH*-Cre) with mice that ubiquitously express Bdnf with flanked loxP sites (*Bdnf*$^{fl/fl}$) results in mice with deficient *Bdnf* expression only in *TH*+ cells.

TH will have the transcriptional machinery to recognize the TH promoter and express Cre. Next, there are two methods for manipulating gene expression in a cell-type-specific manner. The first is to crossbreed two transgenic mice: the one that expresses Cre only in certain cell types (e.g., TH+ neurons) and the other that ubiquitously expresses a LoxP-flanked *Bdnf* gene (i.e., *Bdnf*$^{fl/fl}$). The offspring will no longer express *Bdnf* in TH-expressing cells. A limitation of this technique is that Cre recombination occurs at conception and the transgene is either expressed or deleted permanently. Therefore, changes may occur during development to compensate for the gene modification, making it difficult to know whether subsequent functional differences are due to the gene modification or the compensatory changes that ensued thereafter. Another way to overcome this limitation is to inject a viral vector into a brain region that contains the gene of interest in a plasmid with the gene flanked by inverted LoxP sites. While the virus will infect all the cells in that region, only the cells that are expressing Cre recombinase (e.g., TH+) will recognize the LoxP sites. In this case, Cre recombination will only occur in specific cell types in a particular brain region and, importantly, during a specific time point during development.

Research employing the Cre-Lox recombination approach has shown that the effect of epigenetic mechanisms can be cell-type specific. For instance, the histone methytransferase *G9a* has differential roles in cocaine-related behaviors depending on whether it is expressed in striatal neurons that contain dopamine D1 (D1R) versus D2 (D2R) receptors. *G9a* is downregulated by cocaine in both D1R and D2R-containing neurons; however, Cre-mediated downregulation of *G9a* selectively in D1R-neurons is associated with decreasing cocaine CPP and locomotor behavior in mice, while the opposite effects occur with selective downregulation in D2R-neurons [36]. These effects were observed using both Cre-Lox recombinase procedures described above, providing strong evidence for the cell-type-specific role of *G9a* in cocaine abuse-related behavior.

11. Transgenerational epigenetic inheritance of addiction-like phenotypes

Perhaps the most intriguing discovery in epigenetics is that epigenetic marks acquired due to experience can be passed along to future generations. Unfortunately, this may include epigenetic changes that make one vulnerable to addiction. The phrase "it runs in the family" is often spoken in social circles regarding the seeming ability of addiction to be inherited. While much is known about inheritance based on classical Mendelian genetic inheritance, much less is known about transgenerational epigenetic inheritance.

Several criteria must be met for transgenerational epigenetic inheritance. First, in order to pass down epigenetic changes across generations, the changes need to be present in the germ cells (i.e., sperm or egg). In other words, the epigenetic changes must occur in future generations independent of behavioral and social transfer, relying only on the molecular transmission of epigenetic information [71]. Second, the behavioral phenotypes need to persist across several generations, depending on the sex and pregnancy status of the parent exposed to the initial environmental trigger. In males and nonpregnant females, an environmental trigger that affects the parent generation (i.e., F0) and their germ cells, will directly impact the next (i.e., F1) generation. This is referred to as multi- or inter-generational inheritance [72]. However, if the behavioral phenotype persists into the third generation (i.e., F2), which had no direct exposure to the trigger, it can be regarded as transgenerational inheritance. With pregnant females, not only is the parent and embryo directly affected, but also the germ cells of the embryo that will develop into the F2 generation. Therefore, the F3 generation must exhibit the phenotype to be considered transgenerational. Third, epigenetic modifications present in the parents need to persist into future generations (see **Figure 5**). Interestingly, most epigenetic marks (particularly DNA methylation) are erased immediately in the embryo following fertilization [73]. Very few exceptions are currently known, but some include imprinted genes (i.e., methylation-induced silencing of genes in one parent's allele and not in the others), certain histone and protamine (i.e., histone-like proteins found in sperm) modifications, and reserve pools of coding and noncoding RNA [72]. Although narrowing the field of investigation, the complex pattern of changes required for transgenerational epigenetic inheritance still remains poorly understood [72, 74].

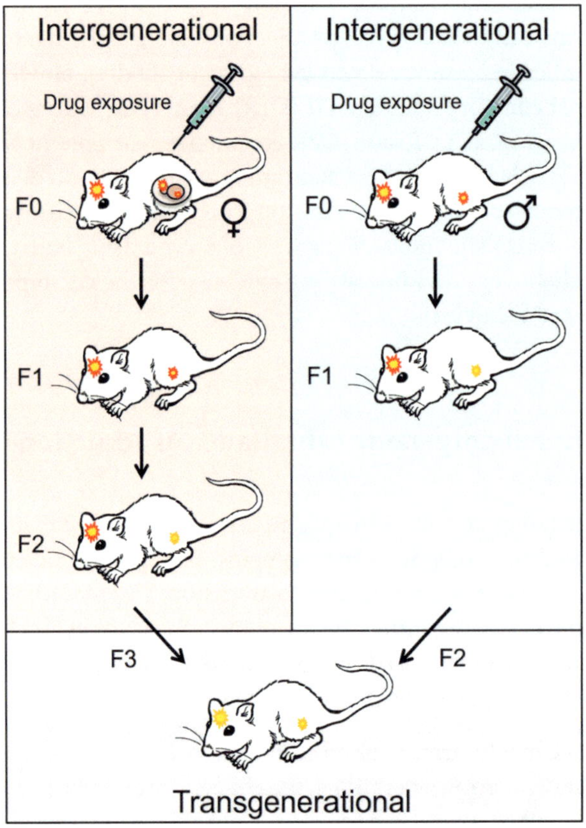

Figure 5. Epigenetic inheritance. For pregnant F0 females (top left panel), drug exposure directly affects (red-outlined symbols) both the F0 female and the fetus, including the brain and germ cells of the upcoming F1 generation. However, the F2 generation also receives direct effects of drug exposure from the F0 generation via the germ cells of the F1 generation. For males (top right panel), drug exposure directly affects both the F0 generation and the germ cells that lead to the F1 generation. Therefore, the F3 and F2 generation of the pregnant female and male, respectively, can receive transgenerational epigenetic inheritance from the F0 generation without having been in direct contact with drugs of abuse (orange-outlined symbols).

11.1. Drug abuse-related traits passed across generations

The idea that addiction-like phenotypes can be passed down across generations based on experiences of the parents is compelling in terms of uncovering potential biomarkers that could be used to predict one's risk of developing drug addiction. Only a few studies have investigated this possibility in the context of drug abuse models. Vassoler and colleagues [75] found that male adult rats with a history of cocaine self-administration passed an addiction-*resistant* phenotype onto male, but not female, offspring. One potential mediator of these effects is mPFC BDNF expression, where both the male F0 generation's sperm and the mPFC of the male, but not female, offspring exhibited increased H3 acetylation at the BDNF promoter, as well as increased BDNF expression in the mPFC of the male offspring. Consistent with this idea, mPFC BDNF is associated with resilience to drug effects [47, 49, 50]. These data are particularly compelling given that it was the father who received the initial trigger (i.e., drug exposure), thereby avoiding potential confounds of maternal care, social/behavioral transfer, and *in utero* environment changes that may occur following drug exposure in the females. Nonetheless, one cannot rule out potential stress effects during copulation. Gapp et al. [76] avoided this potential confound by isolating the sperm of the affected F0 males and artificially inseminating the F0 females. They found that sperm noncoding RNAs from fathers subjected to early life stress sufficiently passed on molecular and behavioral phenotypes to the next two generations. Interestingly, early life stress is also a strong predictor for developing drug addiction [1]. Other studies have shown that repeated morphine administration in F0 female adolescents produces male offspring that are more sensitive to the analgesic and tolerance effects of morphine [77]. Furthermore, ethanol exposure to F0 males decreases ethanol intake and increases sensitivity to the inhibitory effect of ethanol on anxiety-like behavior in F1 offspring [78]. Reduced methylation at the *Bdnf* promoter was also observed in this study in both the F0 male sperm and in the F1 males' VTA. The VTA sends dopaminergic projections to the NAc and BDNF in the VTA has a facilitating effect on drug-abuse-related behavior [79]. These few examples provide some evidence of multi-generational inheritance of drug abuse-related traits and associated changes to the epigenome. However, further research is required to examine if these traits persist into additional generations and whether blocking or reversing the epigenetic changes in the germline will prevent transmission of these traits. The latter effect would have very exciting implications for approaches to prevent the development of addiction in future generations.

12. Concluding remarks

The studies reviewed provide compelling evidence for a link between drug-induced epigenetic regulation of gene expression and drug abuse-related behavior in animals. The epigenetic changes in gene expression occur in brain regions involved in reward learning and motivation. This leads to plasticity-related changes within the neurocircuitries that mediate these processes and is associated with aberrant behaviors that resemble hallmark symptoms of human drug addiction, such as escalation of drug intake [42, 44, 80, 81] and increased willingness to exert effort to obtain drug [46, 82]. Given that epigenetic mechanisms can produce long-lasting changes in gene expression, they are likely candidate explanations for the persistent nature of drug addiction in humans.

Current understanding of experience-dependent epigenetic changes is in its infancy. One notable limitation in this field is the dearth of research on drugs of abuse other than psychostimulants and alcohol. This is a particularly important gap to fill given that regulatory changes in addiction-related genes can have opposite effects on abuse-related behaviors depending on drug class [25, 83, 84]. The field also faces many challenges in discerning the involvement of epigenetic mechanisms in drug addiction given the vast number of molecular regulatory events that are altered by stress and drug experience, the complex interactions that can occur among these regulatory events, and their drug-, region-, and time-specificity. Indeed, high comorbidity exists between drug addiction and stress-related emotional disorders (e.g., PTSD and depression) [85, 86]; therefore, additional work is needed to test whether epigenetic factors underlie the co-occurrence or are specific for one disorder over the other. It will be vital to test the generalizability versus specificity of epigenetic modifications in drug abuse-related behavior.

Despite the challenges that lie ahead, growing knowledge in this field will provide opportunities for novel preventions and interventions of drug abuse and dependence. New technologies for identifying and specifically targeting epigenetic processes hold promise not only for understanding the complex interactions between drug exposure, life experiences, and gene expression, but also as treatment strategies designed to counter epigenetic dysregulation. For instance, the use of synthetic transcription factors may allow drug-induced or inherited epigenetic marks to be erased in order to increase resilience when one is exposed to addictive drugs [69]. Future epigenetics research may also identify biomarkers of vulnerability that may aid prevention strategies. Collectively, these new avenues of drug abuse research are exciting given the urgent need for better treatments of this devastating disorder.

Acknowledgements

This research was supported by the National Institute on Drug Abuse grants DA034097 (JLN) and DA035069 (RMB).

Author details

Ryan M. Bastle and Janet L. Neisewander*

*Address all correspondence to: janet.neisewander@asu.edu

School of Life Sciences, Arizona State University, Tempe, AZ, USA

References

[1] Enoch, M. A., The role of early life stress as a predictor for alcohol and drug dependence. *Psychopharmacology (Berl)* 2011, *214* (1), 17–31.

[2] Enoch, M. A.; Goldman, D., The genetics of alcoholism and alcohol abuse. *Curr Psychiatry Rep* 2001, *3* (2), 144–51.

[3] Reik, W., Stability and flexibility of epigenetic gene regulation in mammalian development. *Nature* 2007, *447* (7143), 425–32.

[4] Milosavljevic, A., Emerging patterns of epigenomic variation. *Trends Genet* 2011, *27* (6), 242–50.

[5] Kauer, J. A.; Malenka, R. C., Synaptic plasticity and addiction. *Nat Rev Neurosci* 2007, *8* (11), 844–58.

[6] Robison, A. J.; Nestler, E. J., Transcriptional and epigenetic mechanisms of addiction. *Nat Rev Neurosci* 2011, *12* (11), 623–37.

[7] Curran, T.; Morgan, J. I., Fos: an immediate-early transcription factor in neurons. *J Neurobiol* 1995, *26* (3), 403–12.

[8] Morgan, J. I.; Curran, T., Stimulus-transcription coupling in the nervous system: involvement of the inducible proto-oncogenes fos and jun. *Annu Rev Neurosci* 1991, *14*, 421–51.

[9] Chaudhuri, A., Neural activity mapping with inducible transcription factors. *Neuroreport* 1997, *8* (13), iii–vii.

[10] Renthal, W.; Nestler, E. J., Epigenetic mechanisms in drug addiction. *Trends Mol Med* 2008, *14* (8), 341–50.

[11] Moore, L. D.; Le, T.; Fan, G., DNA methylation and its basic function. *Neuropsychopharmacology* 2013, *38* (1), 23–38.

[12] Moore, S. P.; Toomire, K. J.; Strauss, P. R., DNA modifications repaired by base excision repair are epigenetic. *DNA Repair (Amst)* 2013, *12* (12), 1152–8.

[13] Branco, M. R.; Ficz, G.; Reik, W., Uncovering the role of 5-hydroxymethylcytosine in the epigenome. *Nat Rev Genet* 2012, *13* (1), 7–13.

[14] Hyman, S. E.; Malenka, R. C.; Nestler, E. J., Neural mechanisms of addiction: the role of reward-related learning and memory. *Annu Rev Neurosci* 2006, *29*, 565–98.

[15] Kelz, M. B.; Nestler, E. J., deltaFosB: a molecular switch underlying long-term neural plasticity. *Curr Opin Neurol* 2000, *13* (6), 715–20.

[16] Anier, K.; Malinovskaja, K.; Aonurm-Helm, A.; Zharkovsky, A.; Kalda, A., DNA methylation regulates cocaine-induced behavioral sensitization in mice. *Neuropsychopharmacology* 2010, *35* (12), 2450–61.

[17] Deng, J. V.; Rodriguiz, R. M.; Hutchinson, A. N.; Kim, I. H.; Wetsel, W. C.; West, A. E., MeCP2 in the nucleus accumbens contributes to neural and behavioral responses to psychostimulants. *Nat Neurosci* 2010, *13* (9), 1128–36.

[18] LaPlant, Q.; Vialou, V.; Covington, H. E., 3rd; Dumitriu, D.; Feng, J.; Warren, B. L.; Maze, I.; Dietz, D. M.; Watts, E. L.; Iniguez, S. D.; Koo, J. W.; Mouzon, E.; Renthal, W.; Hollis, F.; Wang, H.; Noonan, M. A.; Ren, Y.; Eisch, A. J.; Bolanos, C. A.; Kabbaj, M.; Xiao, G.; Neve, R. L.; Hurd, Y. L.; Oosting, R. S.; Fan, G.; Morrison, J. H.; Nestler, E. J.,

Dnmt3a regulates emotional behavior and spine plasticity in the nucleus accumbens. *Nat Neurosci* 2010, *13* (9), 1137–43.

[19] Kriaucionis, S.; Heintz, N., The nuclear DNA base 5-hydroxymethylcytosine is present in Purkinje neurons and the brain. *Science* 2009, *324* (5929), 929–30.

[20] Feng, J.; Shao, N.; Szulwach, K. E.; Vialou, V.; Huynh, J.; Zhong, C.; Le, T.; Ferguson, D.; Cahill, M. E.; Li, Y.; Koo, J. W.; Ribeiro, E.; Labonte, B.; Laitman, B. M.; Estey, D.; Stockman, V.; Kennedy, P.; Courousse, T.; Mensah, I.; Turecki, G.; Faull, K. F.; Ming, G. L.; Song, H.; Fan, G.; Casaccia, P.; Shen, L.; Jin, P.; Nestler, E. J., Role of Tet1 and 5-hydroxymethylcytosine in cocaine action. *Nat Neurosci* 2015, *18* (4), 536–44.

[21] Kumar, A.; Choi, K. H.; Renthal, W.; Tsankova, N. M.; Theobald, D. E.; Truong, H. T.; Russo, S. J.; Laplant, Q.; Sasaki, T. S.; Whistler, K. N.; Neve, R. L.; Self, D. W.; Nestler, E. J., Chromatin remodeling is a key mechanism underlying cocaine-induced plasticity in striatum. *Neuron* 2005, *48* (2), 303–14.

[22] Shen, H. Y.; Kalda, A.; Yu, L.; Ferrara, J.; Zhu, J.; Chen, J. F., Additive effects of histone deacetylase inhibitors and amphetamine on histone H4 acetylation, cAMP responsive element binding protein phosphorylation and DeltaFosB expression in the striatum and locomotor sensitization in mice. *Neuroscience* 2008, *157* (3), 644–55.

[23] Graybiel, A. M.; Moratalla, R.; Robertson, H. A., Amphetamine and cocaine induce drug-specific activation of the c-fos gene in striosome-matrix compartments and limbic subdivisions of the striatum. *Proc Natl Acad Sci U S A* 1990, *87* (17), 6912–6.

[24] Renthal, W.; Carle, T. L.; Maze, I.; Covington, H. E., 3rd; Truong, H. T.; Alibhai, I.; Kumar, A.; Montgomery, R. L.; Olson, E. N.; Nestler, E. J., Delta FosB mediates epigenetic desensitization of the c-fos gene after chronic amphetamine exposure. *J Neurosci* 2008, *28* (29), 7344–9.

[25] Koo, J. W.; Mazei-Robison, M. S.; Chaudhury, D.; Juarez, B.; LaPlant, Q.; Ferguson, D.; Feng, J.; Sun, H.; Scobie, K. N.; Damez-Werno, D.; Crumiller, M.; Ohnishi, Y. N.; Ohnishi, Y. H.; Mouzon, E.; Dietz, D. M.; Lobo, M. K.; Neve, R. L.; Russo, S. J.; Han, M. H.; Nestler, E. J., BDNF is a negative modulator of morphine action. *Science* 2012, *338* (6103), 124–8.

[26] McAllister, A.; Katz, L.; Lo, D., Neurotrophins and synaptic plasticity. *Annu Rev Neurosci* 1999, *22*, 295–318.

[27] Poo, M., Neurotrophins as synaptic modulators. *Nat Rev Neurosci* 2001, *2* (1), 24–32.

[28] Feltenstein, M. W.; See, R. E., The neurocircuitry of addiction: an overview. *Br J Pharmacol* 2008, *154* (2), 261–74.

[29] Pierce, R. C.; Kumaresan, V., The mesolimbic dopamine system: the final common pathway for the reinforcing effect of drugs of abuse? *Neurosci Biobehav Rev* 2006, *30* (2), 215–38.

[30] Pandey, S. C.; Sakharkar, A. J.; Tang, L.; Zhang, H., Potential role of adolescent alcohol exposure-induced amygdaloid histone modifications in anxiety and alcohol intake during adulthood. *Neurobiol Dis* 2015, *82*, 607–19.

[31] Koob, G. F.; Volkow, N. D., Neurocircuitry of addiction. *Neuropsychopharmacology* 2010, *35* (1), 217–38.

[32] Renthal, W.; Kumar, A.; Xiao, G.; Wilkinson, M.; Covington, H. E., 3rd; Maze, I.; Sikder, D.; Robison, A. J.; LaPlant, Q.; Dietz, D. M.; Russo, S. J.; Vialou, V.; Chakravarty, S.; Kodadek, T. J.; Stack, A.; Kabbaj, M.; Nestler, E. J., Genome-wide analysis of chromatin regulation by cocaine reveals a role for sirtuins. *Neuron* 2009, *62* (3), 335–48.

[33] Maze, I.; Covington, H. E., 3rd; Dietz, D. M.; LaPlant, Q.; Renthal, W.; Russo, S. J.; Mechanic, M.; Mouzon, E.; Neve, R. L.; Haggarty, S. J.; Ren, Y.; Sampath, S. C.; Hurd, Y. L.; Greengard, P.; Tarakhovsky, A.; Schaefer, A.; Nestler, E. J., Essential role of the histone methyltransferase G9a in cocaine-induced plasticity. *Science* 2010, *327* (5962), 213–6.

[34] Sun, H.; Maze, I.; Dietz, D. M.; Scobie, K. N.; Kennedy, P. J.; Damez-Werno, D.; Neve, R. L.; Zachariou, V.; Shen, L.; Nestler, E. J., Morphine epigenomically regulates behavior through alterations in histone H3 lysine 9 dimethylation in the nucleus accumbens. *J Neurosci* 2012, *32* (48), 17454–64.

[35] Covington, H. E., 3rd; Maze, I.; Sun, H.; Bomze, H. M.; DeMaio, K. D.; Wu, E. Y.; Dietz, D. M.; Lobo, M. K.; Ghose, S.; Mouzon, E.; Neve, R. L.; Tamminga, C. A.; Nestler, E. J., A role for repressive histone methylation in cocaine-induced vulnerability to stress. *Neuron* 2011, *71* (4), 656–70.

[36] Maze, I.; Chaudhury, D.; Dietz, D. M.; Von Schimmelmann, M.; Kennedy, P. J.; Lobo, M. K.; Sillivan, S. E.; Miller, M. L.; Bagot, R. C.; Sun, H.; Turecki, G.; Neve, R. L.; Hurd, Y. L.; Shen, L.; Han, M. H.; Schaefer, A.; Nestler, E. J., G9a influences neuronal subtype specification in striatum. *Nat Neurosci* 2014, *17* (4), 533–9.

[37] Robison, A. J.; Vialou, V.; Mazei-Robison, M.; Feng, J.; Kourrich, S.; Collins, M.; Wee, S.; Koob, G.; Turecki, G.; Neve, R.; Thomas, M.; Nestler, E. J., Behavioral and structural responses to chronic cocaine require a feedforward loop involving DeltaFosB and calcium/calmodulin-dependent protein kinase II in the nucleus accumbens shell. *J Neurosci* 2013, *33* (10), 4295–307.

[38] Maze, I.; Feng, J.; Wilkinson, M. B.; Sun, H.; Shen, L.; Nestler, E. J., Cocaine dynamically regulates heterochromatin and repetitive element unsilencing in nucleus accumbens. *Proc Natl Acad Sci U S A* 2011, *108* (7), 3035–40.

[39] Bartel, D. P., MicroRNAs: genomics, biogenesis, mechanism, and function. *Cell* 2004, *116* (2), 281–97.

[40] Filipowicz, W.; Bhattacharyya, S. N.; Sonenberg, N., Mechanisms of post-transcriptional regulation by microRNAs: are the answers in sight? *Nat Rev Genet* 2008, *9* (2), 102–14.

[41] Cech, T. R.; Steitz, J. A., The noncoding RNA revolution-trashing old rules to forge new ones. *Cell* 2014, *157* (1), 77–94.

[42] Hollander, J. A.; Im, H. I.; Amelio, A. L.; Kocerha, J.; Bali, P.; Lu, Q.; Willoughby, D.; Wahlestedt, C.; Conkright, M. D.; Kenny, P. J., Striatal microRNA controls cocaine intake through CREB signalling. *Nature* 2010, *466* (7303), 197–202.

[43] Everitt, B. J.; Robbins, T. W., Neural systems of reinforcement for drug addiction: from actions to habits to compulsion. *Nat Neurosci* 2005, *8* (11), 1481–9.

[44] Im, H. I.; Hollander, J. A.; Bali, P.; Kenny, P. J., MeCP2 controls BDNF expression and cocaine intake through homeostatic interactions with microRNA-212. *Nat Neurosci* 2010, *13* (9), 1120–7.

[45] Li, C. Y.; Mao, X.; Wei, L., Genes and (common) pathways underlying drug addiction. *PLoS Comput Biol* 2008, *4* (1), e2.

[46] Bastle, R.; Pentkowski, N.; Oliver, R.; Gardiner, A.; Smith, C.; Taylor, J.; Galles, N.; Perrone-Bizzozero, N.; Neisewander, J., In *Viral-mediated Overexpression of miR-495 in the Nucleus Accumbens Shell Reduces Motivation for Cocaine*, American College of Neuropsychopharmacology, Phoenix, AZ, December; Phoenix, AZ, 2014.

[47] Tapocik, J. D.; Barbier, E.; Flanigan, M.; Solomon, M.; Pincus, A.; Pilling, A.; Sun, H.; Schank, J. R.; King, C.; Heilig, M., microRNA-206 in rat medial prefrontal cortex regulates BDNF expression and alcohol drinking. *J Neurosci* 2014, *34* (13), 4581–8.

[48] Kalivas, P. W.; Volkow, N. D., The neural basis of addiction: a pathology of motivation and choice. *Am J Psychiatry* 2005, *162* (8), 1403–13.

[49] Berglind, W. J.; See, R. E.; Fuchs, R. A.; Ghee, S. M.; Whitfield, T. W., Jr.; Miller, S. W.; McGinty, J. F., A BDNF infusion into the medial prefrontal cortex suppresses cocaine seeking in rats. *Eur J Neurosci* 2007, *26* (3), 757–66.

[50] Sadri-Vakili, G.; Kumaresan, V.; Schmidt, H. D.; Famous, K. R.; Chawla, P.; Vassoler, F. M.; Overland, R. P.; Xia, E.; Bass, C. E.; Terwilliger, E. F.; Pierce, R. C.; Cha, J. H., Cocaine-induced chromatin remodeling increases brain-derived neurotrophic factor transcription in the rat medial prefrontal cortex, which alters the reinforcing efficacy of cocaine. *J Neurosci* 2010, *30* (35), 11735–44.

[51] Michelhaugh, S. K.; Lipovich, L.; Blythe, J.; Jia, H.; Kapatos, G.; Bannon, M. J., Mining Affymetrix microarray data for long non-coding RNAs: altered expression in the nucleus accumbens of heroin abusers. *J Neurochem* 2011, *116* (3), 459–66.

[52] Wright, K. N.; Hollis, F.; Duclot, F.; Dossat, A. M.; Strong, C. E.; Francis, T. C.; Mercer, R.; Feng, J.; Dietz, D. M.; Lobo, M. K.; Nestler, E. J.; Kabbaj, M., Methyl supplementation

attenuates cocaine-seeking behaviors and cocaine-induced c-Fos activation in a DNA methylation-dependent manner. *J Neurosci* 2015, *35* (23), 8948–58.

[53] Massart, R.; Barnea, R.; Dikshtein, Y.; Suderman, M.; Meir, O.; Hallett, M.; Kennedy, P.; Nestler, E. J.; Szyf, M.; Yadid, G., Role of DNA methylation in the nucleus accumbens in incubation of cocaine craving. *J Neurosci* 2015, *35* (21), 8042–58.

[54] Tran-Nguyen, L. T.; Fuchs, R. A.; Coffey, G. P.; Baker, D. A.; O'Dell, L. E.; Neisewander, J. L., Time-dependent changes in cocaine-seeking behavior and extracellular dopamine levels in the amygdala during cocaine withdrawal. *Neuropsychopharmacology* 1998, *19* (1), 48–59.

[55] Grimm, J. W.; Lu, L.; Hayashi, T.; Hope, B. T.; Su, T. P.; Shaham, Y., Time-dependent increases in brain-derived neurotrophic factor protein levels within the mesolimbic dopamine system after withdrawal from cocaine: implications for incubation of cocaine craving. *J Neurosci* 2003, *23* (3), 742–7.

[56] Pentkowski, N. S.; Harder, B. G.; Brunwasser, S. J.; Bastle, R. M.; Peartree, N. A.; Yanamandra, K.; Adams, M. D.; Der-Ghazarian, T.; Neisewander, J. L., Pharmacological evidence for an abstinence-induced switch in 5-HT1B receptor modulation of cocaine self-administration and cocaine-seeking behavior. *ACS Chem Neurosci* 2014, *5* (3), 168–76.

[57] Sanchis-Segura, C.; Lopez-Atalaya, J. P.; Barco, A., Selective boosting of transcriptional and behavioral responses to drugs of abuse by histone deacetylase inhibition. *Neuropsychopharmacology* 2009, *34* (13), 2642–54.

[58] Schroeder, F. A.; Penta, K. L.; Matevossian, A.; Jones, S. R.; Konradi, C.; Tapper, A. R.; Akbarian, S., Drug-induced activation of dopamine D(1) receptor signaling and inhibition of class I/II histone deacetylase induce chromatin remodeling in reward circuitry and modulate cocaine-related behaviors. *Neuropsychopharmacology* 2008, *33* (12), 2981–92.

[59] Sheng, J.; Lv, Z.; Wang, L.; Zhou, Y.; Hui, B., Histone H3 phosphoacetylation is critical for heroin-induced place preference. *Neuroreport* 2011, *22* (12), 575–80.

[60] Sun, J.; Wang, L.; Jiang, B.; Hui, B.; Lv, Z.; Ma, L., The effects of sodium butyrate, an inhibitor of histone deacetylase, on the cocaine- and sucrose-maintained self-administration in rats. *Neurosci Lett* 2008, *441* (1), 72–6.

[61] Malvaez, M.; Sanchis-Segura, C.; Vo, D.; Lattal, K. M.; Wood, M. A., Modulation of chromatin modification facilitates extinction of cocaine-induced conditioned place preference. *Biol Psychiatry* 2010, *67* (1), 36–43.

[62] Qiang, M.; Li, J. G.; Denny, A. D.; Yao, J. M.; Lieu, M.; Zhang, K.; Carreon, S., Epigenetic mechanisms are involved in the regulation of ethanol consumption in mice. *Int J Neuropsychopharmacol* 2015, *18* (2), 1–11.

[63] Simon-O'Brien, E.; Alaux-Cantin, S.; Warnault, V.; Buttolo, R.; Naassila, M.; Vilpoux, C., The histone deacetylase inhibitor sodium butyrate decreases excessive ethanol intake in dependent animals. *Addict Biol* 2015, *20* (4), 676–89.

[64] Warnault, V.; Darcq, E.; Levine, A.; Barak, S.; Ron, D., Chromatin remodeling—a novel strategy to control excessive alcohol drinking. *Transl Psychiatry* 2013, *3*, e231.

[65] Pandey, S. C.; Zhang, H.; Roy, A.; Misra, K., Central and medial amygdaloid brain-derived neurotrophic factor signaling plays a critical role in alcohol-drinking and anxiety-like behaviors. *J Neurosci* 2006, *26* (32), 8320–31.

[66] Jeanblanc, J.; Lemoine, S.; Jeanblanc, V.; Alaux-Cantin, S.; Naassila, M., The class I-specific HDAC inhibitor MS-275 decreases motivation to consume alcohol and relapse in heavy drinking rats. *Int J Neuropsychopharmacol* 2015, *18* (9), 1–9.

[67] Kennedy, P. J.; Feng, J.; Robison, A. J.; Maze, I.; Badimon, A.; Mouzon, E.; Chaudhury, D.; Damez-Werno, D. M.; Haggarty, S. J.; Han, M. H.; Bassel-Duby, R.; Olson, E. N.; Nestler, E. J., Class I HDAC inhibition blocks cocaine-induced plasticity by targeted changes in histone methylation. *Nat Neurosci* 2013, *16* (4), 434–40.

[68] Malvaez, M.; McQuown, S. C.; Rogge, G. A.; Astarabadi, M.; Jacques, V.; Carreiro, S.; Rusche, J. R.; Wood, M. A., HDAC3-selective inhibitor enhances extinction of cocaine-seeking behavior in a persistent manner. *Proc Natl Acad Sci U S A* 2013, *110* (7), 2647–52.

[69] Heller, E. A.; Cates, H. M.; Pena, C. J.; Sun, H.; Shao, N.; Feng, J.; Golden, S. A.; Herman, J. P.; Walsh, J. J.; Mazei-Robison, M.; Ferguson, D.; Knight, S.; Gerber, M. A.; Nievera, C.; Han, M. H.; Russo, S. J.; Tamminga, C. S.; Neve, R. L.; Shen, L.; Zhang, H. S.; Zhang, F.; Nestler, E. J., Locus-specific epigenetic remodeling controls addiction- and depression-related behaviors. *Nat Neurosci* 2014, *17* (12), 1720–7.

[70] van Rooij, E.; Purcell, A. L.; Levin, A. A., Developing microRNA therapeutics. *Circ Res* 2012, *110* (3), 496–507.

[71] Bohacek, J.; Mansuy, I. M., Molecular insights into transgenerational non-genetic inheritance of acquired behaviours. *Nat Rev Genet* 2015, *16* (11), 641–52.

[72] Heard, E.; Martienssen, R. A., Transgenerational epigenetic inheritance: myths and mechanisms. *Cell* 2014, *157* (1), 95–109.

[73] Gapp, K.; von Ziegler, L.; Tweedie-Cullen, R. Y.; Mansuy, I. M., Early life epigenetic programming and transmission of stress-induced traits in mammals: how and when can environmental factors influence traits and their transgenerational inheritance? *Bioessays* 2014, *36* (5), 491–502.

[74] Daxinger, L.; Whitelaw, E., Understanding transgenerational epigenetic inheritance via the gametes in mammals. *Nat Rev Genet* 2012, *13* (3), 153–62.

[75] Vassoler, F. M.; White, S. L.; Schmidt, H. D.; Sadri-Vakili, G.; Pierce, R. C., Epigenetic inheritance of a cocaine-resistance phenotype. *Nat Neurosci* 2013, *16* (1), 42–7.

[76] Gapp, K.; Jawaid, A.; Sarkies, P.; Bohacek, J.; Pelczar, P.; Prados, J.; Farinelli, L.; Miska, E.; Mansuy, I. M., Implication of sperm RNAs in transgenerational inheritance of the effects of early trauma in mice. *Nat Neurosci* 2014, *17* (5), 667–9.

[77] Byrnes, J. J.; Babb, J. A.; Scanlan, V. F.; Byrnes, E. M., Adolescent opioid exposure in female rats: transgenerational effects on morphine analgesia and anxiety-like behavior in adult offspring. *Behav Brain Res* 2011, *218* (1), 200–5.

[78] Finegersh, A.; Homanics, G. E., Paternal alcohol exposure reduces alcohol drinking and increases behavioral sensitivity to alcohol selectively in male offspring. *PLoS One* 2014, *9* (6), e99078.

[79] Lu, L.; Dempsey, J.; Liu, S. Y.; Bossert, J. M.; Shaham, Y., A single infusion of brain-derived neurotrophic factor into the ventral tegmental area induces long-lasting potentiation of cocaine seeking after withdrawal. *J Neurosci* 2004, *24* (7), 1604–11.

[80] Ahmed, S.; Koob, G., Transition from moderate to excessive drug intake: change in hedonic set point. *Science (New York, N.Y.)* 1998, *282* (5387), 298–300.

[81] Everitt, B.; Robbins, T., Neural systems of reinforcement for drug addiction: from actions to habits to compulsion. *Nat Neurosci* 2005, *8* (11), 1481–89.

[82] Roberts, D. C.; Morgan, D.; Liu, Y., How to make a rat addicted to cocaine. *Prog Neuropsychopharmacol Biol Psychiatry* 2007, *31* (8), 1614–24.

[83] Lu, L.; Dempsey, J.; Liu, S.; Bossert, J.; Shaham, Y., A single infusion of brain-derived neurotrophic factor into the ventral tegmental area induces long-lasting potentiation of cocaine seeking after withdrawal. *J Neurosci: Off J Soc Neurosci* 2004, *24* (7), 1604–1611.

[84] Graham, D. L.; Krishnan, V.; Larson, E. B.; Graham, A.; Edwards, S.; Bachtell, R. K.; Simmons, D.; Gent, L. M.; Berton, O.; Bolanos, C. A.; DiLeone, R. J.; Parada, L. F.; Nestler, E. J.; Self, D. W., Tropomyosin-related kinase B in the mesolimbic dopamine system: region-specific effects on cocaine reward. *Biol Psychiatry* 2009, *65* (8), 696–701.

[85] Davis, L.; Uezato, A.; Newell, J. M.; Frazier, E., Major depression and comorbid substance use disorders. *Curr Opin Psychiatry* 2008, *21* (1), 14–8.

[86] Brown, P. J.; Wolfe, J., Substance abuse and post-traumatic stress disorder comorbidity. *Drug Alcohol Depend* 1994, *35* (1), 51–9.

Chapter 3

Alcohol Cues, Craving, and Relapse: Insights from Animal Models

Melanie M. Pina and Amy R. Williams

Additional information is available at the end of the chapter

http://dx.doi.org/10.5772/63105

Abstract

Alcoholism is a chronic relapsing and remitting disorder, where relapse to drinking is often triggered by an intense desire for alcohol (craving) and the consequent motivation to obtain alcohol (seeking). Environmental stimuli (cues) associated with past alcohol use are believed to strongly contribute to relapse, as exposure to these cues can trigger intense feelings of craving and drive alcohol seeking. Over the past several decades, much progress has been made in identifying the neurobiological correlates of alcohol seeking and relapse. Much of this progress is owed to the development of animal models and advanced techniques to manipulate neural activity. In this chapter, we describe some of the most commonly used rodent models of alcohol intake and seeking as well as the methods used to identify the neural structures and circuits involved in alcohol-mediated behavior. Several of the most routinely identified brain structures in alcohol seeking are also described.

Keywords: alcohol, ethanol, relapse, amygdala, accumbens, VTA

1. Introduction

Alcohol use disorders (AUDs) constitute a major global health concern. In 2013 alone, 5.9% of all deaths worldwide were attributed to alcohol intake (WHO, 2015). This statistic combined with the social, emotional, and other physical consequences of excessive alcohol use makes it is difficult to deny the ongoing need for preclinical research. Of greatest interest is identifying the treatments to promote and maintain abstinence in individuals diagnosed with an AUD. Remission, however, is often characterized by a chronic vulnerability to relapse, which is poorly understood. In fact, estimates of long-term relapse rates following remission are as high as 60%, depending on the treatment sought [1]. Lack of information on the neurobiological antecedents and psychological determinates of relapse makes AUDs all the more problematic to address.

Further complicating our understanding of the persistent risk of relapse are the complex interactions between internal processes and the external environment. Most noted are the relationships that develop between environmental stimuli (cues), both contextual and discrete, and the internal states produced by alcohol. Over the course of alcohol use, specific cues become associated with the effects of alcohol through a Pavlovian learning process, whereby an associative (alcohol-cue) relationship is formed. Once the relationship has been acquired, these associative cues are able to autonomously produce psychological and physiological states that are powerful enough to elicit behavior responses. These responses have been suggested to play an important role in the development of AUDs and relapse.

Even after lengthy periods of abstinence, exposure to drug-associated cues can trigger intense feelings of craving and drive drug seeking [2–5], leading to relapse to drug use. When considering alcohol in particular, this lingering sensitivity to related cues is especially problematic given the omnipresent nature of alcohol and alcohol-related cues in society. Therefore, it is important that the neurobiology of this phenomenon be understood so that more effective and durable treatments for alcoholism can be designed.

In the following sections, we describe common methodologies used to probe the neurobiology underlying primary and conditioned ethanol reward. Specifically, these methodological sections detail several commonly used animal models and tools to manipulate the brain. We then discuss the neural substrates that have been identified in ethanol-seeking behavior using these models and tools.

2. Animal models

To gain an understanding of the neurobiological mechanisms underlying AUDs, numerous animal models have been developed. These models are designed to reflect various aspects of alcoholism. The most widely used procedures assess ethanol reward and reinforcement and include drinking, self-administration, and conditioned place preference (CPP). These animal models share significant homology to certain elements of AUDs in humans, such as the patterns of alcohol consumption, responses to alcohol-associated cues, and alcohol-seeking behavior. Note that, in this review, the terms reward and reinforcement are distinguished from one another. Although reward is used to refer to the appetitive nature of a stimulus as indicated by the ability of environmental stimuli to elicit approach behavior, reinforcement will refer to experimental contingencies that increase the likelihood of behavior(s) occurring [6, 7]. It should be noted that no animal model could fully emulate all aspects of human alcoholism. However, animal models allow for unparalleled access to the brain and thus provide a means to evaluate neural mechanisms involved in the aspects of alcohol reward and dependence. These models therefore represent invaluable preclinical tools for identifying potential biological correlates of and treatments for AUDs.

http://dx.doi.org/10.5772/63105

2.1. Drinking

For nearly a century, it has been known that rodents, like humans, will voluntarily consume alcohol [8, 9]. For this reason, rodents have long been used in drinking procedures that involve home-cage access to alcohol (ethanol). This represents the simplest way to gauge ethanol reward, through consumption, which is done simply by providing rodents with a bottle and measuring the amount they drink. Although alcohol is occasionally the only solution provided in drinking studies, two-bottle choice procedures are more commonly used in rodents and yield an additional measure of preference for alcohol. In a two-bottle choice drinking procedure, home-cage access to alcohol and another alcohol-free fluid (typically water) is provided continuously or at temporally controlled intervals. Evidence of ethanol reward is then indicated by the amount consumed and preference for the alcohol-containing solution over the other available fluid. Manipulations that affect alcohol consumption and/or preference but not water or total fluid intake are believed to have interfered with the rewarding properties of ethanol [10].

Although these studies have high face validity (as humans voluntarily consume alcohol orally), they are often limited by the fact that, like humans, rodents are sensitive to the aversive taste of ethanol. At higher concentrations, the aversive taste of ethanol makes it difficult for rodents to drink to the state of intoxication. Therefore, procedures requiring oral intake of ethanol may require water deprivation, slow increases in ethanol concentration, and/or the addition of a sweetener such as sucrose to the ethanol-containing solution to help rodents overcome the aversive taste [11, 12]. For instance, modified sucrose fading techniques [13] are a common strategy that has been used to achieve voluntary consumption of high concentration of ethanol in rodents. With this technique, sweeteners such as sucrose or saccharin are initially added to an ethanol solution then slowly faded out. However, this illustrates a pitfall of these procedures, which is that the underlying motivation for ethanol consumption is not always understood. For example, rodents may freely consume ethanol for the sweetened taste or for its caloric value. Therefore, it is not always evident that ethanol is being consumed in this procedure for its postabsorptive pharmacological effects. Additionally, intervention-induced decreases in alcohol intake in this procedure do not always indicate that a manipulation decreased the ethanol reward. It is possible that a reduced intake may reflect an enhancement of the pharmacological effects of ethanol, resulting in a leftward shift in the dose-response curve, which translates to an increased effect of ethanol at lower amounts. Furthermore, rodents tend to titrate their dose of ethanol consumption and often do not reach blood ethanol concentrations (BECs) of intoxication unless induced to consume greater volumes via sucrose fading or limited access to ethanol [14]. As a result, care must be taken when interpreting results in drinking studies, as the underlying reasons for decreased intake may not always be apparent.

2.2. Self-administration

In self-administration procedures, rodents must successfully perform an operant response (e.g., lever press or nose poke) to receive a small volume of an ethanol solution [15]. With this method, requisite responding is used to assess the reinforcing value of ethanol. A major advantage of self-administration procedures is that they allow for the assessment of ethanol reinforcement at distinct phases. Methodological manipulations in these procedures allow for the evaluation of the development of and enhancement in ethanol responding, including in the absence of drug (extinction) and the reemergence of responding to various environmental stimuli after responding has been extinguished (cue-, stress-, and ethanol-induced reinstatement). Thus, this procedure can be successfully used as a model aspect of alcohol seeking (rate of responding or latency to bar press for alcohol). Also, self-administration studies can be used to assess the animal's motivation to receive ethanol by increasing the difficulty of the requisite responding (a progressive ratio schedule, in which responding requirements are increased after every the delivery of reinforcer) and thus evaluating the willingness of the animal to work for an ethanol reinforcer [16]. As with humans, rodents will exert effort to obtain ethanol and this effort or seeking behavior can be reduced by administration of therapeutic agents indicated for the treatment of AUDs, such as naltrexone [17]. As such, reinstatement procedures have been shown to be highly useful for the preclinical evaluation of pharmacotherapies aimed at reducing ethanol relapse in humans (reviewed in [18]).

In addition to the rate and pattern of responding, self-administration procedures also yield an additional measure of amount of alcohol consumed. However, similar to drinking studies, the aversive taste of ethanol may be difficult to overcome in self-administration procedures. Therefore, liquid deprivation and fading strategies have also been used to establish operant responding for and consumption of ethanol. This similarly compromises straightforward interpretations of the underlying purpose for the behavior. Interpretation of studies using operant oral paradigms may also be complicated because it is difficult to distinguish between the phases of intake. As training procedures are necessary to establish ethanol self-administration and responding or intake serves as the primary dependent variable, it can be challenging to separate acquisition and learning from seeking, for example.

2.3. Place conditioning

Another approach to modeling reward in rodents is the CPP procedure. With this Pavlovian (classical) conditioning procedure, a distinct environmental stimulus [conditioned stimulus (CS)] can acquire incentive salience after being paired with a motivationally significant stimulus [unconditioned stimulus (US)]. Ultimately, the previously neutral stimulus (CS) develops the ability to elicit a conditioned motivational response similar to the response elicited by the US. This mimics the ability of cues or contexts associated with alcohol (e.g., alcohol containers, odors, advertisements, and drinking establishments) to elicit craving and seeking for alcohol in humans with AUDs. In addition, drug-induced CPP can be established in humans in a laboratory setting, further validating this model [19]. As such, the CPP procedure is widely used to study the motivational properties of many abused drugs, and given its numerous benefits, the popularity of this procedure continues to grow. In the last decade alone, there has been a greater than two-fold increase in the total number of publications reporting its use (**Figure 1**). Thus, this procedure is considered one of the most popular models of drug reward [20, 21].

http://dx.doi.org/10.5772/63105

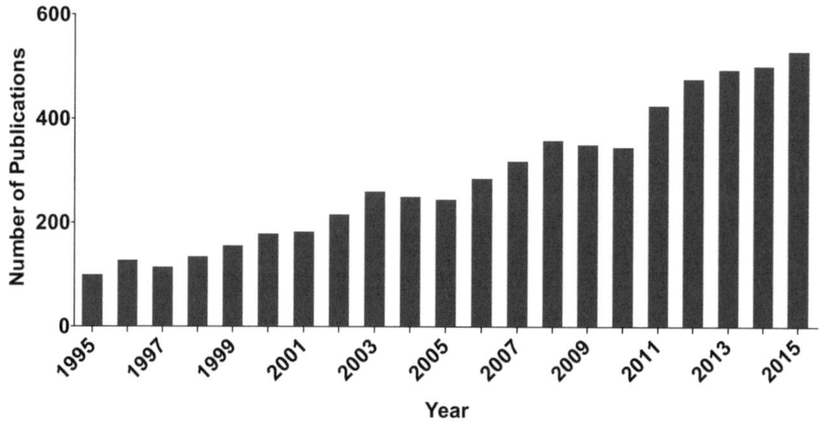

Figure 1. Annual number of CPP studies published over the last 20 years. Values were obtained from PubMed using the search term "CPP" OR "place preference" OR "place conditioning". Adapted from Tzschentke [20, 21].

In a standard ethanol CPP procedure, a discrete cue [e.g., visual or tactile stimulus; referred to as the positive CS (CS+)] presented in one spatial location is repeatedly paired with ethanol, usually administered by the investigator (i.e., noncontingently). On alternating sessions, a different stimulus not paired with ethanol [typically paired with saline, the negative CS (CS-)] is presented in a location adjacent to where the CS+ was presented. During this acquisition phase, an association develops between the CS+ and the subjective effects of ethanol (US). In the subsequent drug-free expression phase, animals are given access to the entire conditioning apparatus and thus to both cues (CS+ and CS-). When given the choice between the CS+ and CS-, animals assess the memory formed in the acquisition phase and will generally approach and maintain contact with (i.e., prefer) the CS+ when a US is rewarding. In other words, if an animal spends a greater amount of time with the ethanol-paired stimulus (CS+) in relation to the nondrug-paired stimulus (CS-), this is taken as an indication of the positive motivational effects of alcohol. Conversely, a greater amount of time spent with the saline-paired stimulus compared to the ethanol-paired stimulus would be considered conditioned place aversion (CPA) and taken to indicate a negative motivational effect of ethanol. The ability of alcohol to produce CPP or CPA depends on many factors, such as past history of ethanol exposure, route of administration, injection timing, and dose (e.g., [22–26]). A result of conditioned reward or aversion can vary by species and strain. Although conditioned ethanol responses have been reported in some strains of rat (e.g., [27–29]), studies overall have shown conflicting results ranging from lack of CPP [30] to CPA [31, 32]. However, ethanol CPP has been found in a wide array of mouse strains [33] and thus has much utility as a model of ethanol reward in this species.

Unlike self-administration, CPP does not require a lengthy training phase. In fact, in an inbred st rain of mouse (DBA/2J) commonly used in ethanol CPP, a significant place preference can be conditioned after only two ethanol-cue pairings [34–36]. Another advantage to this procedure is that it does not involve oral intake of ethanol, which is required in drinking and self-administration procedures. This is highly beneficial in cases where manipulations, such as pharmacology agents, reduce general consummatory behavior in addition to ethanol reward or reinforcement. For example, erroneous conclusions may be made when a drug with anorectic liability reduces the oral intake of ethanol. However, because CPP involves noncontingent ethanol administration, the effect of anorectic drugs on ethanol reward can be assessed more accurately [35]. The place preference paradigm also permits for the evaluation of manipulations on the various phases of learning an ethanol-paired cue that are often difficult to isolate in other procedures, and an understanding of these various phases of learning is important for understanding the progression of alcohol addiction. These phases include the acquisition, conditioned expression, extinction, and reinstatement of the conditioned effects of ethanol. Acquisition and conditioned expression of CPP are described in the paragraph above. Extinction occurs following repeated exposures to the CS+ unpaired with the US (ethanol), which results in a loss of conditioned responding as the animal learns that the CS+ and US are no longer associated and the CS+ loses its rewarding value. Reinstatement, the phase most comparable to relapse in the human condition of addiction, is the reemergence of ethanol-seeking behavior following extinction, usually elicited by a priming injection of a low dose of ethanol (US), stress, or ethanol cues before being placed within the conditioning apparatus. Specifically, when a manipulation disrupts the expression of ethanol CPP, this is generally taken to indicate that it interfered with the conditioned rewarding effect of ethanol or ethanol seeking. Indeed, because CPP can be used to gauge the conditioned rewarding or motivational value of stimuli, it also serves as an effective method to measure cue-induced ethanol-seeking behavior. On the other hand, manipulations that disrupt the development (acquisition) of CPP are thought to impact either associative learning or the primary rewarding effect of ethanol. To distinguish between these two possibilities, this procedure can also be used to assess whether the manipulation also disrupts the acquisition of other associations such as CPA induced by ethanol or other drugs (e.g., [34]). However, if a manipulation specifically affects the extinction of CPP, it is thought to impair the formation of an inhibitory memory, which relies on different neural structures than those required for the acquisition of CPP. If a manipulation impairs the reinstatement of CPP, it is thought to either impair mechanisms that allow for evaluation updating or reemergence of behavior, but manipulations could also prevent access to the original acquisition memory and manipulations must be assessed for specificity to reinstatement.

One disadvantage of the CPP procedure is that the drug is administered by the investigator and therefore delivered noncontingently. Although this may be considered an advantage given the control over the dose it provides, it reduces the face validity of this model. Unlike humans, in this procedure, rodents do not consume alcohol of their own volition. Similarly, humans do not take alcohol via intraperitoneal injections, as is used in this animal model. Moreover, this procedure does not typically involve an escalation in intake, as is usually observed in humans. Comparable to self-administration procedures, manipulations that affect locomotor activity may also nonspecifically impact CPP expression. It has been previously demonstrated that increases in activity may disrupt ethanol CPP expression, thereby obscuring its detection [37]. Hence, results obtained by manipulations that increased or decreased preference test activity must be cautiously interpreted. Despite these drawbacks, this model presents a rapid and efficient method to evaluate the primary and conditioned motivational effects of ethanol in rodents.

2.4. Summary

In summary, animal models have been used extensively in alcohol research, with several models designed to study the various aspects of ethanol-mediated behavior. The most standard used procedures to model ethanol seeking are self-administration and CPP. Although it should be noted that no one procedure is able to mimic all features of human alcohol use, these models allow for the investigation of the underlying neural mechanisms involved in distinct alcohol-related behaviors. Furthermore, the paradigms described here do not encompass all models of AUDs available. Additional models include operant runway models, vapor chamber exposure, intracranial self-stimulation, and locomotor sensitization. In the following sections, several commonly used techniques to probe the neural structures and circuits involved in rodent behavior and their application to animal models of ethanol seeking are described.

3. Tools to manipulate neural structures

Many techniques have been developed to evaluate distinct brain structures. These methods allow for the direct manipulation of a defined brain area to manipulate their activity during behavior. Thus, they require intracranial access typically gained through stereotaxic surgery. Of these methods, the most widely used are lesions and microinjection. However, more modern tools have been developed that harness the capabilities of viral gene transfer to more precisely control cells and circuits. Each of these techniques, classic and contemporary, possesses inherent benefits and drawbacks that are discussed in detail below and summarized in **Table 1**.

3.1. Classical tools

3.1.1. Lesions

A classical method used to study brain function involves the removal or destruction of neural tissue. With this method, experimental lesions are made to defined brain structures through manual, chemical, or electrical means and can also be neurotransmitter specific. Popular neurotransmitter-specific lesioning agents include 6-hydroxydopamine (dopaminergic and noradrenergic neurons), 5,7-dihydroxytryptamine (serotonergic neurons), ibotenic acid [N-methyl-D-aspartate (NMDA) receptor-containing neurons], kainic acid (kainate receptor-containing neurons), and many others. Behavior is then examined in the absence of this tissue, thus providing insight into the involvement of the lesioned structure. Histology, such as simple cresyl violet stains or for markers of neuronal damage, is performed on neural tissue after behavior to confirm the location of damage. One issue that arises is the propensity for other brain structures to compensate for the damaged region. This may severely compromise the interpretation of results obtained from studies using a lesion procedure. Another issue is the difficulty encountered when using lesions to assess the effects at distinct phases of a behavior, as lesions cause irreversible damage to the region. Thus, with many animal models, it is difficult to determine whether ablation of a structure impacted the development (acquisition), performance (expression), extinction, or reinstatement of behavior. To affect a distinct phase of behavior, lesions can be made at specific times in the model. However, phase-specific lesions can unintentionally alter later behavior and can even impair the memory of earlier phases.

Criteria	**Classical tools**						**Contemporary tools**			
	Lesion		**Microinjection**		**Tracing**		**Optogenetic**		**Chemogenetic**	
Spatial resolution	1	Depends on lesion type	1	Spread difficult to determine	2	Labeled spread; targeted to cells	2	Labeled spread; targeted to cells	2	Labeled spread; targeted to cells
Temporal resolution	0	Permanent	1	Minutes to hours depending on drug	0	Permanent	2	Milliseconds	1	Minutes to hours depending on actuator
Non invasive	1	Single i.c. entry but involves intentional tissue damage	0	Permanent hardware, repeated i.c. access	1	Single i.c. entry, but tracers may be toxic	0	Permanent hardware, repeated i.c. access	2	Single i.c. entry, activation by peripheral injection
Cell specificity	0	Marginally possible with chemical lesions	0	Receptors targeted across cell types	1	Increased with viral tracers and transgenic strains	2	Using transgenic strains and viral promoters	2	Using transgenic strains and viral promoters
Minimal need for specialized equipment	0	Current-generating device and electrodes for electrolytic	0	Surgical stainless steel cannula, injectors custom gauge and length	2	Requires micro injectors only	0	Cannula and fiber optics of custom length, multichannel light source	2	Requires microinjectors only
Circuit specificity	0	Indirect with disconnection procedure	0	Indirect with disconnection procedure	1	Labeling of defined projections	2	With axonal light excitation	2	With i.c. actuator infusion or anterograde/retro grade viruses
Bidirectional Modulation Ability	0	Inactivation only	2	Inhibition and activation depend on drug		n/a	2	Depends on opsins and wavelengths	2	Depends on receptors and actuators

0, low; 1, moderate; 2, high; i.c., intracranial.

Table 1. Comparison of commonly used classical and contemporary tools in behavioral neuroscience.

3.1.2. Intracranial microinjections

The local administration of pharmacological agents into discrete brain targets is another strategy to control neural activity. This technique typically requires permanent surgical placement of guide cannula to allow for later access to otherwise inaccessible brain structures while animals are awake and behaving. Small volumes of drug solutions are then administered directly into the brain by threading a smaller gauge injector through the guide cannula. These solutions typically contain drugs that bind to distinct membrane proteins (receptors) expressed within the target brain region to enhance or inhibit local cellular activity during behavior. Similar to lesions, histology is performed afterwards to verify the site of microinjection. This procedure has several major advantages compared to lesions, most of which relate to its ability to produce more temporally specific effects. Unlike lesions, the effects of most pharmacological antagonists and agonists are temporary and can therefore be more precisely controlled and administered during distinct phases of behavioral procedures. This allows for more straightforward interpretation of the effects of this manipulation on behavior. Additionally, this technique can provide insight into the neurochemical signals involved, as agents selective for distinct receptor types can be infused. To a lesser extent than lesions, microinjections also produce damage resulting in reactive gliosis from cannula installation and injector placement. Finally, it is difficult to ascertain the exact extent of diffusion of the administered solution. As diffusion may depend on a variety of factors, such as the volume injected and the nature of the solution (polarity, hydrophobicity), it is difficult to predict. Thus, it is not always clear that the site of infusion is the region directing the observed behavior. For this reason, it is often necessary to include additional groups that receive drug injections in locations proximal to the target structure.

3.2. Contemporary tools

In recent years, there has been a rapid emergence of novel tools engineered to control neuronal activity. Of benefit to these tools have been the advancements in recombinant viruses that are capable of gene transfer in the central nervous system (CNS). For example, viruses with low immunogenicity and cytotoxicity such as adeno-associated virus (AAV) can be delivered directly into the brain to safely and efficiently express recombinant genes [38]. This provides a means to site-specifically express proteins in the CNS that can be used to modulate the activity of cells in target brain tissue. Optogenetics and chemogenetics represent the two most widely used contemporary tools in behavioral neuroscience, as they can be applied in vivo to modulate neural activity in awake behaving mice and rats. As with the classical tools described above, these modern methods have inherent advantages and disadvantages (**Table 1**), which are detailed below.

3.2.1. Optogenetics

In this technique, neurons are genetically modified through intracranial injection of a viral vector to express photosensitive proteins. The most commonly used photosensitive receptors are channelrhodopsin (ChR; excitatory ion channel), halorhodopsin (NpHR; inhibitory ion pump), and archaerhodopsin (ArchT; inhibitory proton pump; reviewed in [39]). These light-gated proteins are activated by targeted illumination, causing rapid (millisecond timescale) depolarization or hyperpolarization of neurons (reviewed in [40]). By evoking or inhibiting spike activity with this light-protein interaction, the activity of distinct brain regions and cell types can be experimentally controlled, including during the performance of behavioral tasks [39]. Because these engineered opsins can be controlled by different light wavelengths, neural activity and behavior can be modulated bidirectionally (i.e., multiplexed), offering a major advantage to this technique. Moreover, the high temporal resolution afforded by this tool makes it ideal to examine the discrete phases of behavior. However, a major issue posed by optogenetics is the possibility of desensitization of the opsin, which can occur within seconds of photoactivation [41]. Thus, this is especially problematic for studies that require inhibition or activation of longer durations, such as is required in certain behavioral tasks that occur on the order of minutes. Repeated stimulation leading to the desensitization of the opsin may even produce opposing results. This is especially problematic in the case of the excitatory opsin ChR, as the desensitization of this receptor and repeated stimulation of the cell may result in a net inhibition, the opposite effect of what is initially intended. The extent of viral diffusion and resulting protein expression is easily measurable with this technique, as most viral constructs contain a fluorescent tag. However, similar to microinjections, implantable hardware is necessary to allow for intracranial insertion of fiber-optic probes. This technique also requires specialized equipment such as fiber-optic probes and programmable light sources, which can be costly. Tethering the animal to the external light source is also necessary, which may restrict the range of apparatuses that can be used and behaviors that can be assessed (although for recent developments in wireless technologies; see [42–46]). Recently, questions regarding the effect of illumination in brain structures have arisen, specifically in regards its thermal effects on neural tissue. It has been suggested that focal illumination, especially when intense and prolonged, can result in phototoxicity, heat-induced cell damage, and oxidative stress that independently alters cellular activity [47]. Even more problematic is evidence indicating that heat alone can increase neuronal firing rates [48]. In fact, even at commonly used intensities, the thermal effect of illumination is sufficient to increase cell firing rates [49]. Overall, optogenetics provides a unique tool to control neuronal activity with high spatiotemporal resolution. However, the required implantable hardware, specialized equipment, tethering, risk of desensitization, and light induction may render this tool less than ideal given the experimental question and design.

3.2.2. Chemogenetics

This relatively new technique involves the engineering of G protein-coupled receptors (GPCRs) to interact exclusively with small molecules that were otherwise unrecognized by the GPCR [50]. The most common of these mutated GPCRs are designer receptors exclusively activated by designer drugs (DREADDs) [51]. The engineered GPCRs possess no detectible constitutive activity and are robustly activated at nanomolar concentrations of otherwise pharmacologically inert compounds. The first established DREADDs were based on excitatory G_q-coupled and inhibitory G_i-coupled human muscarinic receptors M3 (hM3Dq) and M4 (hM4Di), respectively [51–53]. Receptors hM3Dq and hM4Di possess no affinity for the endogenous ligand acetylcholine and are robustly activated by the drug clozapine-N-oxide

(CNO), a pharmacologically inert metabolite of clozapine, which is highly bioavailable and produces no pharmacological effect in rodents [51, 54]. Since their inception, other DREADDs have been engineered, which include a G_s-coupled muscarinic-based (rM3Ds) receptor and G_i-coupled KOR-based DREADD (KORD) [55–57]. Notably, the development of KORD with actuator salvinorin B allows for the bidirectional control of behavior when used in combination with hM3Dq receptors and CNO [57].

Comparable to optogenetics, DREADDs can be ectopically expressed in the CNS by focal infusion of a vector encoding for these receptors. A major advantage of chemogenetics over optogenetics, however, is the lack of required specialized equipment and need for permanently implanted hardware. In fact, DREADDs require just one initial intracranial entry to infuse the viral vector carrying the DREADD-encoding gene. The receptors can then be activated by a relatively noninvasive peripheral injection of an actuator. This is highly advantageous when performing sensitive behavioral procedures that are affected by excessive handling (e.g., CPP and self-administration) [58]. Similar to optogenetics, a more precise detection of viral spread and DREADD expression are possible with this technique, as they are designed to encode for DREADDs as well as a fluorescent marker.

Unlike optogenetics, DREADDs signal through canonical G-protein pathways. Once activated, the duration of the inhibition or activation produced by the DREADD can be long lasting. The duration of effect is also determined by the half-life of actuators, which may remain in central tissue and activate DREADDs for minutes to hours. In some cases, this low temporal resolution may serve as a major shortcoming of this technique. However, a protracted effect is often highly valued in studies where behavioral tasks are of longer duration and long-lasting effects of manipulations are desired. Another issue is that the presence of the receptor does not always indicate that it is a functionality. Additional measures may be necessary to demonstrate the function of these receptors in target tissue. Although it is theoretically possible, no studies have reported DREADD desensitization. However, this presents another reason for including some form of functional confirmation of DREADD effects.

In summary, DREADDs are a useful technique to control neuronal signaling in vivo. Considering the sensitivity and duration of many behavioral tasks, the noninvasive nature of DREADD activation (i.e., peripheral drug injection) and longer time course of inhibition/activation make chemogenetic strategies highly desirable in behavioral research.

3.3. Summary

The above-described tools provide a means through which to target and manipulate brain regions. These tools offer variable degrees of selectivity, with contemporary techniques typically being associated with higher precision in terms of spatial and neuronal targeting. The tools mentioned above do not encapsulate all available methods of discovering the neurobiology behind behaviors. Other commonly used methods not described in this chapter are intracranial electrical or self-stimulation, intracranial microdialysis, electrophysiology, immunohistochemistry (IHC), genetic knockout rodents, and many others that similarly assess the importance of a brain region and specific neurotransmitter systems to behavior.

4. Tools to manipulate specific neural pathways

Historically, the direct manipulation of neural circuits has been a challenging task, with much of the difficulty due to limited methodologies. In the past, many of the tools used possessed relatively low selectivity and provided indirect manipulation. Several strategies, however, have been designed using both classical and contemporary tools to probe the neural circuitry underlying behavior. This section describes several commonly used strategies and includes a discussion of their merits and weaknesses.

4.1. Classical tools

Historically, disconnection procedures involving lesions and pharmacological microinjections have been used to evaluate neural circuitry. This strategy involves the disruption of two directly connected brain regions to assess whether their interaction is involved in behavior (e.g., [59–62]). Typically, a unilateral lesion or inactivating microinjection [e.g., γ-aminobutyric acid (GABA) agonists or channel blocker] is made in source regions and another lesion or microinjection is made in the contralateral hemisphere of its terminal target. Thus, if a behavior is dependent on a source-target interchange, then their contralateral disconnection should be more disruptive to behavior than ipsilateral disconnection or unilateral manipulation of each region individually. However, a major weakness of this strategy is the indirect nature of the manipulation on the circuit. Indeed, the imprecision of this method has at times been proven problematic resulting in significant reductions in behavior with ipsilateral and unilateral manipulations alone (e.g., [60]). This is likely due to the inability of this technique to directly target distinct yet intermixed populations of target-projecting neurons within source regions. Instead, each region is broadly manipulated leading to the inhibition of their overall activity and output throughout the brain.

To help visualize and identify the circuit, neuronal tracing has sometimes been used in conjunction with these classical tools. In these studies, tracing agents are injected into the brain to label neurons in a manner that is retrograde (axon terminal back to the soma), anterograde (soma to axon terminal), or transsynaptic (to adjacent neurons retrogradely or anterogradely). In studies of behavior, circuit involvement is inferred by colabeling of neuronal activity markers such as c-Fos with the tracer through IHC (e.g., [63]). Cells that are immunopositive for both the tracer and activity marker are then used to identify afferent or efferent projection neurons that were activated during behavior. When used in tandem with disconnection procedures, this provides a means to visually assess the impact of disconnection on circuit activity (e.g., [62]). Although these procedures help to label neurons within the circuit and gauge their activity, they still fall short of allowing isolated modulation of the circuit. Overall, this remains a major weakness of classical techniques, as results only offer an indirect measure of neural circuit involvement in behavior.

4.2. Contemporary tools

Optogenetic and chemogenetic strategies have provided a refined and more selective means to directly manipulate neural circuits. This is principally due to viral transduction, as proteins (opsins and DREADDs) are trafficked downstream from soma to axon terminals (anterograde) and therefore expressed on presynaptic boutons as well as to cell bodies [64]. In the case of optogenetics, illumination can then be targeted to axon terminals, which results in the depolarization or hyperpolarization of the neuron. This strategy has been successfully implemented in many behavior studies (reviewed in [64]). However, a concern that arises when using this method is the possibility of antidromic stimulation of the cell. The stimulation of terminals may result in the back-propagation of an action potential that activates the neuron and its collateral inputs to other regions outside the circuit of interest. Therefore, with this strategy, there is a potential for the activation of multiple circuits, which diminishes the selectivity of the manipulation.

Several chemogenetic-based strategies have been used to modulate neural circuit activity. First, a functional disconnection procedure methodologically similar to that used with lesions or microinjections has been reported by Mahler et al. [65]. In this study, hM4Di receptors were unilaterally expressed in ventral tegmental area (VTA) dopamine (DA) cells and contralaterally in rostral ventral pallidum (RVP) cells. The contralateral disconnection of RVP-VTA DA reduced cued reinstatement of cocaine seeking relative to both unilateral RVP inhibition and unilateral VTA DA inhibition. Despite these positive results, it is unclear whether the simultaneous inhibition of RVP and VTA DA, regardless of hemisphere, would have been sufficient to produce a similar effect. Thus, with this technique, it is important to include ipsilateral as well as unilateral controls. In summary, the lack of precision and necessary inclusion of numerous controls renders this a less desirable strategy for the targeted modulation of neural circuits.

Another DREADD-based method that has been used involves the intracranial injection of CNO. The principle behind this strategy is similar to that of the optogenetic circuit-selective method outlined above. Here, like illumination, CNO is targeted to the terminal region of DREADD-expressing cells [65, 66]. The focal infusion of CNO therefore serves to activate/inhibit DREADD-expressing cells and/or presynaptic neurotransmitter release from DREADD-expressing nerve terminals [66]. In this manner, the activity of defined neural circuits can be more precisely controlled. However, given that this strategy requires intracranial microinjections, it also carries with it the disadvantage of requiring permanently indwelling hardware (i.e., guide cannula and obturators), repeated intracranial entries, and a resulting increased risk of tissue damage.

An alternative approach to this involves the intersection of multiple viruses that are injected into serially connected nuclei. Typically, a retrograde virus encoding for cre recombinase is injected in a target region and a cre-inducible virus encoding for DREADD is injected into the source region. In this manner, the activity of a specific source's inputs to the target region (i.e., projection neurons) can be controlled by the systemic injection of CNO. This approach has been successfully implemented using canine adenovirus (CAV-2) to retrogradely infect source region cells and selectively express DREADDs in a specific neural projection [67–69]. Notably, this strategy provides an ideal way to control circuits, especially during behavior. Not only does this method provide a high degree of selectivity, it does not require implantable hardware and can be robustly activated by a simple peripheral injection of an actuator. Theoretically, it is possible for axon collaterals from source region cells to express DREADDs, which given the systemic nature of DREADD activation may lead to activity in sites outside the circuit. Hence, studies using this method should be careful to address this potential caveat.

4.3. Summary

Overall, several techniques involving classical and contemporary tools have been used to manipulate defined neural circuits. On one hand, classical tools provide indirect manipulation and generally require the use of multiple controls to carefully and appropriately interpret results derived using these strategies. Conversely, contemporary tools involving viral-mediated gene transfer confer greater circuit selectivity and have been successfully used to manipulate serial projections form source to target region.

5. Neural structures involved in ethanol-seeking behavior

In the following sections, several neural structures and circuits involved in ethanol-seeking behavior are discussed. Building off of earlier sections, the studies that are described below involved several different animal models and tools to identify the underlying neurobiology of ethanol seeking. Specifically, this chapter will focus on the neural structures involved in ethanol self-administration and CPP, as these models specifically assess ethanol-seeking behavior. A proposed circuit of the key neural structures implicated in cue-induced ethanol seeking as indexed by self-administration and CPP procedures is included in **Figure 2**.

5.1. Findings from ethanol self-administration studies

Studies using ethanol self-administration procedures to evaluate the neural mechanisms underlying ethanol seeking have by and large employed intracranial microinfusions. Most of the neural regions that have been evaluated in self-administration studies are part of the mesocorticolimbic system [70] and are typically situated downstream of the VTA. As with many drugs of abuse, acutely administered ethanol excites DA neurons within the VTA through direct and indirect mechanisms [71–74]. Furthermore, the VTA is robustly activated by ethanol-associated cue exposure [75]. Downstream, the nucleus accumbens (NAc) and amygdala receive dopaminergic input from the VTA [76] and considerable evidence suggests that this dopaminergic input to each region underlies associative learning and motivated behavior [77–81]. As such, NAc and amygdala are two of the most well-characterized structures in terms of their involvement in ethanol seeking and several of these studies are described below.

The NAc has been routinely implicated in the drug-seeking behavior [82, 83]. Many studies have found a differential involvement of core and shell subdivisions in drug seeking depending on the drug of abuse, phase of self-administration, and nature of the procedure and/or stimuli used [84–86]. As with other drugs of abuse, the NAc core and shell have been shown to be differentially involved in cue-induced ethanol seeking. For example, ethanol self-administration studies have shown that transient inactivation of the NAc core but not shell

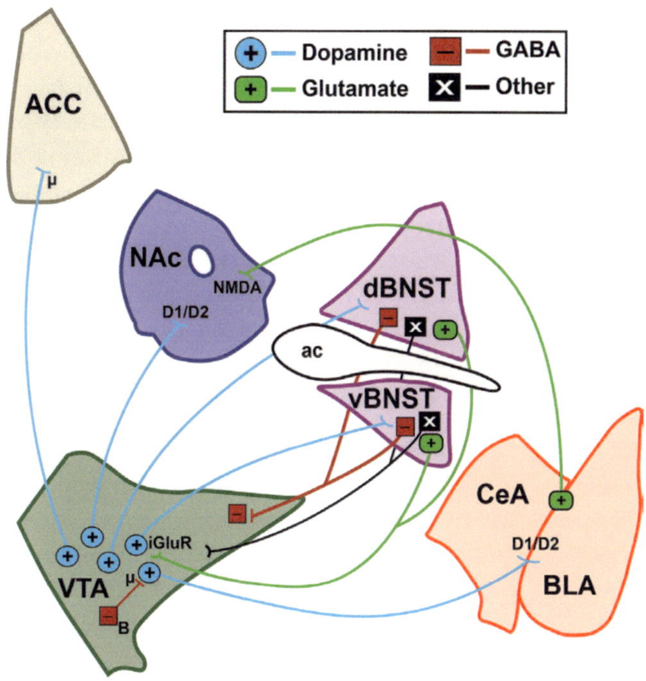

Figure 2. Diagram of the neural circuitry involved in ethanol CPP. Previous studies have demonstrated the involvement of cortex (ACC), amygdala (BLA/CeA), striatum (NAc), and midbrain (VTA) in ethanol CPP. The present work now demonstrates the involvement of the dorsal and ventral BNST (dBNST and vBNST, respectively) and a direct BNST-VTA circuit. Each of these regions receives dopaminergic input from the VTA (indicated by blue arrows) and is part of a broader mesocorticolimbic dopamine system that underlies reward and motivation. Some of the neurochemical signals underlying the involvement of each region in ethanol CPP have also been identified. +, excitatory; -, inhibitory; blue circles, dopamine cells; green rectangles, glutamate cells; red squares, GABA cells; black boxes, unknown neurochemical signal; green arrows, glutamate projections; μ, μ-opioid receptors; B, $GABA_B$ receptor; D1, dopamine D1-like receptor; D2, dopamine D2-like receptor; iGluR, ionotropic glutamate receptors, NMDA, iGluR subtype.

reduces cue-induced reinstatement [87] and context-induced renewal [88] of ethanol seeking. Other studies, however, have demonstrated that NAc shell modulates the expression of cue-induced ethanol seeking [89] and that blockade of DA D1 receptors in the NAc shell but not core reduces the spontaneous recovery of ethanol-seeking behavior following prolonged abstinence [90]. In addition, DA D1 receptor antagonism in NAc core and shell has been reported to block context-induced renewal of extinguished ethanol seeking [91]. These studies vary in their findings of core versus shell involvement in ethanol seeking, likely indicating that the role of NAc subdivisions varies by different phases of self-administration (e.g., acquisition, expression, and reinstatement) and by the use of cues or context. However, this literature overall supports a role for the NAc in general ethanol-seeking behavior and suggests that DA input may underlie its involvement.

The amygdala has also been strongly implicated in drug-seeking behavior, specifically the basolateral amygdala (BLA) and central nucleus of the amygdala (CeA) subdivisions as well as the bed nucleus of the stria terminalis (BNST) of the extended amygdala [92–94]. In ethanol self-administration studies, the inactivation of the BLA has been shown to reduce context-induced renewal of previously extinguished ethanol seeking [95]. The involvement of the BLA in ethanol seeking may involve a glutamatergic mechanism, as intra-BLA ionotropic glutamate receptor antagonism reduced the expression of ethanol seeking elicited by a discrete cue and invigorated by an ethanol-associated context [96]. Notably, the excitatory transmission from the amygdala to the NAc is believed to underlie reward seeking and suggests that an amygdala-NAc circuit may be involved in the expression of reward-seeking behavior. For example, the optical stimulation of BLA glutamate to NAc has been shown to be reinforcing, as mice worked to earn additional stimulation of BLA-NAc synaptic inputs [97]. Conversely, the inhibition of BLA-NAc inputs reduced cue-induced responding for sucrose [97]. In addition, pharmacological disconnection has revealed that an amygdala-NAc interaction underlies a stimulus-controlled expression or maintenance of cocaine seeking [59].

The CeA and BNST have generally been implicated in stress-induced ethanol-seeking reinstatement but may also play a role in cue-induced ethanol reinstatement. For instance, intra-CeA but not intra-BLA infusion of mifepristone, a glucocorticoid receptor antagonist, has been reported to suppress reinstated ethanol seeking induced by the pharmacological stressor yohimbine [98]. Activation of group II metabotropic glutamate receptors blocks stress- and cue-induced reinstatement of ethanol seeking presumably through CeA and BNST actions [99].

Lastly, additional regions that have been implicated in ethanol seeking using self-administration procedures include the dorsomedial striatum [100, 101], medial prefrontal cortex (mPFC) [75], prelimbic cortex, and VTA [102]. Importantly, the VTA, which is the chief source of DA input to NAc, amygdala, and cortical regions, has been shown to be explicitly involved in context- and cue-induced ethanol seeking [103–105]. Overall, self-administration studies have been important in identifying several key neural substrates involved in ethanol-seeking behavior. Several of these structures have also been implicated in cue-induced ethanol seeking through ethanol-induced CPP procedures and thus are discussed in the next section.

5.2. Findings from ethanol CPP studies

Studies on the neural mechanism of ethanol CPP can be grouped into several categories that include acquisition, expression, extinction, and reinstatement. Acquisition studies are those that assess the development of ethanol place preference. These typically include procedures where manipulations occurred during the conditioning or training phase, where animals learn to associate contextual cues with ethanol reward. Conversely, expression studies involve manipulations that occur after the conditioning phase and before preference testing. Expression studies, in particular, are useful in assessing ethanol-seeking behavior and conditioned reward. Below, findings from each of these types of ethanol CPP studies are discussed. Of note, relatively few laboratories study the primary and conditioned rewarding properties of ethanol using a CPP procedure. This is partly due to the difficult and unreliable nature of ethanol place conditioning in rats [21, 106] and the relatively weak ethanol CPP obtained with commonly used inbred mouse strains, such as C57BL/6J [107, 108]. In view of this, many of the studies described below have used male DBA/2J mice. This inbred strain will rapidly and reliably develop and ethanol CPP, even with a minimal amount of conditioning sessions [34, 36, 108].

http://dx.doi.org/10.5772/63105

In this section, we provide an overview of studies that have directly examined the neural areas underlying the acquisition and expression of ethanol place preference.

5.2.1. Acquisition

As with self-administration studies, the NAc and amygdala are the two most evaluated regions in terms of their involvement in ethanol CPP acquisition. Previously, the involvement of the NAc in ethanol place preference acquisition has been investigated. In one study, bilateral electrolytic lesions of the NAc before CPP training disrupted the acquisition of CPP [109]. In a later study, bilateral NAc infusions of the D1-like receptor antagonist SCH-23390 disrupted the development of ethanol CPP [110]. This finding is similar to a finding reported in rats showing that nonselective DA antagonism prevented CPP induced by intracerebroventricular (icv) infusions of ethanol [111]. Combined, these studies indicate that the NAc is necessary for establishing associative relationships between ethanol reward and environmental cues likely through a DA D1-like receptor-dependent mechanism. Other work has looked at the role of the amygdala in ethanol CPP acquisition [109]. Using electrolytic lesions, the amygdala was ablated bilaterally before CPP training. Amygdala lesions disrupted acquisition (and/or expression) of ethanol place preference, suggesting that this region is also involved in ethanol cue learning.

Together, these findings demonstrate that these structures downstream the VTA are necessary for the development of ethanol CPP. Moreover, NAc involvement in ethanol CPP is directly attributed to dopaminergic innervation, as activity at D1-like receptors in this region is necessary for acquisition. One consideration of these results is that acquisition studies involving microinjections can be problematic, as the additional handling required to focally administer a drug can interfere with ethanol CPP [110]. Although they do not require added handling prior, lesions are also problematic when administered preconditioning, as it unclear whether they affected the acquisition or expression phase.

5.2.2. Expression

Over the last decade, studies have investigated the involvement of several brain areas in ethanol place preference expression. These include the VTA, NAc, amygdala, and anterior cingulate cortex (ACC). Each of these structures is thought to be involved in reward and motivation partly through DA mechanisms, and as such, each is part of a broader mesocorticolimbic DA system.

Although VTA DA cells are initially activated by rewarding stimuli, this activation diminishes over time with repeated reward exposures and subsequent learning [112]. Eventually, DA cells are no longer activated by the reward itself and instead become robustly activated by environmental stimuli that have become associated with the reward and predict its delivery [113, 114]. Thus, the involvement of this conditioned DA response in ethanol CPP expression can be supported by studies focusing on the VTA or downstream sites as are described below.

One pharmacological microinjection study separately infused the nonselective opioid receptor antagonist methylnaloxonium and the $GABA_B$ receptor agonist baclofen into the VTA to assess the participation of the VTA in ethanol CPP expression. Methylnaloxonium decreased the magnitude of ethanol CPP, whereas baclofen blocked preference expression entirely. These findings suggested that the VTA activity is necessary for the expression of ethanol place preference. Moreover, GABAergic and opioidergic activity appear to underlie the involvement of the VTA in ethanol CPP expression, presumably through the local modulation of DA cell activity.

Although involvement of the NAc in ethanol place preference acquisition is clear, its involvement in expression is more complicated. In early work, an intra-NAc infusion of methylnaloxonium failed to impact ethanol preference expression, suggesting a lack of NAc opioid receptor involvement in the conditioned ethanol reward [115]. A later study directed bilateral electrolytic lesions at the NAc after ethanol CPP conditioning and before testing to isolate the involvement of this structure in expression [109]. Overall, lesions made at this time point did not affect ethanol place preference, suggesting that the NAc may not be critical in ethanol CPP expression.

However, additional pharmacological procedures have shown a more specific role for the NAc in CPP expression. In one study, intra-NAc antagonism of D1- and D2-like receptors prevented the expression of CPP induced by icv ethanol [111]. In another study, NAc DA (D1- and D2-like) and glutamate (NMDA) receptors were blocked during the CPP expression test using either flupenthixol or AP-5, respectively [116]. Although DA receptor antagonism did not affect ethanol place preference, NMDA receptor antagonism reduced it, suggesting that the involvement of the NAc in expression is specific to activity at NMDA receptors. This effect was reproduced in another study using only unilaterally administered AP5, further indicating the importance of NAc NMDA receptor involvement in ethanol place preference expression [60]. Notably, this study was designed to examine glutamate input to NAc from amygdala. Although findings appeared to demonstrate that amygdala disconnection from NAc blocked ethanol CPP expression, reduced CPP in mice unilaterally infused with AP5 in NAc prevented this interpretation. Overall, these findings have established a role for NAc NMDA, but not DA receptors, in ethanol place preference expression and suggest that glutamatergic input from amygdala may also be involved. Although DA input from VTA to NAc is a hypothesized mechanism underlying drug seeking, these results suggest that it does not underlie ethanol seeking, at least as indexed by CPP. Finally, these studies serve to demonstrate that manipulations more selective than global inactivation or deletion of a structure may be necessary to appropriately gauge that the importance of structure in behavior.

Accordingly, the role of the amygdala in ethanol CPP expression has also been addressed. Like lesions made before conditioning, the bilateral electrolytic lesion of the amygdala made before the test phase blocked ethanol place preference expression [109]. In addition, when bilaterally infused into the amygdala, the D1- and D2-like DA receptor agonist flupenthixol blocked ethanol CPP expression [116]. Together, these results illustrate the role of the amygdala in ethanol-seeking behavior and indicate the importance of dopaminergic input to this structure for ethanol CPP expression.

The BNST also has a role in modulating the expression of ethanol reward. Exposure to ethanol causes changes in glutamate synaptic plasticity [117], increases extracellular DA levels in the

BNST [118], and activates BNST cells [119]. In particular, the inhibition of the BNST during CPP expression using electrolytic lesions, coinfusion of $GABA_A$ and $GABA_B$ receptor agonists muscimol and baclofen, and activation of inhibitory DREADDs (hM4Di-DREADD) lead to a loss or reduction of the expression of ethanol CPP. All of these studies suggest the importance of the BNST to ethanol seeking.

Finally, ACC involvement in expression was assessed by bilaterally infusing the nonspecific opioid receptor antagonist methylnaloxonium into the ACC before the ethanol CPP test [120]. The intra-ACC infusion of methylnaloxonium disrupted ethanol place preference expression, reducing its magnitude at the lowest dose and abolishing it at the highest dose. Hence, the ACC appears to modulate ethanol CPP expression through an opioidergic mechanism.

In summary, findings from expression studies have demonstrated that the VTA, NAc, amygdala, BNST, and ACC are all structures involved in ethanol place preference expression. Infusion of a mixed opioid receptor antagonist into VTA and ACC but not NAc interfered with ethanol CPP expression. Similarly, lesions and mixed DA receptor antagonism disrupted expression when targeted to the amygdala and not NAc. Involvement of the NAc in ethanol CPP expression appeared to be confined to activity NMDA receptors only, suggesting that a more explicit neurochemical mechanism underlies its involvement in ethanol place preference expression.

5.2.3. Extinction and reinstatement

Unlike the acquisition and expression of ethanol CPP, the neural correlates of extinction of ethanol CPP is relatively understudied. The only region consistently studied for its role in ethanol CPP is the mPFC.

The mPFC is known to be involved in the acquisition and extinction of Pavlovian conditioned fear and drug memories [121]; thus, it is not surprising that disruption of its activity impairs the extinction of ethanol CPP. Several studies found that lesions or inhibition of the mPFC, but not the ACC, following acquisition blocks the extinction of CPP [122, 123]. These studies suggest the importance of this mPFC in the formation of inhibitory ethanol seeking memories. Additionally, one study links the NAc core with extinction of ethanol seeking. Lesions of the NAc core were found to have no effect on the expression of ethanol CPP but caused a rapid loss of responding during extinction [109], which suggest that the NAc core is associated with inhibitory ethanol memory, but further research will be needed to confirm the role of the NAc in extinction.

Like extinction, the brain regions involved in the reinstatement of ethanol CPP are not well studied, but there are several studies that implicate particular brain regions. One such study found an increase in c-Fos activity in the BLA of rats following cued reinstatement of ethanol seeking in a discriminative stimulus operant paradigm [75]. Although this is not a direct proof of the necessity of the BLA in ethanol seeking in CPP, another study found that the direct manipulation of the BLA alters cued reinstatement of cocaine seeking [59]. Together, these studies suggest the importance of the BLA in ethanol reinstatement and likely in the reinstatement of ethanol CPP. Other regions, such as the VTA, amygdala, and BNST, are likely involved in the extinction and reinstatement of ethanol CPP, as they are important for the extinction and reinstatement of CPP of other addictive substances. Investigating the involvement of these regions in extinction and reinstatement of ethanol CPP will be an important step for understanding the circuitry of relapse.

5.3. Summary

In summary, these studies show the importance of several brain regions heavily implicated in drug reward to ethanol seeking as well. Most of these studies evaluated the structures situated downstream the VTA that have been implicated in drug seeking based on their efferent dopaminergic input. In addition to these studies demonstrating that downstream sites are involved, findings from Bechtholt and Cunningham [115] further illustrate the importance of the VTA in ethanol-seeking behavior. As opioid receptors are situated presynaptically on local GABAergic inputs to DA cells, the authors hypothesized that methylnaloxonium disinhibited VTA GABAergic interneurons. This likely inhibited VTA DA activity, thereby reducing ethanol place preference expression. Conversely, baclofen presumably reduced CPP by acting directly on VTA DA cells, as they express $GABA_B$ receptors. Thus, the VTA is a critical structure for drug and, specifically, ethanol cue associations. Although these findings and proposed mechanisms underscore the importance of VTA DA in ethanol CPP expression, they provide little information on the inputs to the VTA that modulate DA cell activity. Thus, the origins and neurochemical sources of VTA DA cell innervation involved in ethanol-seeking behavior remain unknown. Accordingly, the next section discusses the involvement of VTA input in reward and identifies several inputs that may be of importance and deserve further study for their role in ethanol CPP.

5.4. Inputs to the VTA

Excitatory (glutamatergic) afferents of the VTA arise from virtually all structures to which this region projects, with the exception of the NAc and lateral septum (LS), which provide strong GABAergic inputs [124]. This suggests that there is a broad network of excitatory reciprocal projections to and from the VTA, with much of the glutamatergic input to VTA neurons arising from subcortical regions that include but are not limited to amygdala, mesopontine nuclei, lateral habenula, and hypothalamus [125]. Although this reciprocal flow of neurotransmission is also found between the VTA and cortex, the PFC serves as the only cortical source of glutamate to the VTA [126]. Importantly, these glutamatergic afferents play a critical role in regulating VTA neuron firing. Specifically, glutamatergic input to the VTA appears to be critical for behaviorally relevant burst firing of VTA DA neurons [127]. The resulting phasic release of DA from the VTA is intimately associated with goal-directed behaviors and drug reward [128].

In addition to the contemporary methods described earlier, recent advances in immunohistological techniques have facilitated a more precise mapping of afferent and efferent projections of the VTA. As a result, an updated view on the role of broad neural circuit activity (including that of the VTA) in relation to behavior has been formed. In this current view, the net result of cell-specific projections onto cell-specific targets is accounted for and the subsequent plotting of these circuits suggests a complex topographical map. This map indicates the existence of an intricate network of connectivity designed to tightly regulate the activity of neuronal ensembles, which in turn orchestrate complex and divergent behaviors, even from within the same circuits. In the VTA specifically, not all inputs are alike in their behavioral consequences. Here, DA activity is governed by a complex network of cell-type-specific neuron-to-neuron connections, the net effect of which can result in vastly different motivational states [129, 130].

Several lines of evidence suggest the importance of monosynaptic inputs to VTA DA neurons (one-step inputs) in governing motivational behaviors. For example, investigation of the laterodorsal tegmental (LDT) nucleus has revealed that 80% of its glutamatergic afferents synapse onto VTA DA neurons directly [131]. The importance of these glutamatergic inputs have been corroborated through electrophysiological analysis, which has shown that this region is essential to VTA DA cell burst firing [132]. Moreover, in vivo stimulation of LDT glutamate afferents has been reported to selectively terminate on and stimulate a distinct population of VTA DA neurons, which thereby generate reward [130].

The BNST is another region upstream the VTA that has been identified as critically involved in regulating the activity of DA cell activity [133–135]. Specifically, the BNST positively modulates VTA DA activity putatively through two primary and distinct mechanisms: (1) a direct glutamate projection to VTA DA and (2) a direct GABA projection to VTA GABA [129, 135–137]. Of note, more recent evidence derived from studies using more advanced and selective tools suggests that a BNST GABA input to VTA GABA is the predominant source of the modulation of the BNST of the VTA [129]. Of relevance, behavior in rodents has demonstrated that the BNST underlies cue-elicited drug seeking. For example, transient inactivation of the BNST has been shown to prevent cue-induced reinstatement of cocaine seeking [138]. Direct projections from BNST to VTA appear to be important for cocaine-related behaviors. For example, disconnection of the BNST-VTA pathway has been shown to reduce expression of cocaine CPP [62], but the role of that projection in ethanol seeking still remains unknown and further study of this projection and other VTA inputs will advance our understanding of the larger neural network driving ethanol seeking.

6. Conclusion

Alcohol is a widely used legal intoxicant that produces a huge financial toll ($223.5 billion in 2006 alone) on the United States (Centers for Disease Control and Prevention, 2014) due to the workplace, healthcare, legal, and criminal consequences of excessive consumption of alcohol. Despite the prevalent societal knowledge of the detriment of excessive alcohol use, AUDs continue to be a common disorder that is difficult to treat. The primary challenge of providing lasting treatments for AUDs is the high propensity for those with AUDs to relapse into alcohol use. Relapse is often caused when a cue associated with alcohol (i.e., a bar, alcohol advertisement) or alcohol itself is presented to a person with an AUD. This cue recalls the associative effects of ethanol and induces a craving and an internal drive to seek and consume alcohol. Thus, it is critical to understand how alcohol cue associations are formed and maintained despite receiving treatment for alcohol abuse. This chapter has outlined the animal models that are being used by preclinical researchers to better understand the formation, expression, extinction, and reinstatement (relapse) of alcohol cue associations that promote ethanol seeking and has summarized each of their advantages and disadvantages. Of particular use is the CPP paradigm. CPP allows the experimenter to separate distinct phases of acquiring, expressing, extinguishing, and reexpressing conditioned ethanol seeking and thus can easily study the neural mechanisms involved in each. This chapter also presented the classical and contemporary tools that can be used separately and in conjunction to probe the exact neural structures and circuitry involved in alcohol cues and seeking. Although classical tools have given us the greatest insight into the neurobiology of ethanol seeking thus far, contemporary tools have been and will allow for a much clearer and specific understanding of the structures involved in animal models of alcohol seeking. Finally, this chapter presented evidence from ethanol self-administration and ethanol CPP studies of the modulation of ethanol seeking by the mesolimbic structures (VTA, NAc), the limbic system (amygdala, BNST, ACC), and cortical structures (mPFC). Of particular importance is the VTA that sends vast dopaminergic input to many of these structures. The challenge of future research is to identify more structures critical for the acquisition and expression, and especially the extinction and reinstatement, of ethanol CPP and the inputs of the VTA that modulate dopaminergic tone and thus ethanol-seeking behavior (such as the BNST-VTA projection). A better understanding of the whole circuit driving every aspect of ethanol seeking will improve our knowledge of AUDs and treatment options.

Author details

Melanie M. Pina* and Amy R. Williams

*Address all correspondence to: melareaoftsai@gmail.com

Oregon Health & Science University, 3181 SW Sam Jackson Park Rd, Portland, United States

References

[1] Moos RH, Moos BS. Rates and predictors of relapse after natural and treated remission from alcohol use disorders. Addiction 2006 Feb;101(2):212–22.

[2] Ciccocioppo R, Martin-Fardon R, Weiss F. Stimuli associated with a single cocaine experience elicit long-lasting cocaine-seeking. Nat Neurosci. 2004 Mar 28;7(5):495–6.

[3] Ciccocioppo R, Sanna PP, Weiss F. Cocaine-predictive stimulus induces drug-seeking behavior and neural activation in limbic brain regions after multiple months of abstinence: reversal by D(1) antagonists. Proc Natl Acad Sci U S A 2001 Feb;98(4):1976–81.

[4] Ciccocioppo R, Angeletti S, Weiss F. Long-lasting resistance to extinction of response reinstatement induced by ethanol-related stimuli: role of genetic ethanol preference. Alcohol Clin Exp Res. 2001 Oct;25(10):1414–9.

[5] Weiss F, Martin-Fardon R, Ciccocioppo R, Kerr TM, Smith DL, Ben-Shahar O. Enduring resistance to extinction of cocaine-seeking behavior induced by drug-related cues. Neuropsychopharmacology 2001 Sep;25(3):361–72.

[6] Bardo MT, Bevins RA. Conditioned place preference: what does it add to our preclinical understanding of drug reward? Psychopharmacology (Berl). 2000 Dec;153(1):31–43.

[7] White NM. Reward or reinforcement: what's the difference? Neurosci Biobehav Rev. 1989 Jun;13(2–3):181–6.

[8] Richter CP. A study of the effect of moderate doses of alcohol on the growth and behavior of the rat. J Exp Zool. 1926 Apr;44(1):397–418.

[9] Richter CP, Campbell KH. Alcohol taste thresholds and concentrations of solution preferred by rats. Science 1940 May 24;91(2369):507–8.

[10] Gill K, Amit Z. Serotonin uptake blockers and voluntary alcohol consumption. In: Galanter M, editor. Recent Developments in Alcoholism. Boston, MA: Springer; 1989. pp. 225–48.

[11] Meisch RA. Ethanol Self-Administration: Infrahuman Studies. In: Thompson, T and Dews P., editors. Advances in Behavioral Pharmacology. NY: Academic Press; 1977. pp. 35–84.

[12] Samson HH, Tolliver GA, Lumeng L, Li TK. Ethanol reinforcement in the alcohol nonpreferring rat: initiation using behavioral techniques without food restriction. Alcohol Clin Exp Res. 1989 Jun;13(3):378–85.

[13] Samson HH. Initiation of ethanol reinforcement using a sucrose-substitution procedure in food- and water-sated rats. Alcohol Clin Exp Res. 1986 Aug;10(4):436–42.

[14] Rhodes JS, Best K, Belknap JK, Finn DA, Crabbe JC. Evaluation of a simple model of ethanol drinking to intoxication in C57BL/6J mice. Physiol Behav. 2005 Jan 31;84(1):53–63.

[15] Samson HH, Pfeffer AO, Tolliver GA. Oral ethanol self-administration in rats: models of alcohol-seeking behavior. Alcohol Clin Exp Res. 1988 Oct;12(5):591–8.

[16] Stafford D, LeSage MG, Glowa JR. Progressive-ratio schedules of drug delivery in the analysis of drug self-administration: a review. Psychopharmacology (Berl). 1998 Oct; 139(3):169–84.

[17] Lê AD, Poulos CX, Harding S, Watchus J, Juzytsch W, Shaham Y. Effects of naltrexone and fluoxetine on alcohol self-administration and reinstatement of alcohol seeking induced by priming injections of alcohol and exposure to stress. Neuropsychopharmacology 1999 Sep;21(3):435–44.

[18] Epstein DH, Preston KL, Stewart J, Shaham Y. Toward a model of drug relapse: an assessment of the validity of the reinstatement procedure. Psychopharmacology (Berl). 2006 Sep 22;189(1):1–16.

[19] Childs E, de Wit H. Amphetamine-induced place preference in humans. Biol Psychiatry 2009 May 15;65(10):900–4.

[20] Tzschentke TM. Measuring reward with the conditioned place preference paradigm: a comprehensive review of drug effects, recent progress and new issues. Prog Neurobiol. 1998 Dec;56(6):613–72.

[21] Tzschentke TM. Measuring reward with the conditioned place preference (CPP) paradigm: update of the last decade. Addict Biol. 2007 Sep;12(3–4):227–462.

[22] Bormann NM, Cunningham CL. Ethanol-induced conditioned place aversion in rats: effect of interstimulus interval. Pharmacol Biochem Behav. 1998 Feb;59(2):427–32.

[23] Cunningham CL, Henderson CM. Ethanol-induced conditioned place aversion in mice. Behav Pharmacol. 2000 Nov;11(7–8):591–602.

[24] Cunningham CL, Clemans JM, Fidler TL. Injection timing determines whether intragastric ethanol produces conditioned place preference or aversion in mice. Pharmacol Biochem Behav. 2002 Jun;72(3):659–68.

[25] Cunningham CL, Ferree NK, Howard MA. Apparatus bias and place conditioning with ethanol in mice. Psychopharmacology (Berl). 2003 Dec;170(4):409–22.

[26] Cunningham CL, Okorn DM, Howard CE. Interstimulus interval determines whether ethanol produces conditioned place preference or aversion in mice. Anim Learn Behav. 1997;25:31–42.

[27] Grahame NJ, Chester JA, Rodd-Henricks K. Alcohol place preference conditioning in high-and low-alcohol preferring selected lines of mice. Pharmacol Biochem Behav. 2001 Apr;68(4):805–14.

[28] Ciccocioppo R, Panocka I, Froldi R, Quitadamo E, Massi M. Ethanol induces conditioned place preference in genetically selected alcohol-preferring rats. Psychopharmacology (Berl). 1999 Jan;141(3):235–41.

[29] Morales M, Varlinskaya EI, Spear LP. Evidence for conditioned place preference to a moderate dose of ethanol in adult male Sprague-Dawley rats. Alcohol 2012 Nov;46(7): 643–8.

[30] Asin KE, Wirtshafter D, Tabakoff B. Failure to establish a conditioned place preference with ethanol in rats. Pharmacol Biochem Behav. 1985 Feb;22(2):169–73.

[31] Cunningham CL. Flavor and location aversions produced by ethanol. Behav Neural Biol. 1979 Nov;27(3):362–7.

[32] van der Kooy D, O'Shaughnessy M, Mucha RF, Kalant H. Motivational properties of ethanol in naive rats as studied by place conditioning. Pharmacol Biochem Behav. 1983 Sep;19(3):441–5.

[33] Cunningham CL. Genetic relationship between ethanol-induced conditioned place preference and other ethanol phenotypes in 15 inbred mouse strains. Behav Neurosci. 2014 Aug;128(4):430–45.

[34] Pina MM, Cunningham CL. Effects of dopamine receptor antagonists on the acquisition of ethanol-induced conditioned place preference in mice. Psychopharmacology (Berl). 2014 Feb;231(3):459–68.

[35] Pina MM, Cunningham CL. Effects of the novel cannabinoid CB1 receptor antagonist PF 514273 on the acquisition and expression of ethanol conditioned place preference. Alcohol 2014 Aug;48(5):427–31.

[36] Pina MM, Young EA, Ryabinin AE, Cunningham CL. The bed nucleus of the stria terminalis regulates ethanol-seeking behavior in mice. Neuropharmacology 2015 Dec; 99:627–38.

[37] Gremel CM, Cunningham CL. Role of test activity in ethanol-induced disruption of place preference expression in mice. Psychopharmacology (Berl). 2007 Apr;191(2):195–202.

[38] Mastakov MY, Baer K, Symes CW, Leichtlein CB, Kotin RM, During MJ. Immunological aspects of recombinant adeno-associated virus delivery to the mammalian brain. J Virol. 2002 Aug;76(16):8446–54.

[39] Han X. In vivo application of optogenetics for neural circuit analysis. ACS Chem Neurosci. 2012 Aug 15;3(8):577–84.

[40] Fenno L, Yizhar O, Deisseroth K. The development and application of optogenetics. Annu Rev Neurosci. 2011;34(1):389–412.

[41] Mattis J, Tye KM, Ferenczi EA, Ramakrishnan C, O'Shea DJ, Prakash R, et al. Principles for applying optogenetic tools derived from direct comparative analysis of microbial opsins. Nat Methods 2012 Feb;9(2):159–72.

[42] Jeong J-W, McCall JG, Shin G, Zhang Y, Al-Hasani R, Kim M, et al. Wireless optofluidic systems for programmable in vivo pharmacology and optogenetics. Cell 2015 Jul 30;162(3):662–74.

[43] Kim T-I. Injectable, unusual electronics for wireless optogenetics. Brain Stimul. 2015 Mar;8(2):437.

[44] Kim T-I, McCall JG, Jung YH, Huang X, Siuda ER, Li Y, et al. Injectable, cellular-scale optoelectronics with applications for wireless optogenetics. Science 2013 Apr 12;340(6129):211–6.

[45] McCall JG, Kim T-I, Shin G, Huang X, Jung YH, Al-Hasani R, et al. Fabrication and application of flexible, multimodal light-emitting devices for wireless optogenetics. Nat Protoc. 2013 Dec;8(12):2413–28.

[46] Park SI, Shin G, Banks A, McCall JG, Siuda ER, Schmidt MJ, et al. Ultraminiaturized photovoltaic and radio frequency powered optoelectronic systems for wireless optogenetics. J Neural Eng. 2015 Oct;12(5):056002.

[47] Gysbrechts B, Wang L, Trong NND, Cabral H, Navratilova Z, Battaglia F, et al. Light distribution and thermal effects in the rat brain under optogenetic stimulation. J Biophoton. 2015 Jul;(Epub ahead of print)

[48] Reig R, Mattia M, Compte A, Belmonte C, Sanchez-Vives MV. Temperature modulation of slow and fast cortical rhythms. J Neurophysiol. 2010 Mar;103(3):1253–61.

[49] Stujenske JM, Spellman T, Gordon JA. Modeling the spatiotemporal dynamics of light and heat propagation for in vivo optogenetics. Cell Rep. 2015 Jul 21;12(3):525–34.

[50] Sternson SM, Roth BL. Chemogenetic tools to interrogate brain functions. Annu Rev Neurosci. 2014 Jun;37(1):387–407.

[51] Armbruster BN, Li X, Pausch MH, Herlitze S, Roth BL. Evolving the lock to fit the key to create a family of G protein-coupled receptors potently activated by an inert ligand. Proc Natl Acad Sci U S A 2007 Mar 20;104(12):5163–8.

[52] Alexander GM, Rogan SC, Abbas AI, Armbruster BN, Pei Y, Allen JA, et al. Remote control of neuronal activity in transgenic mice expressing evolved G protein-coupled receptors. Neuron 2009 Jul 16;63(1):27–39.

[53] Nichols CD, Roth BL. Engineered G-protein coupled receptors are powerful tools to investigate biological processes and behaviors. Front Mol Neurosci. 2009;2:16.

[54] Bender D, Holschbach M, Stöcklin G. Synthesis of n.c.a. carbon-11 labelled clozapine and its major metabolite clozapine-N-oxide and comparison of their biodistribution in mice. Nucl Med Biol. 1994 Oct;21(7):921–5.

[55] Farrell MS, Roth BL. Pharmacosynthetics: reimagining the pharmacogenetic approach. Brain Res. 2013 May;1511:6–20.

[56] Guettier J-M, Gautam D, Scarselli M, Ruiz de Azua I, Li JH, Rosemond E, et al. A chemical-genetic approach to study G protein regulation of beta cell function in vivo. Proc Natl Acad Sci U S A 2009 Nov 10;106(45):19197–202.

[57] Vardy E, Robinson JE, Li C, Olsen RHJ, DiBerto JF, Giguere PM, et al. A New DREADD facilitates the multiplexed chemogenetic interrogation of behavior. Neuron 2015 May 20;86(4):936–46.

[58] Bechtholt AJ, Gremel CM, Cunningham CL. Handling blocks expression of conditioned place aversion but not conditioned place preference produced by ethanol in mice. Pharmacol Biochem Behav. 2004 Dec;79(4):739–44.

[59] Di Ciano P, Everitt BJ. Direct interactions between the basolateral amygdala and nucleus accumbens core underlie cocaine-seeking behavior by rats. J Neurosci. 2004 Aug 11;24(32):7167–73.

[60] Gremel CM, Cunningham CL. Effects of disconnection of amygdala dopamine and nucleus accumbens N-methyl-D-aspartate receptors on ethanol-seeking behavior in mice. Eur J Neurosci. 2010 Jan;31(1):148–55.

[61] Parkinson JA, Willoughby PJ, Robbins TW, Everitt BJ. Disconnection of the anterior cingulate cortex and nucleus accumbens core impairs Pavlovian approach behavior: further evidence for limbic cortical-ventral striatopallidal systems. Behav Neurosci. 2000 Feb;114(1):42–63.

[62] Sartor GC, Aston-Jones GS. Regulation of the ventral tegmental area by the bed nucleus of the stria terminalis is required for expression of cocaine preference. Eur J Neurosci. 2012 Dec;36(11):3549–58.

[63] Mahler SV, Aston-Jones GS. Fos activation of selective afferents to ventral tegmental area during cue-induced reinstatement of cocaine seeking in rats. J Neurosci. 2012 Sep; 32(38):13309–26.

[64] Tye KM, Deisseroth K. Optogenetic investigation of neural circuits underlying brain disease in animal models. Nat Rev Neurosci. 2012 Apr 1;13(4):251–66.

[65] Mahler SV, Vazey EM, Beckley JT, Keistler CR, McGlinchey EM, Kaufling J, et al. Designer receptors show role for ventral pallidum input to ventral tegmental area in cocaine seeking. Nat Neurosci. 2014 Apr;17(4):577–85.

[66] Zhu H, Roth BL. Silencing synapses with DREADDs. Neuron 2014 May 21;82(4):723–5.

[67] Boender AJ, de Jong JW, Boekhoudt L, Luijendijk MCM, van der Plasse G, Adan RAH. Combined use of the canine adenovirus-2 and DREADD-technology to activate specific neural pathways in vivo. PLoS ONE 2014 Jan;9(4):e95392.

[68] Carter ME, Soden ME, Zweifel LS, Palmiter RD. Genetic identification of a neural circuit that suppresses appetite. Nature 2013 Nov 7;503(7474):111–4.

[69] Nair SG, Strand NS, Neumaier JF. DREADDing the lateral habenula: a review of methodological approaches for studying lateral habenula function. Brain Res. 2013 May;1511:93–101.

[70] Gardner EL, Ashby CR. Heterogeneity of the mesotelencephalic dopamine fibers: physiology and pharmacology. Neurosci Biobehav Rev. 2000 Jan;24(1):115–8.

[71] Brodie MS, Pesold C, Appel SB. Ethanol directly excites dopaminergic ventral tegmental area reward neurons. Alcohol Clin Exp Res. 1999 Nov;23(11):1848–52.

[72] McDaid J, McElvain MA, Brodie MS. Ethanol effects on dopaminergic ventral tegmental area neurons during block of Ih: involvement of barium-sensitive potassium currents. J Neurophysiol. 2008 Jun 25;100(3):1202–10.

[73] Morikawa H, Morrisett RA. Ethanol action on dopaminergic neurons in the ventral tegmental area: interaction with intrinsic ion channels and neurotransmitter inputs. Int Rev Neurobiol. 2010;91:235–88.

[74] Mrejeru A, Martí-Prats L, Avegno EM, Harrison NL, Sulzer D. A subset of ventral tegmental area dopamine neurons responds to acute ethanol. Neuroscience 2015 Apr 2;290:649–58.

[75] Dayas CV, Liu X, Simms JA, Weiss F. Distinct patterns of neural activation associated with ethanol seeking: effects of naltrexone. Biol Psychiatry 2007 Apr;61(8):979–89.

[76] Swanson LW. The projections of the ventral tegmental area and adjacent regions: a combined fluorescent retrograde tracer and immunofluorescence study in the rat. Brain Res Bull. 1982 Jul;9(1–6):321–53.

[77] Cador M, Robbins TW, Everitt BJ. Involvement of the amygdala in stimulus-reward associations: interaction with the ventral striatum. Neuroscience 1989;30(1):77–86.

[78] Clark JJ, Collins AL, Sanford CA, Phillips PEM. Dopamine encoding of Pavlovian incentive stimuli diminishes with extended training. J Neurosci. 2013 Feb 20;33(8):3526–32.

[79] Di Chiara G, Bassareo V, Fenu S, De Luca MA, Spina L, Cadoni C, et al. Dopamine and drug addiction: the nucleus accumbens shell connection. Neuropharmacology 2004;47(Suppl. 1):227–41.

[80] Ikemoto S, Panksepp J. The role of nucleus accumbens dopamine in motivated behavior: a unifying interpretation with special reference to reward-seeking. Brain Res Brain Res Rev. 1999 Dec;31(1):6–41.

[81] Wise RA. Dopamine, learning and motivation. Nat Rev Neurosci. 2004 Jun;5(6):483–94.

[82] Everitt BJ, Robbins TW. Neural systems of reinforcement for drug addiction: from actions to habits to compulsion. Nat Neurosci. 2005 Nov;8(11):1481–9.

[83] McFarland K, Kalivas PW. The circuitry mediating cocaine-induced reinstatement of drug-seeking behavior. J Neurosci. 2001 Nov 1;21(21):8655–63.

[84] Alderson HL, Parkinson JA, Robbins TW, Everitt BJ. The effects of excitotoxic lesions of the nucleus accumbens core or shell regions on intravenous heroin self-administration in rats. Psychopharmacology (Berl). 2000 Dec 21;153(4):455–63.

[85] Fuchs RA, Evans KA, Parker MC, See RE. Differential involvement of the core and shell subregions of the nucleus accumbens in conditioned cue-induced reinstatement of cocaine seeking in rats. Psychopharmacology (Berl). 2004 Nov;176(3–4):459–65.

[86] Fuchs RA, Ramirez DR, Bell GH. Nucleus accumbens shell and core involvement in drug context-induced reinstatement of cocaine seeking in rats. Psychopharmacology (Berl). 2008 Nov;200(4):545–56.

[87] Chaudhri N, Sahuque LL, Cone JJ, Janak PH. Reinstated ethanol-seeking in rats is modulated by environmental context and requires the nucleus accumbens core. Eur J Neurosci. 2008 Dec;28(11):2288–98.

[88] Chaudhri N, Sahuque LL, Schairer WW, Janak PH. Separable roles of the nucleus accumbens core and shell in context- and cue-induced alcohol-seeking. Neuropsychopharmacology 2010 Feb;35(3):783–91.

[89] Millan EZ, Reese RM, Grossman CD, Chaudhri N, Janak PH. Nucleus accumbens and posterior amygdala mediate cue-triggered alcohol seeking and suppress behavior during the omission of alcohol-predictive cues. Neuropsychopharmacology 2015 Oct; 40(11):2555–65.

[90] Hauser SR, Deehan GA, Dhaher R, Knight CP, Wilden JA, McBride WJ, et al. D1 receptors in the nucleus accumbens-shell, but not the core, are involved in mediating ethanol-seeking behavior of alcohol-preferring (P) rats. Neuroscience 2015 Jun 4;295:243–51.

[91] Chaudhri N, Sahuque LL, Janak PH. Ethanol seeking triggered by environmental context is attenuated by blocking dopamine D1 receptors in the nucleus accumbens core and shell in rats. Psychopharmacology (Berl). 2009 Dec;207(2):303–14.

[92] Crombag HS, Bossert JM, Koya E, Shaham Y. Review. Context-induced relapse to drug seeking: a review. Philos Trans R Soc Lond Ser B Biol Sci. 2008 Oct;363(1507):3233–43.

[93] Erb S, Stewart J. A role for the bed nucleus of the stria terminalis, but not the amygdala, in the effects of corticotropin-releasing factor on stress-induced reinstatement of cocaine seeking. J Neurosci. 1999 Oct 15;19(20):RC35.

[94] Shaham Y, Erb S, Stewart J. Stress-induced relapse to heroin and cocaine seeking in rats: a review. Brain Res Brain Res Rev. 2000 Aug;33(1):13–33.

[95] Chaudhri N, Woods CA, Sahuque LL, Gill TM, Janak PH. Unilateral inactivation of the basolateral amygdala attenuates context-induced renewal of Pavlovian-conditioned alcohol-seeking. Eur J Neurosci. 2013 Sep;38(5):2751–61.

[96] Sciascia JM, Reese RM, Janak PH, Chaudhri N. Alcohol-seeking triggered by discrete Pavlovian cues is invigorated by alcohol contexts and mediated by glutamate signaling in the basolateral amygdala. Neuropsychopharmacology 2015 Nov;40(12):2801–12.

[97] Stuber GD, Sparta DR, Stamatakis AM, van Leeuwen WA, Hardjoprajitno JE, Cho S, et al. Excitatory transmission from the amygdala to nucleus accumbens facilitates reward seeking. Nature 2011 Jul 21;475(7356):377–80.

[98] Simms JA, Haass-Koffler CL, Bito-Onon J, Li R, Bartlett SE. Mifepristone in the central nucleus of the amygdala reduces yohimbine stress-induced reinstatement of ethanol-seeking. Neuropsychopharmacology 2012 Mar;37(4):906–18.

[99] Zhao Y, Dayas CV, Aujla H, Baptista MAS, Martin-Fardon R, Weiss F. Activation of group II metabotropic glutamate receptors attenuates both stress and cue-induced ethanol-seeking and modulates c-fos expression in the hippocampus and amygdala. J Neurosci. 2006 Sep 27;26(39):9967–74.

[100] Corbit LH, Nie H, Janak PH. Habitual alcohol seeking: time course and the contribution of subregions of the dorsal striatum. Biol Psychiatry 2012 Sep;72(5):389–95.

[101] Corbit LH, Nie H, Janak PH. Habitual responding for alcohol depends upon both AMPA and D2 receptor signaling in the dorsolateral striatum. Front Behav Neurosci. 2014;8:301.

[102] Brown RM, Kim AK, Khoo SY-S, Kim JH, Jupp B, Lawrence AJ. Orexin-1 receptor signalling in the prelimbic cortex and ventral tegmental area regulates cue-induced reinstatement of ethanol-seeking in iP rats. Addict Biol. 2015 May;21(3):603–12.

[103] Hauser SR, Deehan GA, Toalston JE, Bell RL, McBride WJ, Rodd ZA. Enhanced alcohol-seeking behavior by nicotine in the posterior ventral tegmental area of female alcohol-preferring (P) rats: modulation by serotonin-3 and nicotinic cholinergic receptors. Psychopharmacology (Berl). 2014 Mar 6;231(18):3745–55.

[104] Hauser SR, Ding Z-M, Getachew B, Toalston JE, Oster SM, McBride WJ, et al. The posterior ventral tegmental area mediates alcohol-seeking behavior in alcohol-preferring rats. J Pharmacol Exp Ther. 2011 Mar;336(3):857–65.

[105] Löf E, Olausson P, deBejczy A, Stomberg R, McIntosh JM, Taylor JR, et al. Nicotinic acetylcholine receptors in the ventral tegmental area mediate the dopamine activating and reinforcing properties of ethanol cues. Psychopharmacology (Berl). 2007 Aug 17;195(3):333–43.

[106] Fidler TL, Bakner L, Cunningham CL. Conditioned place aversion induced by intra-gastric administration of ethanol in rats. Pharmacol Biochem Behav. 2004 Apr;77(4): 731–43.

[107] Cunningham CL. Localization of genes influencing ethanol-induced conditioned place preference and locomotor activity in BXD recombinant inbred mice. Psychopharmacology (Berl). 1995 Jul;120(1):28–41.

[108] Cunningham CL, Niehus DR, Malott DH, Prather LK. Genetic differences in the rewarding and activating effects of morphine and ethanol. Psychopharmacology (Berl). 1992 Jun;107(2–3):385–93.

[109] Gremel CM, Cunningham CL. Roles of the nucleus accumbens and amygdala in the acquisition and expression of ethanol-conditioned behavior in mice. J Neurosci. 2008;28(5):1076–84.

[110] Young EA, Dreumont SE, Cunningham CL. Role of nucleus accumbens dopamine receptor subtypes in the learning and expression of alcohol-seeking behavior. Neurobiol Learn Mem. 2014 Jun;108:28–37.

[111] Walker BM, Ettenberg A. Intracerebroventricular ethanol-induced conditioned place preferences are prevented by fluphenazine infusions into the nucleus accumbens of rats. Behav Neurosci. 2007;121(2):401–10.

[112] Schultz W. Responses of midbrain dopamine neurons to behavioral trigger stimuli in the monkey. J Neurophysiol. 1986;56(5):1439–61.

[113] Ljungberg T, Apicella P, Schultz W. Responses of monkey dopamine neurons during learning of behavioral reactions. J Neurophysiol. 1992 Jan;67(1):145–63.

[114] Schultz W. A neural substrate of prediction and reward. Science 1997 Mar;275(5306): 1593–9.

[115] Bechtholt AJ, Cunningham CL. Ethanol-induced conditioned place preference is expressed through a ventral tegmental area dependent mechanism. Behav Neurosci. 2005 Feb;119(1):213–23.

[116] Gremel CM, Cunningham CL. Involvement of amygdala dopamine and nucleus accumbens NMDA receptors in ethanol-seeking behavior in mice. Neuropsychopharmacology 2009 May;34(6):1443–53.

[117] Wills TA, Klug JR, Silberman Y, Baucum AJ, Weitlauf C, Colbran RJ, et al. GluN2B subunit deletion reveals key role in acute and chronic ethanol sensitivity of glutamate synapses in bed nucleus of the stria terminalis. Proc Natl Acad Sci U S A 2012 Jan 31;109(5):E278–87.

[118] Carboni E, Silvagni A, Rolando MT, Di Chiara G. Stimulation of in vivo dopamine transmission in the bed nucleus of stria terminalis by reinforcing drugs. J Neurosci. 2000 Oct 15;20(20):RC102.

[119] Chang SL, Patel NA, Romero AA. Activation and desensitization of Fos immunoreactivity in the rat brain following ethanol administration. Brain Res. 1995 May;679(1):89–98.

[120] Gremel CM, Young EA, Cunningham CL. Blockade of opioid receptors in anterior cingulate cortex disrupts ethanol-seeking behavior in mice. Behav Brain Res. 2011 Jun; 219(2):358–62.

[121] Peters J, Kalivas PW, Quirk GJ. Extinction circuits for fear and addiction overlap in prefrontal cortex. Learn Mem. 2009 May;16(5):279–88.

[122] Groblewski PA, Cunningham CL. Repeated microinjections into the medial prefrontal cortex (mPFC) impair extinction of conditioned place preference in mice. Behav Brain Res. 2012 Apr;230(1):299–303.

[123] Groblewski PA, Ryabinin AE, Cunningham CL. Activation and role of the medial prefrontal cortex (mPFC) in extinction of ethanol-induced associative learning in mice. Neurobiol Learn Mem. 2012 Jan;97(1):37–46.

[124] Geisler S, Derst C, Veh RW, Zahm DS. Glutamatergic afferents of the ventral tegmental area in the rat. J Neurosci. 2007 May;27(21):5730–43.

[125] Omelchenko N, Sesack SR. Glutamate synaptic inputs to ventral tegmental area neurons in the rat derive primarily from subcortical sources. Neuroscience 2007;146(3): 1259–74.

[126] Carr DB, Sesack SR. Projections from the rat prefrontal cortex to the ventral tegmental area: target specificity in the synaptic associations with mesoaccumbens and meso-cortical neurons. J Neurosci. 2000;20(10):3864–73.

[127] Overton PG, Clark D. Burst firing in midbrain dopaminergic neurons. Brain Res Brain Res Rev. 1997 Dec;25(3):312–34.

[128] Wanat MJ, Willuhn I, Clark JJ, Phillips PEM. Phasic dopamine release in appetitive behaviors and drug addiction. Curr Drug Abuse Rev. 2009;2(2):195–213.

[129] Jennings JH, Sparta DR, Stamatakis AM, Ung RL, Pleil KE, Kash TL, et al. Distinct extended amygdala circuits for divergent motivational states. Nature 2013 Apr 11;496(7444):224–8.

[130] Lammel S, Lim BK, Ran C, Huang KW, Betley MJ, Tye KM, et al. Input-specific control of reward and aversion in the ventral tegmental area. Nature 2012 Nov;491(7423):212–7.

[131] Omelchenko N, Sesack SR. Laterodorsal tegmental projections to identified cell populations in the rat ventral tegmental area. J Comp Neurol. 2005;483(2):217–35.

[132] Lodge DJ, Grace AA. The laterodorsal tegmentum is essential for burst firing of ventral tegmental area dopamine neurons. Proc Natl Acad Sci U S A 2006;103(13):5167–72.

[133] Georges F, Aston-Jones GS. Potent regulation of midbrain dopamine neurons by the bed nucleus of the stria terminalis. J Neurosci. 2001 Aug 15;21(16):RC160.

[134] Georges F, Aston-Jones GS. Activation of ventral tegmental area cells by the bed nucleus of the stria terminalis: a novel excitatory amino acid input to midbrain dopamine neurons. J Neurosci. 2002 Jun;22(12):5173–87.

[135] Jalabert M, Aston-Jones GS, Herzog E, Manzoni O, Georges F. Role of the bed nucleus of the stria terminalis in the control of ventral tegmental area dopamine neurons. Prog Neuro-Psychopharmacol Biol Psychiatry 2009 Nov 13;33(8):1336–46.

[136] Kudo T, Uchigashima M, Miyazaki T, Konno K, Yamasaki M, Yanagawa Y, et al. Three types of neurochemical projection from the bed nucleus of the stria terminalis to the ventral tegmental area in adult mice. J Neurosci. 2012 Dec;32(50):18035–46.

[137] Kudo T, Konno K, Uchigashima M, Yanagawa Y, Sora I, Minami M, et al. GABAergic neurons in the ventral tegmental area receive dual GABA/enkephalin-mediated inhibitory inputs from the bed nucleus of the stria terminalis. Eur J Neurosci. Jun;39(11): 1796–809.

[138] Buffalari DM, See RE. Inactivation of the bed nucleus of the stria terminalis in an animal model of relapse: effects on conditioned cue-induced reinstatement and its enhancement by yohimbine. Psychopharmacology (Berl). 2011 Jan;213(1):19–27.

Chapter 4

Dopamine and Alcohol Dependence: From Bench to Clinic

Nitya Jayaram-Lindström, Mia Ericson,
Pia Steensland and Elisabet Jerlhag

Additional information is available at the end of the chapter

http://dx.doi.org/10.5772/63144

Abstract

Alcohol dependence, a chronic relapsing psychiatric disorder, is a major cause of mortality and morbidity. The role of dopamine in alcohol-induced reward as well in the development of alcohol dependence is reviewed herein. Both preclinical and clinical studies have suggested that alcohol activates the mesolimbic dopamine system (defined as a dopamine projection from the ventral tegmental area (VTA) to the nucleus accumbens (NAc, i.e. ventral striatum)) leading to a euphoric sensation. Alcohol dependence is characterized by a disruption in the reward-related brain areas including fewer dopamine D2 receptors in ventral striatum. Investigations of the underlying dopaminergic mechanisms involved during the development and maintenance of alcohol dependence could identify novel targets. Human and rodent experimental studies show that dopamine receptor antagonists, agonists and partial agonists as well as dopamine stabilizers influencing dopamine transmission, alter alcohol-mediated behaviours and thus may be potential treatment targets for alcohol dependence. Although there exists promising preclinical results, the majority of placebo-controlled randomized clinical trials with traditional dopamine antagonists and agonists have so far have been discouraging. Furthermore, the severe side-effect profiles of many of these compounds may limit their clinical use. Newer dopamine agents, such as partial agonists and dopamine stabilizers, attenuate alcohol-mediated behaviours in rodents as well as humans. Preclinical as well as clinical studies have shown that substances indirectly targeting the mesolimbic dopamine system may be potential targets for attenuation of alcohol reward. Collectively, the data reviewed herein may contribute to further understanding the complex mechanisms involved in development of alcohol dependence and we suggest that the newer dopamine agents as well as indirect modulators of dopamine signalling deserve to be further evaluated for treatment of alcohol dependence.

Keywords: alcohol-use disorder, mesocorticolimbic dopamine system, nucleus accumbens, dopamine stabilizer, antipsychotic drugs

1. Introduction

Alcohol dependence is a chronic relapsing psychiatric disorder significantly contributing to the global burden of disease [1] and affects about four percent of the world's population over the age of 15 (WHO). In the fifth edition of the diagnostic and statistical manual of mental disorders (DSM), the term alcohol use disorder was introduced and grossly defined as problem drinking that has become severe. The characteristics of this disorder include loss of control over alcohol intake, impaired cognitive functioning, negative social consequences, physical tolerance, withdrawal and craving for alcohol. To date, there are three medications approved by both the European Medicines Agency (EMA) and the Food and Drug Administration (FDA) for the treatment of alcohol dependence; disulfiram, naltrexone and acamprosate. The FDA has also approved the use of a long-acting injectable naltrexone. More recently, the EMA granted authorization also for nalmefene, a compound intended for the reduction of alcohol consumption in adults with alcohol dependence (EMA 2012). Details regarding the mechanism of action of these compounds are outside the scope of this review. In brief, the pharmacological profile is established for disulfiram (an aldehydedehydrogenase inhibitor), naltrexone (an opioid receptor antagonist) and nalmefene (an opioid receptor modulator), whereas the mechanism of action of the anti-alcohol relapse drug acamprosate is not fully understood. An indirect activation of mesolimbic dopamine via accumbal glycine receptors and ventral tegmental nicotinic acetylcholine receptors (nAChRs) appears likely [2, 3], but additional targets has been suggested (for review see [4]). Finally, the clinical efficacy of these agents is limited [5], possibly due to the heterogeneous nature of the disorder and the complex neurochemical mechanisms underlying alcohol dependence. Thus, the need for novel and efficacious medications remains.

The mesocorticolimbic dopamine system (or the so-called brain reward system, **Figure 1**) is one of the established neurobiological systems involved during the development and maintenance of alcohol dependence and thus one potential treatment target. Here, we aim to review the animal and human data describing the role of dopamine and the mesolimbic dopamine system during acute and chronic alcohol exposure. Finally, preclinical and clinical studies evaluating the potential of available dopaminergic agents as well as indirect dopamine modulators as novel medications for alcohol dependence are discussed.

1.1. The brain reward system: the mesocorticolimbic dopamine system

The mesocorticolimbic dopamine system has an established role in driving the rewarding sensations from natural rewards such as food, sex and exercise, which are important behaviours to ensure our survival [6, 7] as well as among drugs of abuse, including alcohol (for review see [8]). The physiological importance of the mesocorticolimbic dopamine system is highlighted by its evolutionary stability and conservation in primitive invertebrates, such as, flatworms, all the way up to primates, including humans. It was identified serendipitously in the 1950s when Olds and Milner found that rats self-administer electrical currents into certain specific brain regions [9]. These findings were later corroborated by studies showing that rats favoured electrical stimulation in the same specific brain regions, over natural rewards [10]. The primary neurotransmitter regulating the rewarding sensation was determined to be dopamine [11]. Furthermore, the specific neuronal circuitries were progressively mapped with major projections from the ventral tegmental area (VTA) to the nucleus accumbens (NAc, i.e. the ventral striatum), the prefrontal cortex (PFC) and amygdala. Collectively, this network of neurons was denominated the mesocorticolimbic dopamine system [12, 13]. The system was later divided into two distinct projections [12], modulating different dopamine-mediated behavioural effects; the mesolimbic pathway (from the VTA to the NAc) thought to be responsible for the rewarding and pleasurable effects of natural as well as substances of abuse including alcohol (e.g. [14–16]), and the mesocortical pathway (from the VTA to the PFC) believed to be responsible for the motivational and emotional effects [15]. In addition, there are dopamine projections from the VTA to the amygdala and the hippocampus, respectively, involved in reward associative learning and declarative memory formation [15, 17].

In healthy controls, alcohol consumption stimulates dopamine release mediating its reinforcing effects. Repeated bouts of intoxications will overtime downregulate the dopamine activity in the mesocorticolimbic pathway, leading to an increased risk of developing alcohol dependence and other impulse control disorders. [18, 13]. It has also been hypothesized that in vulnerable individuals (e.g. those with a family history of alcohol dependence), the proneness

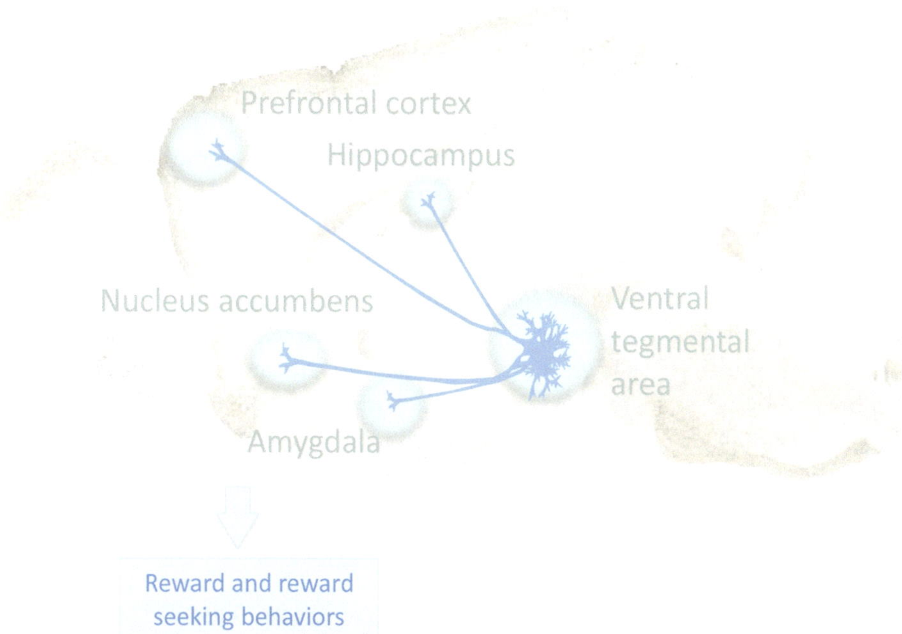

Figure 1. Representative illustration of the mesocorticolimbic dopamine system in rat brain.

to develop an addiction is higher since they are born with a reduced number of dopamine D2 receptors in mesocorticolimbic pathway, leading to the alcohol dependence [18, 13]. Further, it has been speculated that this dopamine deficiency is responsible for driving craving and compulsive drinking and contributes to relapse even after a period of protracted abstinence [18, 19]. The preclinical and clinical evidence of the underlying interaction between alcohol and the dopamine D2 receptors within the mesocorticolimbic dopamine system during the acute as well as during chronic intake is reviewed below. The involvement of the dopamine D1, D3, D4 and D5 receptors falls outside the scope of the present review but has previously been reviewed elsewhere [20].

1.2. Interaction between alcohol and the mesocorticolimbic dopamine system

1.2.1. Preclinical evidence: acute alcohol exposure and dopamine

Dopamine's importance for alcohol-induced reward was first identified in studies showing that the catecholamine-synthesis inhibitor, α-methyltyrosine (an agent with the ability to inhibit the formation of dopamine in the cytosol of terminals of dopaminergic neurons [21]) blocked alcohol-induced euphoria, social interaction and talkativeness in humans [22] as well as attenuated alcohol-induced locomotor activity in rats [23]. *Ex vivo* and *in vivo* voltammetry studies in rats found that alcohol increases the dopamine levels in NAc [24]. In addition, *in vivo* microdialysis studies have since shown that systemic administration of alcohol and other drugs of abuse, including amphetamine, cocaine, opiate and nicotine, increases the accumbal dopamine levels in freely moving rats [25–35], strengthening the hypothesis of an association between the rewarding or euphoric sensation and dopamine release in the NAc. This hypothesis is further supported by studies showing that drugs that are not rewarding or abused by humans do not modify synaptic accumbal dopamine levels in rat [27]. In addition, voluntary alcohol consumption causes a dose-dependent [36] release of dopamine in the NAc in rat [37–39]. Finally, intravenous administration of alcohol, as well as other drugs of abuse, increases the firing rate of dopamine neurons in the VTA in rats [40, 41]. Further support for the role of dopamine D2 receptors in the reinforcing effects of alcohol is given by a study showing that dopamine receptor D2 knockout mice self-administer less alcohol than the wild-type mice [42]. In addition to the extensive literature showing a link between accumbal dopamine and alcohol-induced reinforcement, it has been shown that the pure anticipation of alcohol (i.e. without alcohol being present) increases the release of dopamine in NAc in rodents trained to self-administer alcohol [43–45, 36] and that accumbal dopamine release is associated with associative learning, rather than exposure to the reward itself [46]. Moreover, this anticipation effect is more noticeable in high compared to low-alcohol-preferring rats [47]. Studies have also shown that the anticipation of a reward increases the firing of accumbal dopamine neurons [41]. It should, however, be mentioned that results from studies with lesion of the mesocorticolimbic dopamine pathways have shown contradicting results with both decreased [48–50] and unaltered alcohol intake [51–56]. These inconsistent results indicate that the role of accumbal dopamine in reinforcement is complex and highlights that the rewarding properties of alcohol may extend beyond direct or indirect effects on dopamine, involving interactions with several other neurotransmitters including acetylcholine, glutamate, GABA, serotonin (5HT), noradrenaline, taurine and opioids, as well as hormones and peptides [24, 57, 58].

To further elucidate the role of the NAc and the VTA in alcohol-mediated dopamine regulation, extensive rodent studies, with for example intra-cranial alcohol infusions and electrophysiological techniques, have been conducted. With regards to the NAc, rodent studies confirm that intra-NAc alcohol perfusions increase the release of dopamine in the same brain region (e.g. [59, 38, 60–62]). An effect that is suggested to be regulated via a neuronal circuitry involving glycine receptors in the NAc as well as anterior ventral tegmental nAChR [59, 63, 64]. Interestingly, the NAc is a heterogeneous region most often divided into two distinct anatomically and functionally different regions, that is the central core and the surrounding shell compartment [65–69] and it has been suggested that dopaminergic innervation of the NAc core is associated with the nigrostriatal system, while that of the NAc shell is related to the mesolimbic system [70]. Alcohol has been shown to increase the release of dopamine in NAc shell, but not in the core [71–73]. Studies are also emerging suggesting the need for further division of this brain region since it was demonstrated that a borderline region between the core and shell of the NAc is the region most responsive to alcohol [74].

With regards to the VTA, both *in vitro* and *in vivo* studies show that alcohol increases the firing of dopamine neurons in the VTA projecting to NAc [75–79, 40]. Similarly, in a situation of synaptic transmission blockade, alcohol has been found to increase the firing of dissociated VTA dopamine neurons [76, 77] implying that alcohol activates ventral tegmental dopamine neurons independent of afferent signalling. Furthermore, studies with intra-VTA alcohol infusions highlight that different subregions within the heterogeneous VTA might have different ability to modulate the alcohol-induced dopamine response. Specifically, rats voluntarily self-administer alcohol, as well as acetaldehyde (an alcohol metabolite) into the posterior, but not anterior, part of the VTA [80–85], indicating that alcohol is reinforcing only within the posterior VTA. The suggestion is further supported by a study showing that intracranial infusions into the posterior VTA of the D2 agonist quinpirole (in doses that activate local D2 autoreceptors, thereby reducing the firing rate of VTA dopamine neurons [86, 87]), attenuates alcohol self-administration, which can be restored when the D2 agonist is removed or blocked with administration of a D2 antagonist [84]. In corroboration are the findings that the sensitivity of the posterior VTA to the reinforcing effects of alcohol is enhanced in alcohol-preferring rats [88]. There are, however, some contradicting results indicating that these subregion-specific effects might be related to the administered dose of alcohol, the use of various methods, the rat strains across the studies as well as differences in coordinates used for local injections (within the anterior VTA). For example, it has been demonstrated that perfusion of a low, but not a high dose of alcohol into the anterior, but not posterior part of the VTA increased accumbal dopamine in rats [89], and a recent study indicates that additional VTA subregions might be involved as alcohol increases the firing frequency of a subset of dopamine neurons in the medial, but not lateral, part of the VTA [90]. It should also be noted that in both outbreed as well as alcohol-preferring rats, there are studies showing no influence on the accumbal dopamine levels regardless of dose of alcohol or location in the VTA [59, 91]. Collectively, these data suggest that VTA is a heterogeneous area that differs in morphology and topography (for review, see [92]), and the anterior/posterior and lateral/medial part have different functions regarding alcohol and its activation of the mesolimbic dopamine system.

1.2.2. Clinical evidence: acute alcohol consumption and dopamine

The development of positron imaging technique (PET) and the radiotracer ^{11}C-raclopride in the 1990s made it possible to study *in vivo* dopamine function in humans. A series of human imaging studies over the last decade have demonstrated that alcohol [93, 94] as well as other drugs of abuse [95] increase striatal dopamine release. This is further corroborated by the findings that self-reported behavioural measures of stimulation, euphoria or drug wanting by alcohol correlates with the magnitude and rate of ventral striatum dopamine release [96–98, 94, 99, 100]. These studies clearly substantiated the involvement of dopamine in the reinforcing effects of alcohol and closely mimicked the findings of the preclinical studies.

1.2.3. Preclinical evidence: chronic alcohol exposure and dopamine

As mentioned above, it has been hypothesized that the chronic intake of alcohol induces a dopamine deficit state in the brain reward system and that this dysfunction may drive craving and relapse to drinking [101, 18, 19]. In outbred rodents, however, the effects on the mesolimbic dopamine system following chronic alcohol treatment are inconsistent [102]. One possible explanation for these discrepancies may be that most preclinical studies to-date have used forced alcohol administration which introduces an element of stress and artefact into the experiment, casting doubt on the applicability to our understanding of human alcohol dependence. In this review, we will therefore focus on studies with clear face validity to the human condition, that is those using voluntary self-administration.

The dopamine deficiency hypothesis is supported by a study showing decreased dopamine receptor gene expression after several months of voluntary alcohol drinking [103]. In addition, microdialysis studies in freely moving outbred rats show a decreased dopamine output in the NAc, compared to age-matched alcohol-naïve controls, following 7 weeks [104] and 10 months [29] of voluntary alcohol consumption. Furthermore, after 10 months of drinking, a blunted dopamine response following a systemic alcohol challenge has been found in long-term drinking, compared to alcohol-naïve rats [29]. These results indicate that long-term drinking attenuates the responsiveness of the system to external dopamine stimulation, in addition to decreasing baseline levels of dopamine. It should, however, be noted that acute administration of alcohol induces a twofold increase in dopamine output in the NAc shell in high compared to low-alcohol-preferring rats [105], indicating that there might be a difference in these aspects between outbred standard laboratory rats and inbred alcohol-preferring rats.

The selectively inbred alcohol-preferring and non-alcohol-preferring rat strains have been extensively used to investigate the neurochemical mechanisms underlying alcohol dependence. In line with the dopamine deficiency hypothesis, the baseline accumbal dopamine levels appear to be lower [105] and the dopamine D2 receptors in NAc are fewer [106] in high-preferring compared to low-preferring rats. In fact, neurochemical data show that high-alcohol-seeking behaviour is associated with 10–15% lower accumbal dopamine content compared with low-alcohol-seeking rats [107]. In addition, overexpression of accumbal dopamine D2 receptors reduces alcohol in non-preferring as well as high-preferring rats [108, 109]. These results highlight that not only chronic alcohol consumption, but also genetic factors, influence the dopaminergic response to alcohol. Furthermore, it has been suggested that more dorsal parts of the striatum is recruited once the dependence develops [110, 111] although until now this has been investigated only in other drugs of abuse than alcohol.

1.2.4. Clinical evidence: alcohol dependence and dopamine

As mentioned earlier, in vulnerable individuals (related to genetic and environmental factors) as well as healthy individuals, repeated administration of alcohol can lead to perturbations in the dopamine-regulated circuitry, leading to the development of alcohol dependence. For instance, a human laboratory study has demonstrated that intravenous administration of alcohol causes an increase in dopamine in the ventral striatum in non-treatment-seeking alcohol-dependent individuals [112]. Further, imaging studies have shown that the number of dopamine D2 receptors is lower in individuals with alcohol or drug dependence, compared to healthy controls [113, 114] and there is considerable evidence that the low levels of D2 receptors levels contribute to the excessive urges/craving for alcohol and subsequently to relapse [115]. In addition, decreased dopamine transmission in the mesolimbic regions, such as the ventral striatum, likely contributes to anhedonia and decreased reward sensitivity in alcohol-dependent individuals. Further, in abstinent high-risk drinkers as well as alcohol-dependent individuals, alcohol-associated cues activate the ventral striatum, which further contribute to the high risk of relapse in these individuals [116, 117].

A recent PET study [118] demonstrated for the first time that, in addition to the ventral striatum, the long-term consumption of alcohol leads to lowered dopamine levels also in prefrontal cortical structures. These findings support the extensive clinical findings demonstrating that alcohol-dependent individuals have significant impairments in executive functions such as working memory, impulsivity and decision-making; functions governed by the cortical brain structures. The fact that there is also less dopamine in the prefrontal cortex, governing these executive functions, is of significance as it could impair the alcohol-dependent individual's capacity to utilize behavioural treatment strategies, which are critical to relapse prevention.

Collectively, these data indicate that dopamine plays a central role in reward, motivation and planning. Given the relevance of dopamine in the chronic phase of alcohol use and in the development of alcohol dependence, there is considerable interest in evaluating medications that can specifically modify dopamine, thereby serving as potential pharmacotherapies to treat alcohol dependence.

1.2.5. Human genetic evidence: alcohol dependence and dopamine

The preclinical and clinical evidence presented above suggest that dopamine regulates alcohol-mediated behaviours. Numerous human genetic studies have therefore investigated associations between alcohol dependence and genes related to dopamine function. As early as the

1990s, a polymorphism in the dopamine D2 receptor gene was found to be associated with alcohol dependence [119]. Several studies have since then tried to replicate this association, but the outcome has been inconsistent (for review, see [120]). Although associations have been found between polymorphism of the dopamine D4 gene and alcohol craving, binge drinking as well as novelty seeking (which is a known personality trait important for drinking behaviour in patients with alcohol dependence) [121–123], no positive associations between dopamine D4 receptor genes and alcohol dependence *per se* have been established (for review, see [120]).

Released dopamine into the synaptic cleft is eliminated by catechol-O-methyltransferase (COMT) metabolism as well as reuptake by dopamine transporter (DAT). Studies have shown that DAT polymorphism is associated with alcohol withdrawal symptoms as well as with paternal history of alcohol dependence rather than alcohol dependence *per se* [124, 125]. The risk of developing late onset alcohol dependence (especially in males) as well as the co-dependence of alcohol and nicotine is associated with polymorphism in COMT [126–128]. Albeit cumulative evidence shows association between polymorphisms in various dopamine-related genes and behaviours associated with alcohol dependence, the findings are inconclusive and therefore, the conclusions from these human genetic studies are limited and remain controversial.

2. The dopamine system: a potential treatment target for alcohol dependence

2.1. Dopamine D2 receptor antagonists

Traditional dopamine D2 receptor antagonists (so-called neuroleptics, first-generation antipsychotic drugs or typical antipsychotic drugs) are primary used for the treatment of psychosis, schizophrenia and bipolar disorder [11] based on their ability to counteract a heightened dopamine activity in the brain. It should also be mentioned that these typical antipsychotic agents might have effects on other receptors including dopamine D1, $5HT_2$ and alpha1 receptors. As reviewed above, the acute reinforcing effects of addictive drugs, including alcohol, could be mediated by increased dopamine release in the NAc, activating dopamine D2 receptors [71, 27, 30]. Thus, traditional dopamine D2 receptor antagonists have been evaluated as potential treatment targets for alcohol dependence based on the hypothesis that they are expected to block the rewarding effects of alcohol.

2.1.1. Preclinical evidence for the use of dopamine D2 receptor antagonists to attenuate alcohol-mediated behaviours

The hypothesis that dopamine D2 receptor antagonists have the ability to attenuate alcohol-mediated behaviours is supported by rodent studies showing that both haloperidol and pimozide attenuate alcohol-induced locomotor stimulation [129] and that these compounds as well as fluphenazine, decrease alcohol-seeking behaviour and operant self-administration [130–132]. These findings are further substantiated by the data showing that peripheral administration of the dopamine D2 receptor antagonist fluphenazine decreased responding for alcohol, without affecting responses for water in rats [133]. In addition, haloperiodol dose-dependently reduced operant self-administration of alcohol in rats [134] as well as decreased alcohol presentations in the self-administration model [132]. Supportively, low doses of dopamine D2 receptor antagonists inhibit the rewarding properties of other drugs of abuse in rats [135, 42, 136]. It should be noted that some studies have shown contradicting effects [137–139], indicating that the role of dopamine in alcohol-mediated behaviours in complex.

Studies elucidating the underlying mechanism of action of the complex dopamine–alcohol interaction have been conducted. Experiments exploring the role of accumbal dopamine receptors in alcohol-mediated behaviours showed that intra-NAc administration of first-generation antipsychotic drugs including fluphenazine or raclopride decreased alcohol self-administration in rats [133] as well as the total responding for alcohol [140] and reduced the total responding by decreasing time course and response rate for alcohol self-administration in rats [141]. On the other hand, local administration of the dopamine D2 receptor antagonist, sulpiride, into the anterior VTA did not alter alcohol nor sucrose intake in high-alcohol-preferring rats [142]. It should also be mentioned that accumbal dopamine D1 receptor might regulate alcohol-induced reward. Indeed, intra-NAc infusion of a dopamine D1 receptor antagonist (SCH23390 or ecopipam) decreased alcohol-mediated behaviours in rats [141, 143]. Collectively, these data indicate that the dopamine D2 as well as D1 receptors within the NAc regulate alcohol reinforcement.

2.1.2. Clinical evidence for the use of dopamine D2 antagonists for the treatment of alcohol dependence

Based on the preclinical evidence of a reduction in alcohol consumption via blockade of dopamine D2 receptors, the potential of dopamine D2 antagonists as a pharmacotherapy for alcohol dependence has been investigated in clinical populations.

Dopamine D2 receptor antagonists have been studied in human laboratory studies involving alcohol administration in dependent individuals and found to be effective in reducing craving. In a laboratory study involving 16 individuals with alcohol abuse and/or dependence, the D2 antagonist haloperidol was compared to placebo. The results of this small study demonstrated that haloperidol significantly decreased measures of craving, reduced impulsivity, and the amounts of alcohol ingested [144]. The dopamine D2 antagonist flupenthixol has also been evaluated in a clinical study of 281 recently detoxified alcohol-dependent patients [145]. The results demonstrated that treatment with the depot formulation of flupenthixol led to a significant increase in rates of relapse (85.2% on active treatment compared with 62.5% on placebo). A major concern with flupenthixol is results from studies demonstrating an increase in the risk of relapse in rodents as well as humans [146], an effect preferentially observed in males [147]. Overall, the clinical utility of atypical antipsychotics has shown to be of some benefit in patients suffering from alcohol dependence and a concomitant psychiatric diagnosis including schizophrenia [148, 149]. A major challenge, however, with the first-generation antipsychotic drugs is their severe side effect profile including extrapyramidal symptoms, sedation, cognitive impairment, neuroleptic malignant syndrome, which have limited their use in research and in turn its clinical utility in treating alcohol dependence [150, 151].

2.2. Atypical dopamine D2 receptor antagonists

The newer generations of dopamine D2 receptor antagonists (so-called atypical antipsychotics or second generation antipsychotic drugs) have a broader pharmacological profile since they target several dopamine receptors, including D1, D3, D4 and D5, as well as various other neurotransmitter systems including 5-HT, muscarinic acetylcholine and histamine receptors. These atypical antipsychotics have a significantly improved side effect profile compared to the traditional first generation of dopamine D2 antagonists. Thus, there has been a renewed interest in evaluating these medications as potential treatment for alcohol dependence with the assumption that the atypical antipsychotics might reduce craving and consumption of alcohol without the substantial adverse effect profile [152]. Furthermore, they are clinically used for alcohol-dependent patients during the acute detoxification phase to prevent agitation, hallucinations and delirium tremens [153].

2.2.1. Preclinical evidence for the use of atypical dopamine D2 receptor antagonists (i.e. atypical antipsychotics) to attenuate alcohol-mediated behaviours

The hypothesis that atypical antipsychotics may decrease alcohol intake are supported by two separate studies with risperidone and olanzapine in high-alcohol-preferring rats [154, 155]. Furthermore, remoxipride decreases the number of alcohol presentations per session in rats by inducing an early termination of the alcohol-drinking bout during the self-administration session [132] and repeated systemic administration of paliperidone decreased the acquisition of alcohol consumption in high-alcohol-preferring P rats [156]. In addition, a recent study, comparing the effect of the atypical antipsychotic drug clozapine to that of the traditional dopamine D2 receptor antagonist haloperidol, showed that clozapine but not haloperidol attenuated the initiation of alcohol drinking and development of alcohol preference in high-alcohol-preferring rats [157]. Neither compound had an effect on maintenance of chronic alcohol drinking [157], which is in line with a study showing that clozapine did not reduce alcohol consumption in alcohol-preferring rats [155].

2.2.2. Clinical evidence for the use of atypical dopamine D2 antagonists for the treatment of alcohol dependence

The atypical antipsychotic tiapride has been found to be efficacious in reducing alcohol drinking two placebo-controlled clinical trials [158, 159]. A small study in twenty alcohol-dependent individuals, with significant levels of anxiety or depression, showed that tiapride treatment causes a reduced alcohol intake as well as prolonged periods of abstinence [158]. In the largest of the studies [159], 100 recently abstinent alcohol-dependent patients were randomized to 300 mg of tiapride or placebo for a 3-month treatment period. This study showed that patients receiving medication had higher rates of abstinence and improved on an array of health care outcomes.

Another atypical antipsychotic drug, quetiapine, has been evaluated in a case study [160] and an open-label study [161] in patients with alcohol dependence and comorbid psychiatric diagnosis. Both studies demonstrated that quetiapine was well tolerated and in the latter study, the medication not only reduced alcohol consumption and overall psychiatric symptom intensity but also significantly reduced craving. A double-blind placebo-controlled study by Kampman and colleagues evaluated the effect of quetiapine and found that the medication was well tolerated and clinically effective in reducing drinking [162]. The effect of medication was found to be stronger in individuals with a more severe disease phenotype. It should, however, be noted that more recent clinical trials using the extended release formulation of quetiapine [163, 164] failed to replicate the clinical findings of the previous studies.

In a retrospective study of 151 schizophrenic patients with alcohol dependence, 36 patients received the atypical antipsychotic medication clozapine. At the 6-month follow-up, 79% of the patients on clozapine were in remission from a diagnosis of alcohol dependence, while approximately 33% of those not taking clozapine were in remission [148].

Olanzapine, another example of a second generation of antipsychotics, has been evaluated in a human cue-craving study, where the compound reduced the urge to drink post-exposure to alcohol cues, without affecting the rewarding effects of alcohol following the consumption of a priming dose of alcohol [152]. Based on this clinical finding and the knowledge that olanzapine also has a high affinity for the D4 receptors, it was hypothesized whether the dopamine receptor D4 gene maybe involved in meditating its clinical effects. In a subsequent pharmacogenetic, 12-weeks placebo-controlled trial in heavy social drinker olanzapine was evaluated in 67 individuals [165] showing that those individuals with the dopamine D4 receptor 7 repeat allele (a polymorphism of the dopamine D4 receptor gene) reported a greater reduction in cue-induced craving and alcohol consumption compared to individuals with the short allele. These data are supported by the findings that olanzapine reduces craving for alcohol at baseline for both individuals with the DRD4 shorter and longer allele, but only reduces craving after exposure to alcohol cues and after a priming dose of alcohol for individuals with the DRD4 longer allele [166]. Overall, the results from studies evaluating olanzapine as a potential medication for alcohol dependence have provided evidence of a marginal effect restricted to a sub population of patients (with the longer dopamine D4 receptor allele).

In conclusion, although some clinical trials with atypical antipsychotics in alcohol-dependent patients show promising results, a recent systemic review of atypical antipsychotics, a heterogeneous class of drugs [167] has demonstrated inconsistent clinical response across studies on these compounds effects on alcohol-related parameters. The clinical use of atypical antipyschotics for treatment of alcohol dependence might also be limited by their side effects profile, even though it is substantially improved compared to the typical antipsychotics (for review see [168]).

2.3. Dopamine D2 agonists

As described previously, in vivo microdialysis studies rodent and imaging studies in individuals with alcohol dependence have demonstrated that chronic exposure to alcohol induce a dopamine deficit state. Thus, it is logical to hypothesize that a dopamine agonist would substitute for this dopaminergic dysfunction during alcohol dependence and alleviate the associated depression-like symptoms and craving for alcohol.

2.3.1. Preclinical evidence for the use of dopamine agonists to attenuate alcohol-mediated behaviours

The potential of dopamine D2 agonists to regulate alcohol-mediated behaviours is supported by a study showing that apomorphine, dose-dependently reduces operant self-administration as well as decreases momentary response rates for alcohol in rats [134] and that SDZ-205-152, a synthetic-mixed D1/D2 dopamine receptor agonist dose-dependently reduces self-administration of alcohol, but not water, in rats [169]. Moreover, cabergoline, a dopamine D2 receptor agonist, decreased alcohol intake, relapse drinking as well as alcohol-seeking behaviour in rodents [170]. In addition, low doses of bromocriptine produced a significant, dose-dependent shift in decreasing the preference for alcohol while enhancing water consumption [171], indicating that the compound at lower doses preferentially augment autoreceptor function, leading to decreased dopamine turnover with a blunted response to the rewarding effects of alcohol as a result. Studies with intra-NAc administration of quinpirole, further indicating that D2 receptors are involved in a biphasic effect on alcohol self-administration, by showing that low doses of the agonist increase, whereas higher doses decrease, self-administration of alcohol [141] (but see also [140]). A study has also investigated the effect of dopamine D2 receptor agonist administration into VTA on alcohol intake. This study showed that microinjection of either quinpirole or quinelorane, into the anterior part of the VTA dose-dependently decreased alcohol, but not sucrose, intake in alcohol-preferring rats [142]. In support are the data showing that local administration of cabergoline into the VTA reduced alcohol-seeking behaviour in rats [170]. These data are contradictory to the findings showing that the dopamine D2 receptor antagonist into the anterior VTA did not alter alcohol intake in high-alcohol-preferring rats [142]. Therefore, mechanisms regulating alcohol reinforcement might be different in selectively breed high alcohol-consuming rats compared to outbreed rats, and this should be investigated in more detail. It should also be mentioned that infusion of the dopamine D1-like agonist SKF 38393 into NAc had no effect on alcohol self-administration in rats [141]. Albeit the data are somewhat contradictory, it might be hypothesized that accumbal as well as ventral tegmental dopamine D2 receptors may regulate alcohol reinforcement in rodents.

2.3.2. Clinical evidence for the use of dopamine agonists for the treatment of alcohol dependence

Bromocriptine, a dopamine agonist has been used clinically for Parkinson's disease. At low doses, bromocriptine can reduce alcohol consumption in animals [171]; it is possible that low-dose dopamine agonists preferentially augment autoreceptor function, thereby decreasing dopamine turnover and blunting the rewarding effects of alcohol. An early double-blinded study [172] reported that bromocriptine reduced alcohol craving in alcohol-dependent patients with a specific genotype of the dopamine D2 receptor gene (i.e. the A1/A1 and A1/A2 genotypes). However, subsequent double-blind placebo-controlled trials found no effect on relapse or related behaviours [173, 174]. Currently, due to the knowledge of the addictive potential of dopamine agonists, combined with the lack of consistent findings from clinical studies, it is suggested that dopamine receptor agonists do not hold promise as a treatment for alcohol dependence.

2.4. Partial dopamine agonists

Based on the knowledge that alcohol can both stimulate dopamine activity as well as induce a hypo-dopaminergic state, it has been suggested that partial agonists might have potential as novel medications for alcohol dependence. A partial agonist, such as aripiprazole, has a lower intrinsic activity at the receptor than a full agonist (e.g. dopamine), meaning that when it binds to the receptor, it will activate the receptor but produce a less potent biological response than the full agonist [175–177]. In the presence of high levels of the full agonist, a partial agonist will have functional antagonistic activity by binding to the receptor and preventing the response from the full agonist. Partial dopamine D2 agonists, therefore, offer the opportunity to treat the dysregulated dopamine activity during acute alcohol consumption as well as alcohol dependence.

2.4.1. Preclinical evidence for the use of partial dopamine agonists to attenuate alcohol-mediated behaviours

In line with the hypothesis that a partial dopamine D2 agonist would block the reinforcing effects of alcohol, aripiprazole attenuates alcohol's ability to increase the locomotor activity in mice [178, 179](an indirect measure of activation of the mesolimbic dopamine system). On the other hand, aripiprazole did not interfere with the alcohol-induced impairment in motor balance as measured by rotarod test [179]. Furthermore, repeated systemic aripiprazole administration decreases alcohol intake in alcohol-preferring rats [180], while single oral administration dose-dependently decreases alcohol self-administration in outbred rats [181]. In addition, aripiprazole has been shown to reverse alcohol-induced place preference and anxiety-like behaviour in mice [182].

2.4.2. Clinical evidence for the use of dopamine partial agonists for the treatment of alcohol dependence

Clinically, the partial dopamine D2 agonist aripiprazole has been evaluated in a few randomized placebo-controlled trials and human laboratory studies. A pilot study showed that aripiprazole reduces the rate of relapse and craving in patients with alcohol dependence [183]. In a subsequent larger 12-weeks, double-blind, placebo-controlled study of 295 alcohol-dependent patients aripiprazole was initiated at 2 mg/day, titrated to a maximum dose of 20 mg/day [184]. This study showed that aripiprazole decreased heavy drinking days compared to placebo during week four and eight; however, the effect was lost by the maximum dose at week twelve [184]. The effects of aripiprazole were also evaluated in a human laboratory study in non-treatment seeking alcohol-dependent individuals (n = 30), showing that the compound was well-tolerated and reduced drinking, especially in impulsive individuals [185]. Voronin and colleagues also showed that aripiprazole decreased the number of drinks in a bar–lab environment after consumption of a priming drink, as well as weakened the association between the priming-induced stimulation and further drinking. In another double-blind comparison trial, aripiprazole was shown to reduce craving [186] but to a lesser extent than the FDA-approved medication naltrexone [187]. Finally, a brain imaging study demonstrated that aripiprazole attenuated cue-induced activation as evidenced by a reduced activation of the right ventral striatum with a corresponding reduction in drinking in individuals with alcohol dependence [188]. Thus far, early results with aripiprazole appear promising, although whether this or similar compounds might be useful to treat alcohol dependence or be positioned as a medication with a specific profile, that is as targeted intervention in more impulsive alcohol-dependent individuals needs to be evaluated further.

2.5. Dopamine stabilizers

As a further development of the partial agonist concept, Nobel Laureate Arvid Carlsson and co-workers, developed a novel family of compounds based on their ability to stabilize, that is to stimulate, suppress or show no effect on the dopamine activity depending on the prevailing dopaminergic tone [189]. This stabilizing concept was postulated based on a PET study in rhesus monkeys where infusions with the compound (-)-OSU6162 (OSU6162) induced a dopaminergic tone-dependent effect with a reduction in the striatal L-[11C]DOPA influx rate in monkeys with high baseline values and an increased striatal L-[11C]DOPA influx rate in animals with low baseline values [190]. The mechanism of action is, however, not completely understood, and although *in vitro* studies indicate that OSU6162, like aripiprazole, acts as a partial agonist at D2 receptors [191, 192], behavioural studies have failed to demonstrate any intrinsic activity of the compound ([195]). Instead it has been suggested that OSU6162 produces functionally opposite effects by acting as an antagonist at both presynaptic autoreceptors and postsynaptic D2 receptors [189, 193–195]. Based on the hypothesis that OSU6162 can counteract both hyper- and hypo-dopaminergic states, the compound has recently been evaluated in both animal models modulating alcohol-mediated behaviours as well as in a placebo-controlled human laboratory study in alcohol-dependent patients.

2.5.1. Preclinical evidence for the use of dopamine stabilizers to attenuate alcohol-mediated behaviours

A series of experiments in outbred rats show that the dopamine stabilizer OSU6162 attenuates several alcohol-mediated behaviours including voluntary alcohol intake, alcohol withdrawal symptoms and cue/priming-induced reinstatement of alcohol seeking in long-term drinking rats [196]. Furthermore, OSU6162 blunted alcohol-induced dopamine output in the NAc of alcohol-naïve rats [196], indicating that OSU6162 has the ability to attenuate the rewarding effects of alcohol. In contrast, a more recent microdialysis study conducted in long-term drinking rats, showed that OSU6162, compared to vehicle-pretreatment, had no significant effect on the alcohol-induced dopamine peak [29]. The contrasting microdialysis results in alcohol-drinking versus alcohol-naïve rats highlight OSU6162′s ability to modulate the dopamine output dependent on the prevailing dopaminergic tone. Furthermore, these results indicate that OSU6162 might have the ability to attenuate alcohol-mediated behaviours by counteracting the hypo-dopaminergic state induced by long-term drinking. Collectively, together with the finding that OSU6162 did not induce conditioned place preference [29] (an indication that the compound has no rewarding properties of its own), these results indicate that OSU6162 has many of the favourable characteristics of a potential medication for alcohol dependence.

2.5.2. Clinical evidence for the use of a dopamine stabilizer for the treatment of alcohol dependence

The dopamine stabilizer OSU6162 was recently evaluated in a placebo-controlled human laboratory alcohol craving study in 56 alcohol dependent individuals [197]. Two weeks of OSU6162 treatment significantly attenuated priming-induced craving and induced significantly lower subjective "liking" of the consumed alcohol, compared to placebo. Interestingly, the treatment effects of OSU6162 were driven by those individuals with high level of baseline impulsivity, corroborating previous results with the partial dopamine D2 agonist aripiprazole [185]. These results suggest that pharmacological stabilization of the dopamine system might prove as an effective target for alleviating some of the reward driven behaviours during alcohol dependence. Together with OSU6162's favourable side effect profile [198, 197, 199], these results render support for a larger placebo-controlled efficacy trial in alcohol-dependent patients to evaluate OSU6162's effect on drinking outcomes.

2.6. Pharmacological agents inducing indirect modulation of dopamine

As mentioned previously, in addition the affecting the dopamine system directly, alcohol interacts with the mesolimbic dopamine system indirectly via several other neurotransmitters. There is a wide range of such compounds, and here, we will only mention a few, specifically targeting glycine receptors and nAChRs, with a clear interaction with dopamine transmission in the mesolimbic dopamine system [64].

2.6.1. Preclinical evidence for the use of compounds that indirectly targets dopamine to attenuate alcohol-mediated behaviours

Rodent studies exploring the potential of targeting the glycine system as a medication for alcohol dependence showed that systemic administration of the glycine transporter-1 inhibitor Org25935 increased extracellular glycine in the NAc, which prevented alcohol-induced dopamine release [200, 201] as well as decreased alcohol intake and prevented relapse drinking [202, 203]. These results provided rational for a randomized placebo-controlled clinical trial in alcohol-dependent individuals.

Emerging data suggests that the activity of dopamine neurons in the VTA projecting to the NAc is regulated by several afferents, such as, for example the cholinergic neurons projecting from the laterodorsal tegmental nucleus (LDTg) (for review see [204]). Although alcohol's direct interaction with this cholinergic-dopaminergic reward link remains to be fully elucidated, a study show that voluntary alcohol intake in high-alcohol-consuming rats causes a concomitant release of ventral tegmental acetylcholine and accumbal dopamine [39]. Several rodent studies with nAChR antagonists such as mecamylamine or selective nAChRs antagonists such as alpha-conotoxin MII highlight the potential of nAChRs as novel medications for alcohol dependence by showing that these compounds prevent alcohol from increasing dopamine and reduce alcohol consumption behaviour [28, 38, 32, 34, 35]. These nAChR antagonists are limited in a clinical setting due to low blood–brain barrier permeability and an unfavourable side effect profile. The potential of nAChR's as novel treatment target was revived with the marketing of the partial nAChR agonist varenicline as a smoking cessation agent. It has been shown that varenicline reduce alcohol intake and alcohol-seeking behaviour in long-term drinking rats [205] and modulate NAc dopamine after systemic administrations of alcohol alone and in combination with nicotine [206].

2.6.2. Clinical evidence for the use of indirect modulation of dopamine for the treatment of alcohol dependence

Albeit the preclinical data look promising regarding the glycine transporter-1 inhibitor Org25935, the multicenter randomized clinical trial produced a negative outcome on alcohol intake, but did not discard the potential importance of the mechanism [207]. More promising clinical studies with varenicline show that this agent decreased alcohol consumption and craving in an experimental setting in heavy-drinking smokers [208–210]. Moreover, data from a randomized clinical trial in alcohol-dependent individuals show that the smoking cessation agent reduced the weekly percent heavy drinking days drinks, decreased the drinks per drinking day as well as prevented alcohol craving [211]. It should, however, be noted that recent clinical trials in alcohol-dependent individuals were unable to find a beneficial effect of varenicline based on self-reported alcohol consumption [212, 213]. Nevertheless, when also monitoring the selective alcohol biomarker phosphatidylethanol (PEth) in the blood of the subjects in the above-mentioned clinical trial [212], it was found that varenicline indeed had effect on this objective measure of alcohol consumption [214] strengthening the potential of varenicline as potential novel medication for alcohol dependence. Besides glycine receptors and nAChR, there are various signalling systems indirectly targeting the mesolimbic dopamine system with promising preclinical findings on alcohol-mediated behaviours. Collectively, these data indicate that indirect modulation of dopamine signalling might be a potential target for novel treatment strategies for alcohol dependence and that these targets should be investigated in more detail in human laboratory studies as well as randomized clinical trials.

3. Conclusion

Extensive preclinical and clinical research support the hypothesis that alcohol's acute reinforcing effects are mediated through a dopamine surge in the mesocorticolimbic dopamine system and that the chronic and excessive alcohol consumption, in contrast, induces a dopamine deficient state driving the processes of craving and relapse. In addition, it is well substantiated that alcohol affects dopamine directly via the NAc and VTA as well as through indirect activation of the mesolimbic pathway via interaction with other reward-related brain regions and neurotransmitters. These complex relationships need to be investigated further. Given dopamine's pivotal role in the development and maintenance of alcohol dependence, medications targeting dopamine does constitute an important area of research. Although promising preclinical results, the majority of results from the clinical studies with dopamine-acting medications have thus far been discouraging. The side effects profile of many of the evaluated compounds, including typical antipsychotic drugs, render them clinically unfav-

http://dx.doi.org/10.5772/63144

ourable. On the other hand, newer dopamine agents, without complete antagonism or agonism, especially the dopamine stabilizers show promise and deserve further investigation in alcohol-dependent patients.

Acknowledgements

The study is supported by grants from the Swedish Research Council (2009-2782, 2014-3887 and 2015-03219), Swedish Society for Medical Research, Swedish Alcohol Monopoly Foundation for Alcohol Research.

Author details

Nitya Jayaram-Lindström[1], Mia Ericson[2], Pia Steensland[1] and Elisabet Jerlhag[3*]

*Address all correspondence to: Elisabet.Jerlhag@pharm.gu.se

1 Centre for Psychiatry Research, Department of Clinical Neuroscience, Karolinska Institutet and Stockholm Health Care Services, Stockholm County Council, Stockholm, Sweden

2 Department of Psychiatry and Neurochemistry, Institute of Neuroscience and Physiology, The Sahlgrenska Academy, University of Gothenburg, Gothenburg, Sweden

3 Department of Pharmacology, Institute of Neuroscience and Physiology, The Sahlgrenska Academy, University of Gothenburg, Gothenburg, Sweden

References

[1] Rehm J, Mathers C, Popova S, Thavorncharoensap M, Teerawattananon Y, and Patra J. Global burden of disease and injury and economic cost attributable to alcohol use and alcohol-use disorders. Lancet. 2009;373:2223–33.

[2] Chau P, Hoifodt-Lido H, Lof E, Soderpalm B, and Ericson M. Glycine receptors in the nucleus accumbens involved in the ethanol intake-reducing effect of acamprosate. Alcohol Clin Exp Res. 2010;34:39–45.

[3] Chau P, Stomberg R, Fagerberg A, Soderpalm B, and Ericson M. Glycine receptors involved in acamprosate's modulation of accumbal dopamine levels: an in vivo microdialysis study. Alcohol Clin Exp Res. 2010;34:32–8.

[4] De Witte P, Littleton J, Parot P, and Koob G. Neuroprotective and abstinence-promoting effects of acamprosate: elucidating the mechanism of action. CNS Drugs. 2005;19:517–37.

[5] Heilig M and Egli M. Pharmacological treatment of alcohol dependence: target symptoms and target mechanisms. Pharmacol Ther. 2006;111:855–76.

[6] Hansen S, Harthon C, Wallin E, Lofberg L, and Svensson K. Mesotelencephalic dopamine system and reproductive behavior in the female rat: effects of ventral tegmental 6-hydroxydopamine lesions on maternal and sexual responsiveness. Behav Neurosci. 1991;105:588–98.

[7] Schultz W, Dayan P, and Montague PR. A neural substrate of prediction and reward. Science. 1997;275:1593–9.

[8] Everitt BJ, Belin D, Economidou D, Pelloux Y, Dalley JW, and Robbins TW. Review. Neural mechanisms underlying the vulnerability to develop compulsive drug-seeking habits and addiction. Philos Trans R Soc Lond B Biol Sci. 2008;363:3125–35.

[9] Olds J and Milner P. Positive reinforcement produced by electrical stimulation of septal area and other regions of rat brain. J Comp Physiol Psychol. 1954;47:419–27.

[10] Phillips A and Fieberger HC, *Neruochemical correlates of brain-stimulation. Untangeling the Gordian knot.*, in *The neurochemical basis of reward*, J.M. Liebman and S.J. Cooper, Editors. 1989, Clarendon Press: Oxford, England. pp. 67–104.

[11] Carlsson A. Thirty years of dopamine research. Adv Neurol. 1993;60:1–10.

[12] Dahlstrom A and Fuxe K. Localization of monoamines in the lower brain stem. Experientia. 1964;20:398–9.

[13] Wise RA and Rompre PP. Brain dopamine and reward. Annu Rev Psychol. 1989;40:191–225.

[14] Koob GF. Drugs of abuse: anatomy, pharmacology and function of reward pathways. Trends Pharmacol Sci. 1992;13:177–84.

[15] Robinson TE and Berridge KC. The neural basis of drug craving: an incentive-sensitization theory of addiction. Brain Res Brain Res Rev. 1993;18:247–91.

[16] Wise RA. The role of reward pathways in the development of drug dependence. Pharmacol Ther. 1987;35:227–63.

[17] Russo SJ and Nestler EJ. The brain reward circuitry in mood disorders. Nat Rev Neurosci. 2013;14:609–25.

[18] Diana M. The dopamine hypothesis of drug addiction and its potential therapeutic value. Front Psychiatry. 2011;2:64.

[19] Koob GF. Theoretical frameworks and mechanistic aspects of alcohol addiction: alcohol addiction as a reward deficit disorder. Curr Top Behav Neurosci. 2013;13:3–30.

[20] Le Foll B, Gallo A, Le Strat Y, Lu L, and Gorwood P. Genetics of dopamine receptors and drug addiction: a comprehensive review. Behav Pharmacol. 2009;20:1–17.

[21] Watanabe S, Fusa K, Takada K, Aono Y, Saigusa T, Koshikawa N, and Cools AR. Effects of alpha-methyl-p-tyrosine on extracellular dopamine levels in the nucleus accumbens and the dorsal striatum of freely moving rats. J Oral Sci. 2005;47:185–90.

[22] Ahlenius S, Carlsson A, Engel J, Svensson T, and Sodersten P. Antagonism by alpha methyltyrosine of the ethanol-induced stimulation and euphoria in man. Clin Pharmacol Ther. 1973;14:586–91.

[23] Engel J, Strombom U, Svensson TH, and Waldeck B. Suppression by alpha-methyltyrosine of ethanol-induced locomotor stimulation: partial reversal by L-dopa. Psychopharmacologia. 1974;37:275–9.

[24] Engel JA, Fahlke C, Hulthe P, Hard E, Johannessen K, Snape B, and Svensson L. Biochemical and behavioral evidence for an interaction between ethanol and calcium channel antagonists. J Neural Transm. 1988;74:181–93.

[25] Blomqvist O, Engel JA, Nissbrandt H, and Soderpalm B. The mesolimbic dopamine-activating properties of ethanol are antagonized by mecamylamine. Eur J Pharmacol. 1993;249:207–13.

[26] Blomqvist O, Ericson M, Engel JA, and Soderpalm B. Accumbal dopamine overflow after ethanol: localization of the antagonizing effect of mecamylamine. Eur J Pharmacol. 1997;334:149–56.

[27] Di Chiara G and Imperato A. Preferential stimulation of dopamine release in the nucleus accumbens by opiates, alcohol, and barbiturates: studies with transcerebral dialysis in freely moving rats. Ann N Y Acad Sci. 1986;473:367–81.

[28] Ericson M, Blomqvist O, Engel JA, and Soderpalm B. Voluntary ethanol intake in the rat and the associated accumbal dopamine overflow are blocked by ventral tegmental mecamylamine. Eur J Pharmacol. 1998;358:189–96.

[29] Feltmann K, Fredriksson I, Wirf M, Schilstrom B, and Steensland P. The monoamine stabilizer (-)-OSU6162 counteracts downregulated dopamine output in the nucleus accumbens of long-term drinking Wistar rats. Addict Biol. 2016;21:438-49.

[30] Imperato A and Di Chiara G. Preferential stimulation of dopamine release in the nucleus accumbens of freely moving rats by ethanol. J Pharmacol Exp Ther. 1986;239:219–28.

[31] Jerlhag E, Egecioglu E, Landgren S, Salome N, Heilig M, Moechard D, Datta R, Perissoud D, Dickson SL, and Engel JA. Requirement of central ghrelin signaling for alcohol reward. PNAS. 2009;106:11318–11323.

[32] Jerlhag E, Grotli M, Luthman K, Svensson L, and Engel JA. Role of the subunit composition of central nicotinic acetylcholine receptors for the stimulatory and dopamine-enhancing effects of ethanol. Alcohol Alcohol. 2006;41:486–93.

[33] Jonsson S, Adermark L, Ericson M, and Soderpalm B. The involvement of accumbal glycine receptors in the dopamine-elevating effects of addictive drugs. Neuropharmacology. 2014;82:69–75.

[34] Larsson A, Jerlhag E, Svensson L, Soderpalm B, and Engel JA. Is an alpha-conotoxin MII-sensitive mechanism involved in the neurochemical, stimulatory, and rewarding effects of ethanol? Alcohol. 2004;34:239–50.

[35] Larsson A, Svensson L, Soderpalm B, and Engel JA. Role of different nicotinic acetylcholine receptors in mediating behavioral and neurochemical effects of ethanol in mice. Alcohol. 2002;28:157–67.

[36] Weiss F, Lorang MT, Bloom FE, and Koob GF. Oral alcohol self-administration stimulates dopamine release in the rat nucleus accumbens: genetic and motivational determinants. J Pharmacol Exp Ther. 1993;267:250–8.

[37] Doyon WM, York JL, Diaz LM, Samson HH, Czachowski CL, and Gonzales RA. Dopamine activity in the nucleus accumbens during consummatory phases of oral ethanol self-administration. Alcohol Clin Exp Res. 2003;27:1573–82.

[38] Ericson M, Molander A, Lof E, Engel JA, and Soderpalm B. Ethanol elevates accumbal dopamine levels via indirect activation of ventral tegmental nicotinic acetylcholine receptors. Eur J Pharmacol. 2003;467:85–93.

[39] Larsson A, Edstrom L, Svensson L, Soderpalm B, and Engel JA. Voluntary ethanol intake increases extracellular acetylcholine levels in the ventral tegmental area in the rat. Alcohol Alcohol. 2005;40:349–58.

[40] Gessa GL, Muntoni F, Collu M, Vargiu L, and Mereu G. Low doses of ethanol activate dopaminergic neurons in the ventral tegmental area. Brain Res. 1985;348:201–3.

[41] Martin PD and Ono T. Effects of reward anticipation, reward presentation, and spatial parameters on the firing of single neurons recorded in the subiculum and nucleus accumbens of freely moving rats. Behav Brain Res. 2000;116:23–38.

[42] Risinger FO, Freeman PA, Rubinstein M, Low MJ, and Grandy DK. Lack of operant ethanol self-administration in dopamine D2 receptor knockout mice. Psychopharmacology (Berl). 2000;152:343–50.

[43] Gonzales RA and Weiss F. Suppression of ethanol-reinforced behavior by naltrexone is associated with attenuation of the ethanol-induced increase in dialysate dopamine levels in the nucleus accumbens. J Neurosci. 1998;18:10663–71.

[44] Katner SN and Weiss F. Ethanol-associated olfactory stimuli reinstate ethanol-seeking behavior after extinction and modify extracellular dopamine levels in the nucleus accumbens. Alcohol Clin Exp Res. 1999;23:1751–60.

[45] Melendez RI, Rodd-Henricks ZA, Engleman EA, Li TK, McBride WJ, and Murphy JM. Microdialysis of dopamine in the nucleus accumbens of alcohol-preferring (P) rats during anticipation and operant self-administration of ethanol. Alcohol Clin Exp Res. 2002;26:318–25.

[46] Spanagel R and Weiss F. The dopamine hypothesis of reward: past and current status. Trends Neurosci. 1999;22:521–7.

[47] Katner SN, Kerr TM, and Weiss F. Ethanol anticipation enhances dopamine efflux in the nucleus accumbens of alcohol-preferring (P) but not Wistar rats. Behav Pharmacol. 1996;7:669–674.

[48] Brown ZW and Amit Z. The effects of selective catecholamine depletions by 6-hydroxydopamine on ethanol preference in rats. Neurosci Lett. 1977;5:333–6.

[49] Myers RD and Melchior CL. Alcohol drinking in the rat after destruction of serotonergic and catecholaminergic neurons in the brain. Res Commun Chem Pathol Pharmacol. 1975;10:363–78.

[50] Richardson JS and Novakovski DM. Brain monoamines and free choice ethanol consumption in rats. Drug Alcohol Depend. 1978;3:253–64.

[51] Fahlke C, Hansen S, Engel JA, and Hard E. Effects of ventral striatal 6-OHDA lesions or amphetamine sensitization on ethanol consumption in the rat. Pharmacol Biochem Behav. 1994;47:345–9.

[52] Hansen S, Fahlke C, Hard E, and Thomasson R. Effects of ibotenic acid lesions of the ventral striatum and the medial prefrontal cortex on ethanol consumption in the rat. Alcohol. 1995;12:397–402.

[53] Kiianmaa K and Attila LM. Alcohol intake, ethanol-induced narcosis and intoxication in rats following neonatal 6-hydroxydopamine or 5, 7-dihydroxytryptamine treatment. Naunyn Schmiedebergs Arch Pharmacol. 1979;308:165–70.

[54] Koistinen M, Tuomainen P, Hyytia P, and Kiianmaa K. Naltrexone suppresses ethanol intake in 6-hydroxydopamine-treated rats. Alcohol Clin Exp Res. 2001;25:1605–12.

[55] Quarfordt SD, Kalmus GW, and Myers RD. Ethanol drinking following 6-OHDA lesions of nucleus accumbens and tuberculum olfactorium of the rat. Alcohol. 1991;8:211–7.

[56] Rassnick S, Stinus L, and Koob GF. The effects of 6-hydroxydopamine lesions of the nucleus accumbens and the mesolimbic dopamine system on oral self-administration of ethanol in the rat. Brain Res. 1993;623:16–24.

[57] Ericson M, Chau P, Clarke RB, Adermark L, and Soderpalm B. Rising taurine and ethanol concentrations in nucleus accumbens interact to produce dopamine release after ethanol administration. Addict Biol. 2011;16:377–85.

[58] Little HJ. The contribution of electrophysiology to knowledge of the acute and chronic effects of ethanol. Pharmacol Ther. 1999;84:333–53.

[59] Ericson M, Lof E, Stomberg R, Chau P, and Soderpalm B. Nicotinic acetylcholine receptors in the anterior, but not posterior, ventral tegmental area mediate ethanol-induced elevation of accumbal dopamine levels. J Pharmacol Exp Ther. 2008;326:76–82.

[60] Lof E, Olausson P, deBejczy A, Stomberg R, McIntosh JM, Taylor JR, and Soderpalm B. Nicotinic acetylcholine receptors in the ventral tegmental area mediate the dopamine activating and reinforcing properties of ethanol cues. Psychopharmacology (Berl). 2007;195:333–43.

[61] Wozniak KM and Linnoila M. Recent advances in pharmacological research on alcohol. Possible relations with cocaine. Recent Dev Alcohol. 1992;10:235–72.

[62] Yoshimoto K, McBride WJ, Lumeng L, and Li TK. Alcohol stimulates the release of dopamine and serotonin in the nucleus accumbens. Alcohol. 1992;9:17–22.

[63] Molander A and Soderpalm B. Glycine receptors regulate dopamine release in the rat nucleus accumbens. Alcohol Clin Exp Res. 2005;29:17–26.

[64] Soderpalm B, Lof E, and Ericson M. Mechanistic studies of ethanol's interaction with the mesolimbic dopamine reward system. Pharmacopsychiatry. 2009;42 Suppl 1:S87–94.

[65] Graybiel AM and Ragsdale CW, Jr. Histochemically distinct compartments in the striatum of human, monkeys, and cat demonstrated by acetylthiocholinesterase staining. Proc Natl Acad Sci USA. 1978;75:5723–6.

[66] Heimer L, Zahm DS, Churchill L, Kalivas PW, and Wohltmann C. Specificity in the projection patterns of accumbal core and shell in the rat. Neuroscience. 1991;41:89–125.

[67] Voorn P, Gerfen CR, and Groenewegen HJ. Compartmental organization of the ventral striatum of the rat: immunohistochemical distribution of enkephalin, substance P, dopamine, and calcium-binding protein. J Comp Neurol. 1989;289:189–201.

[68] Zahm DS. Functional-anatomical implications of the nucleus accumbens core and shell subterritories. Ann N Y Acad Sci. 1999;877:113–28.

[69] Zahm DS and Brog JS. On the significance of subterritories in the "accumbens" part of the rat ventral striatum. Neuroscience. 1992;50:751–67.

[70] Deutch AY and Cameron DS. Pharmacological characterization of dopamine systems in the nucleus accumbens core and shell. Neuroscience. 1992;46:49–56.

[71] Bassareo V, De Luca MA, Aresu M, Aste A, Ariu T, and Di Chiara G. Differential adaptive properties of accumbens shell dopamine responses to ethanol as a drug and as a motivational stimulus. Eur J Neurosci. 2003;17:1465–72.

[72] Cadoni C, Solinas M, and Di Chiara G. Psychostimulant sensitization: differential changes in accumbal shell and core dopamine. Eur J Pharmacol. 2000;388:69–76.

[73] Iyaniwura TT, Wright AE, and Balfour DJ. Evidence that mesoaccumbens dopamine and locomotor responses to nicotine in the rat are influenced by pretreatment dose and strain. Psychopharmacology (Berl). 2001;158:73–9.

[74] Howard EC, Schier CJ, Wetzel JS, and Gonzales RA. The dopamine response in the nucleus accumbens core-shell border differs from that in the core and shell during operant ethanol self-administration. Alcohol Clin Exp Res. 2009;33:1355–65.

[75] Brodie MS and Appel SB. The effects of ethanol on dopaminergic neurons of the ventral tegmental area studied with intracellular recording in brain slices. Alcohol Clin Exp Res. 1998;22:236–44.

[76] Brodie MS, Pesold C, and Appel SB. Ethanol directly excites dopaminergic ventral tegmental area reward neurons. Alcohol Clin Exp Res. 1999;23:1848–52.

[77] Brodie MS, Shefner SA, and Dunwiddie TV. Ethanol increases the firing rate of dopamine neurons of the rat ventral tegmental area in vitro. Brain Res. 1990;508:65–9.

[78] Brodie MS, Trifunovic RD, and Shefner SA. Serotonin potentiates ethanol-induced excitation of ventral tegmental area neurons in brain slices from three different rat strains. J Pharmacol Exp Ther. 1995;273:1139–46.

[79] Bunney EB, Appel SB, and Brodie MS. Electrophysiological effects of cocaethylene, cocaine, and ethanol on dopaminergic neurons of the ventral tegmental area. J Pharmacol Exp Ther. 2001;297:696–703.

[80] Gatto GJ, McBride WJ, Murphy JM, Lumeng L, and Li TK. Ethanol self-infusion into the ventral tegmental area by alcohol-preferring rats. Alcohol. 1994;11:557–64.

[81] Ikemoto S, Murphy JM, and McBride WJ. Regional differences within the rat ventral tegmental area for muscimol self-infusions. Pharmacol Biochem Behav. 1998;61:87–92.

[82] Ikemoto S and Wise RA. Rewarding effects of the cholinergic agents carbachol and neostigmine in the posterior ventral tegmental area. J Neurosci. 2002;22:9895–904.

[83] Rodd ZA, Bell RL, Zhang Y, Murphy JM, Goldstein A, Zaffaroni A, Li TK, and McBride WJ. Regional heterogeneity for the intracranial self-administration of ethanol and acetaldehyde within the ventral tegmental area of alcohol-preferring (P) rats: involvement of dopamine and serotonin. Neuropsychopharmacology. 2005;30:330–8.

[84] Rodd ZA, Melendez RI, Bell RL, Kuc KA, Zhang Y, Murphy JM, and McBride WJ. Intracranial self-administration of ethanol within the ventral tegmental area of male

Wistar rats: evidence for involvement of dopamine neurons. J Neurosci. 2004;24:1050–7.

[85] Rodd-Henricks ZA, McKinzie DL, Crile RS, Murphy JM, and McBride WJ. Regional heterogeneity for the intracranial self-administration of ethanol within the ventral tegmental area of female Wistar rats. Psychopharmacology (Berl). 2000;149:217–24.

[86] Congar P, Bergevin A, and Trudeau LE. D2 receptors inhibit the secretory process downstream from calcium influx in dopaminergic neurons: implication of K+ channels. J Neurophysiol. 2002;87:1046–56.

[87] Jeziorski M and White FJ. Dopamine agonists at repeated "autoreceptor-selective" doses: effects upon the sensitivity of A10 dopamine autoreceptors. Synapse. 1989;4:267–80.

[88] Rodd ZA, Bell RL, McQueen VK, Davids MR, Hsu CC, Murphy JM, Li TK, Lumeng L, and McBride WJ. Chronic ethanol drinking by alcohol-preferring rats increases the sensitivity of the posterior ventral tegmental area to the reinforcing effects of ethanol. Alcohol Clin Exp Res. 2005;29:358–66.

[89] Jerlhag E and Engel JA. Local infusion of low, but not high, doses of alcohol into the anterior ventral tegmental area causes release of accumbal dopamine. Open J Psychiatry. 2013;4:53-59.

[90] Mrejeru A, Marti-Prats L, Avegno EM, Harrison NL, and Sulzer D. A subset of ventral tegmental area dopamine neurons responds to acute ethanol. Neuroscience. 2015;290:649–58.

[91] Tuomainen P, Patsenka A, Hyytia P, Grinevich V, and Kiianmaa K. Extracellular levels of dopamine in the nucleus accumbens in AA and ANA rats after reverse microdialysis of ethanol into the nucleus accumbens or ventral tegmental area. Alcohol. 2003;29:117–24.

[92] Ikemoto S. Dopamine reward circuitry: two projection systems from the ventral midbrain to the nucleus accumbens-olfactory tubercle complex. Brain Res Rev. 2007;56:27–78.

[93] Boileau I, Assaad JM, Pihl RO, Benkelfat C, Leyton M, Diksic M, Tremblay RE, and Dagher A. Alcohol promotes dopamine release in the human nucleus accumbens. Synapse. 2003;49:226–31.

[94] Urban NB, Kegeles LS, Slifstein M, Xu X, Martinez D, Sakr E, Castillo F, Moadel T, O'Malley SS, Krystal JH, and Abi-Dargham A. Sex differences in striatal dopamine release in young adults after oral alcohol challenge: a positron emission tomography imaging study with [(1)(1)C]raclopride. Biol Psychiatry. 2010;68:689–96.

[95] Volkow ND, Fowler JS, Wang GJ, and Swanson JM. Dopamine in drug abuse and addiction: results from imaging studies and treatment implications. Mol Psychiatry. 2004;9:557–69.

[96] Drevets WC, Gautier C, Price JC, Kupfer DJ, Kinahan PE, Grace AA, Price JL, and Mathis CA. Amphetamine-induced dopamine release in human ventral striatum correlates with euphoria. Biol Psychiatry. 2001;49:81–96.

[97] Leyton M, Boileau I, Benkelfat C, Diksic M, Baker G, and Dagher A. Amphetamine-induced increases in extracellular dopamine, drug wanting, and novelty seeking: a PET/[11C]raclopride study in healthy men. Neuropsychopharmacology. 2002;27:1027–35.

[98] Ramchandani VA, Umhau J, Pavon FJ, Ruiz-Velasco V, Margas W, Sun H, Damadzic R, Eskay R, Schoor M, Thorsell A, Schwandt ML, Sommer WH, George DT, Parsons LH, Herscovitch P, Hommer D, and Heilig M. A genetic determinant of the striatal dopamine response to alcohol in men. Mol Psychiatry. 2011;16:809–17.

[99] Volkow ND, Wang GJ, Fowler JS, Logan J, Angrist B, Hitzemann R, Lieberman J, and Pappas N. Effects of methylphenidate on regional brain glucose metabolism in humans: relationship to dopamine D2 receptors. Am J Psychiatry. 1997;154:50–5.

[100] Yoder KK, Constantinescu CC, Kareken DA, Normandin MD, Cheng TE, O'Connor SJ, and Morris ED. Heterogeneous effects of alcohol on dopamine release in the striatum: a PET study. Alcohol Clin Exp Res. 2007;31:965–73.

[101] Becker HC and Mulholland PJ. Neurochemical mechanisms of alcohol withdrawal. Handb Clin Neurol. 2014;125:133–56.

[102] Tupala E and Tiihonen J. Dopamine and alcoholism: neurobiological basis of ethanol abuse. Prog Neuropsychopharmacol Biol Psychiatry. 2004;28:1221–47.

[103] Jonsson S, Ericson M, and Soderpalm B. Modest long-term ethanol consumption affects expression of neurotransmitter receptor genes in the rat nucleus accumbens. Alcohol Clin Exp Res. 2014;38:722–9.

[104] Barak S, Carnicella S, Yowell QV, and Ron D. Glial cell line-derived neurotrophic factor reverses alcohol-induced allostasis of the mesolimbic dopaminergic system: implications for alcohol reward and seeking. J Neurosci. 2011;31:9885–94.

[105] Bustamante D, Quintanilla ME, Tampier L, Gonzalez-Lira V, Israel Y, and Herrera-Marschitz M. Ethanol induces stronger dopamine release in nucleus accumbens (shell) of alcohol-preferring (bibulous) than in alcohol-avoiding (abstainer) rats. Eur J Pharmacol. 2008;591:153–8.

[106] Stefanini E, Frau M, Garau MG, Garau B, Fadda F, and Gessa GL. Alcohol-preferring rats have fewer dopamine D2 receptors in the limbic system. Alcohol Alcohol. 1992;27:127–30.

[107] McBride WJ, Murphy JM, Lumeng L, and Li TK. Serotonin, dopamine and GABA involvement in alcohol drinking of selectively bred rats. Alcohol. 1990;7:199–205.

[108] Thanos PK, Taintor NB, Rivera SN, Umegaki H, Ikari H, Roth G, Ingram DK, Hitzemann R, Fowler JS, Gatley SJ, Wang GJ, and Volkow ND. DRD2 gene transfer into the

nucleus accumbens core of the alcohol preferring and nonpreferring rats attenuates alcohol drinking. Alcohol Clin Exp Res. 2004;28:720–8.

[109] Thanos PK, Volkow ND, Freimuth P, Umegaki H, Ikari H, Roth G, Ingram DK, and Hitzemann R. Overexpression of dopamine D2 receptors reduces alcohol self-administration. J Neurochem. 2001;78:1094–103.

[110] Everitt BJ and Robbins TW. Neural systems of reinforcement for drug addiction: from actions to habits to compulsion. Nat Neurosci. 2005;8:1481–9.

[111] Volkow ND, Fowler JS, Wang GJ, Swanson JM, and Telang F. Dopamine in drug abuse and addiction: results of imaging studies and treatment implications. Arch Neurol. 2007;64:1575–9.

[112] Yoder KK, Albrecht DS, Dzemidzic M, Normandin MD, Federici LM, Graves T, Herring CM, Hile KL, Walters JW, Liang T, Plawecki MH, O'Connor S, and Kareken DA. Differences in IV alcohol-induced dopamine release in the ventral striatum of social drinkers and nontreatment-seeking alcoholics. Drug Alcohol Depend. 2016; 160:163-69.

[113] Dettling M, Heinz A, Dufeu P, Rommelspacher H, Graf KJ, and Schmidt LG. Dopaminergic responsivity in alcoholism: trait, state, or residual marker? Am J Psychiatry. 1995;152:1317–21.

[114] Volkow ND, Wang GJ, Fowler JS, Logan J, Ding YS, Gatley J, Hitzemann R, and Pappas N. Decreases in dopamine receptors but not in dopamine transporters in alcoholics. J Nucl Med. 1996;37:122–122.

[115] Heinz A, Siessmeier T, Wrase J, Hermann D, Klein S, Grusser SM, Flor H, Braus DF, Buchholz HG, Grunder G, Schreckenberger M, Smolka MN, Rosch F, Mann K, and Bartenstein P. Correlation between dopamine D(2) receptors in the ventral striatum and central processing of alcohol cues and craving. Am J Psychiatry. 2004;161:1783–9.

[116] Braus DF, Wrase J, Grusser S, Hermann D, Ruf M, Flor H, Mann K, and Heinz A. Alcohol-associated stimuli activate the ventral striatum in abstinent alcoholics. J Neural Transm. 2001;108:887–94.

[117] Kareken DA, Claus ED, Sabri M, Dzemidzic M, Kosobud AE, Radnovich AJ, Hector D, Ramchandani VA, O'Connor SJ, Lowe M, and Li TK. Alcohol-related olfactory cues activate the nucleus accumbens and ventral tegmental area in high-risk drinkers: preliminary findings. Alcohol Clin Exp Res. 2004;28:550–7.

[118] Narendran R, Mason NS, Paris J, Himes ML, Douaihy AB, and Frankle WG. Decreased prefrontal cortical dopamine transmission in alcoholism. Am J Psychiatry. 2014;171:881–8.

[119] Blum K, Noble EP, Sheridan PJ, Montgomery A, Ritchie T, Jagadeeswaran P, Nogami H, Briggs AH, and Cohn JB. Allelic association of human dopamine D2 receptor gene in alcoholism. JAMA. 1990;263:2055–60.

[120] Kimura M and Higuchi S. Genetics of alcohol dependence. Psychiatry Clin Neurosci. 2011;65:213–25.

[121] Hutchison KE, McGeary J, Smolen A, Bryan A, and Swift RM. The DRD4 VNTR polymorphism moderates craving after alcohol consumption. Health Psychol. 2002;21:139–46.

[122] Laucht M, Becker K, Blomeyer D, and Schmidt MH. Novelty seeking involved in mediating the association between the dopamine D4 receptor gene exon III polymorphism and heavy drinking in male adolescents: results from a high-risk community sample. Biol Psychiatry. 2007;61:87–92.

[123] Vaughn MG, Beaver KM, DeLisi M, Howard MO, and Perron BE. Dopamine D4 receptor gene exon III polymorphism associated with binge drinking attitudinal phenotype. Alcohol. 2009;43:179–84.

[124] Gorwood P, Limosin F, Batel P, Hamon M, Ades J, and Boni C. The A9 allele of the dopamine transporter gene is associated with delirium tremens and alcohol-withdrawal seizure. Biol Psychiatry. 2003;53:85–92.

[125] Vaske J, Beaver KM, Wright JP, Boisvert D, and Schnupp R. An interaction between DAT1 and having an alcoholic father predicts serious alcohol problems in a sample of males. Drug Alcohol Depend. 2009;104:17–22.

[126] Enoch MA, Waheed JF, Harris CR, Albaugh B, and Goldman D. Sex differences in the influence of COMT Val158Met on alcoholism and smoking in plains American Indians. Alcohol Clin Exp Res. 2006;30:399–406.

[127] Tiihonen J, Hallikainen T, Lachman H, Saito T, Volavka J, Kauhanen J, Salonen JT, Ryynanen OP, Koulu M, Karvonen MK, Pohjalainen T, Syvalahti E, and Hietala J. Association between the functional variant of the catechol-O-methyltransferase (COMT) gene and type 1 alcoholism. Mol Psychiatry. 1999;4:286–9.

[128] Wang T, Franke P, Neidt H, Cichon S, Knapp M, Lichtermann D, Maier W, Propping P, and Nothen MM. Association study of the low-activity allele of catechol-O-methyltransferase and alcoholism using a family-based approach. Mol Psychiatry. 2001;6:109–11.

[129] Liljequist S, Berggren U, and Engel J. The effect of catecholamine receptor antagonists on ethanol-induced locomotor stimulation. J Neural Transm. 1981;50:57–67.

[130] Czachowski CL, Chappell AM, and Samson HH. Effects of raclopride in the nucleus accumbens on ethanol seeking and consumption. Alcohol Clin Exp Res. 2001;25:1431–40.

[131] Czachowski CL, Santini LA, Legg BH, and Samson HH. Separate measures of ethanol seeking and drinking in the rat: effects of remoxipride. Alcohol. 2002;28:39–46.

[132] Files FJ, Denning CE, and Samson HH. Effects of the atypical antipsychotic remoxipride on alcohol self-administration. Pharmacol Biochem Behav. 1998;59:281–5.

[133] Rassnick S, Pulvirenti L, and Koob GF. SDZ-205,152, a novel dopamine receptor agonist, reduces oral ethanol self-administration in rats. Alcohol. 1993;10:127–32.

[134] Pfeffer AO and Samson HH. Haloperidol and apomorphine effects on ethanol reinforcement in free feeding rats. Pharmacol Biochem Behav. 1988;29:343–50.

[135] Maldonado R, Saiardi A, Valverde O, Samad TA, Roques BP, and Borrelli E. Absence of opiate rewarding effects in mice lacking dopamine D2 receptors. Nature. 1997;388:586–9.

[136] Wise RA. Neurobiology of addiction. Curr Opin Neurobiol. 1996;6:243–51.

[137] Brown ZW, Gill K, Abitbol M, and Amit Z. Lack of effect of dopamine receptor blockade on voluntary ethanol consumption in rats. Behav Neural Biol. 1982;36:291–4.

[138] Linseman MA. Effects of dopaminergic agents on alcohol consumption by rats in a limited access paradigm. Psychopharmacology (Berl). 1990;100:195–200.

[139] Pfeffer AO and Samson HH. Effect of pimozide on home cage ethanol drinking in the rat: dependence on drinking session length. Drug Alcohol Depend. 1986;17:47–55.

[140] Samson HH, Hodge CW, Tolliver GA, and Haraguchi M. Effect of dopamine agonists and antagonists on ethanol-reinforced behavior: the involvement of the nucleus accumbens. Brain Res Bull. 1993;30:133–41.

[141] Hodge CW, Samson HH, and Chappelle AM. Alcohol self-administration: further examination of the role of dopamine receptors in the nucleus accumbens. Alcohol Clin Exp Res. 1997;21:1083–91.

[142] Nowak KL, McBride WJ, Lumeng L, Li TK, and Murphy JM. Involvement of dopamine D2 autoreceptors in the ventral tegmental area on alcohol and saccharin intake of the alcohol-preferring P rat. Alcohol Clin Exp Res. 2000;24:476–83.

[143] Price KL and Middaugh LD. The dopamine D1 antagonist reduces ethanol reward for C57BL/6 mice. Alcohol Clin Exp Res. 2004;28:1666–75.

[144] Modell JG, Mountz JM, Glaser FB, and Lee JY. Effect of haloperidol on measures of craving and impaired control in alcoholic subjects. Alcohol Clin Exp Res. 1993;17:234–40.

[145] Wiesbeck GA, Weijers HG, Lesch OM, Glaser T, Toennes PJ, and Boening J. Flupenthixol decanoate and relapse prevention in alcoholics: results from a placebo-controlled study. Alcohol Alcohol. 2001;36:329–34.

[146] Walter H, Ramskogler K, Semler B, Lesch OM, and Platz W. Dopamine and alcohol relapse: D1 and D2 antagonists increase relapse rates in animal studies and in clinical trials. J Biomed Sci. 2001;8:83–8.

[147] Wiesbeck GA, Weijers HG, Wodarz N, Lesch OM, Glaser T, and Boening J. Gender-related differences in pharmacological relapse prevention with flupenthixol decanoate in detoxified alcoholics. Arch Womens Ment Health. 2003;6:259–62.

[148] Drake RE, Xie H, McHugo GJ, and Green AI. The effects of clozapine on alcohol and drug use disorders among patients with schizophrenia. Schizophr Bull. 2000;26:441–9.

[149] Soyka M, Aichmuller C, v Bardeleben U, Beneke M, Glaser T, Hornung-Knobel S, and Wegner U. Flupenthixol in relapse prevention in schizophrenics with comorbid alcoholism: results from an open clinical study. Eur Addict Res. 2003;9:65–72.

[150] Osser DN, Najarian DM, and Dufresne RL. Olanzapine increases weight and serum triglyceride levels. J Clin Psychiatry. 1999;60:767–70.

[151] Sussman N. The implications of weight changes with antipsychotic treatment. J Clin Psychopharmacol. 2003;23:S21–6.

[152] Hutchison KE, Swift R, Rohsenow DJ, Monti PM, Davidson D, and Almeida A. Olanzapine reduces urge to drink after drinking cues and a priming dose of alcohol. Psychopharmacology (Berl). 2001;155:27–34.

[153] Peters DH and Faulds D. Tiapride. A review of its pharmacology and therapeutic potential in the management of alcohol dependence syndrome. Drugs. 1994;47:1010–32.

[154] Ingman K, Honkanen A, Hyytia P, Huttunen MO, and Korpi ER. Risperidone reduces limited access alcohol drinking in alcohol-preferring rats. Eur J Pharmacol. 2003;468:121–7.

[155] Ingman K and Korpi ER. Alcohol drinking of alcohol-preferring AA rats is differentially affected by clozapine and olanzapine. Eur J Pharmacol. 2006;534:133–40.

[156] Chau DT, Khokhar JY, Gulick D, Dawson R, and Green AI. Desipramine enhances the ability of paliperidone to decrease alcohol drinking. J Psychiatr Res. 2015;69:9–18.

[157] Chau DT, Khokhar JY, Dawson R, Ahmed J, Xie H, and Green AI. The comparative effects of clozapine versus haloperidol on initiation and maintenance of alcohol drinking in male alcohol-preferring P rat. Alcohol. 2013;47:611–8.

[158] Shaw GK, Majumdar SK, Waller S, MacGarvie J, and Dunn G. Tiapride in the long-term management of alcoholics of anxious or depressive temperament. Br J Psychiatry. 1987;150:164–8.

[159] Shaw GK, Waller S, Majumdar SK, Alberts JL, Latham CJ, and Dunn G. Tiapride in the prevention of relapse in recently detoxified alcoholics. Br J Psychiatry. 1994;165:515–23.

[160] Croissant B, Klein O, Gehrlein L, Kniest A, Hermann D, Diehl A, and Mann K. Quetiapine in relapse prevention in alcoholics suffering from craving and affective symptoms: a case series. Eur Psychiatry. 2006;21:570–3.

[161] Martinotti G, Di Nicola M, Romanelli R, Andreoli S, Pozzi G, Moroni N, and Janiri L. High and low dosage oxcarbazepine versus naltrexone for the prevention of relapse in alcohol-dependent patients. Hum Psychopharmacol. 2007;22:149–56.

[162] Kampman KM, Pettinati HM, Lynch KG, Whittingham T, Macfadden W, Dackis C, Tirado C, Oslin DW, Sparkman T, and O'Brien CP. A double-blind, placebo-controlled pilot trial of quetiapine for the treatment of Type A and Type B alcoholism. J Clin Psychopharmacol. 2007;27:344–51.

[163] Brown ES, Davila D, Nakamura A, Carmody TJ, Rush AJ, Lo A, Holmes T, Adinoff B, Caetano R, Swann AC, Sunderajan P, and Bret ME. A randomized, double-blind, placebo-controlled trial of quetiapine in patients with bipolar disorder, mixed or depressed phase, and alcohol dependence. Alcohol Clin Exp Res. 2014;38:2113–8.

[164] Litten RZ, Fertig JB, Falk DE, Ryan ML, Mattson ME, Collins JF, Murtaugh C, Ciraulo D, Green AI, Johnson B, Pettinati H, Swift R, Afshar M, Brunette MF, Tiouririne NA, Kampman K, Stout R, and Group NS. A double-blind, placebo-controlled trial to assess the efficacy of quetiapine fumarate XR in very heavy-drinking alcohol-dependent patients. Alcohol Clin Exp Res. 2012;36:406–16.

[165] Hutchison KE, Ray L, Sandman E, Rutter MC, Peters A, Davidson D, and Swift R. The effect of olanzapine on craving and alcohol consumption. Neuropsychopharmacology. 2006;31:1310–7.

[166] Hutchison KE, Wooden A, Swift RM, Smolen A, McGeary J, Adler L, and Paris L. Olanzapine reduces craving for alcohol: a DRD4 VNTR polymorphism by pharmacotherapy interaction. Neuropsychopharmacology. 2003;28:1882–8.

[167] Kishi T, Sevy S, Chekuri R, and Correll CU. Antipsychotics for primary alcohol dependence: a systematic review and meta-analysis of placebo-controlled trials. J Clin Psychiatry. 2013;74:e642–54.

[168] Ucok A and Gaebel W. Side effects of atypical antipsychotics: a brief overview. World Psychiatry. 2008;7:58–62.

[169] Rassnick S, Krechman J, and Koob GF. Chronic ethanol produces a decreased sensitivity to the response-disruptive effects of GABA receptor complex antagonists. Pharmacol Biochem Behav. 1993;44:943–50.

[170] Carnicella S, Ahmadiantehrani S, He DY, Nielsen CK, Bartlett SE, Janak PH, and Ron D. Cabergoline decreases alcohol drinking and seeking behaviors via glial cell line-derived neurotrophic factor. Biol Psychiatry. 2009;66:146–53.

[171] Weiss F, Mitchiner M, Bloom FE, and Koob GF. Free-choice responding for ethanol versus water in alcohol preferring (P) and unselected Wistar rats is differentially modified by naloxone, bromocriptine, and methysergide. Psychopharmacology (Berl). 1990;101:178–86.

[172] Lawford BR, Young RM, Rowell JA, Qualichefski J, Fletcher BH, Syndulko K, Ritchie T, and Noble EP. Bromocriptine in the treatment of alcoholics with the D2 dopamine receptor A1 allele. Nat Med. 1995;1:337–41.

[173] Naranjo CA, Dongier M, and Bremner KE. Long-acting injectable bromocriptine does not reduce relapse in alcoholics. Addiction. 1997;92:969–78.

[174] Powell BJ, Campbell JL, Landon JF, Liskow BI, Thomas HM, Nickel EJ, Dale TM, Penick EC, Samuelson SD, and Lacoursiere RB. A double-blind, placebo-controlled study of nortriptyline and bromocriptine in male alcoholics subtyped by comorbid psychiatric disorders. Alcohol Clin Exp Res. 1995;19:462–8.

[175] Burris KD, Molski TF, Xu C, Ryan E, Tottori K, Kikuchi T, Yocca FD, and Molinoff PB. Aripiprazole, a novel antipsychotic, is a high-affinity partial agonist at human dopamine D2 receptors. J Pharmacol Exp Ther. 2002;302:381–9.

[176] Carlsson A, Waters N, Holm-Waters S, Tedroff J, Nilsson M, and Carlsson ML. Interactions between monoamines, glutamate, and GABA in schizophrenia: new evidence. Annu Rev Pharmacol Toxicol. 2001;41:237–60.

[177] Yokoi F, Grunder G, Biziere K, Stephane M, Dogan AS, Dannals RF, Ravert H, Suri A, Bramer S, and Wong DF. Dopamine D2 and D3 receptor occupancy in normal humans treated with the antipsychotic drug aripiprazole (OPC 14597): a study using positron emission tomography and [11C]raclopride. Neuropsychopharmacology. 2002;27:248–59.

[178] Jerlhag E. The antipsychotic aripiprazole antagonizes the ethanol- and amphetamine-induced locomotor stimulation in mice. Alcohol. 2008;42:123–7.

[179] Viana TG, Almeida-Santos AF, Aguiar DC, and Moreira FA. Effects of aripiprazole, an atypical antipsychotic, on the motor alterations induced by acute ethanol administration in mice. Basic Clin Pharmacol Toxicol. 2013;112:319–24.

[180] Ingman K, Kupila J, Hyytia P, and Korpi ER. Effects of aripiprazole on alcohol intake in an animal model of high-alcohol drinking. Alcohol Alcohol. 2006;41:391–8.

[181] Nirogi R, Kandikere V, Jayarajan P, Bhyrapuneni G, Saralaya R, Muddana N, and Abraham R. Aripiprazole in an animal model of chronic alcohol consumption and dopamine D(2) receptor occupancy in rats. Am J Drug Alcohol Abuse. 2013;39:72–9.

[182] Shibasaki M, Kurokawa K, Mizuno K, and Ohkuma S. Effect of aripiprazole on anxiety associated with ethanol physical dependence and on ethanol-induced place preference. J Pharmacol Sci. 2012;118:215–24.

[183] Janiri L, Martinotti G, and Di Nicola M. Aripiprazole for relapse prevention and craving in alcohol-dependent subjects: results from a pilot study. J Clin Psychopharmacol. 2007;27:519–20.

[184] Anton RF, Kranzler H, Breder C, Marcus RN, Carson WH, and Han J. A randomized, multicenter, double-blind, placebo-controlled study of the efficacy and safety of

aripiprazole for the treatment of alcohol dependence. J Clin Psychopharmacol. 2008;28:5–12.

[185] Voronin K, Randall P, Myrick H, and Anton R. Aripiprazole effects on alcohol consumption and subjective reports in a clinical laboratory paradigm—possible influence of self-control. Alcohol Clin Exp Res. 2008;32:1954–61.

[186] Martinotti G, Di Nicola M, and Janiri L. Efficacy and safety of aripiprazole in alcohol dependence. Am J Drug Alcohol Abuse. 2007;33:393–401.

[187] Martinotti G, Di Nicola M, Di Giannantonio M, and Janiri L. Aripiprazole in the treatment of patients with alcohol dependence: a double-blind, comparison trial vs. naltrexone. J Psychopharmacol. 2009;23:123–9.

[188] Myrick H, Li X, Randall PK, Henderson S, Voronin K, and Anton RF. The effect of aripiprazole on cue-induced brain activation and drinking parameters in alcoholics. J Clin Psychopharmacol. 2010;30:365–72.

[189] Carlsson ML, Carlsson A, and Nilsson M. Schizophrenia: from dopamine to glutamate and back. Curr Med Chem. 2004;11:267–77.

[190] Tedroff J, Torstenson R, Hartvig P, Sonesson C, Waters N, Carlsson A, Neu H, Fasth KJ, and Langstrom B. Effects of the substituted (S)-3-phenylpiperidine (-)-OSU6162 on PET measurements in subhuman primates: evidence for tone-dependent normalization of striatal dopaminergic activity. Synapse. 1998;28:280–7.

[191] Kara E, Lin H, Svensson K, Johansson AM, and Strange PG. Analysis of the actions of the novel dopamine receptor-directed compounds (S)-OSU6162 and ACR16 at the D2 dopamine receptor. Br J Pharmacol. 2010;161:1343–50.

[192] Seeman P and Guan HC. Dopamine partial agonist action of (-)OSU6162 is consistent with dopamine hyperactivity in psychosis. Eur J Pharmacol. 2007;557:151–3.

[193] Lahti RA, Tamminga CA, and Carlsson A. Stimulating and inhibitory effects of the dopamine "stabilizer" (-)-OSU6162 on dopamine D2 receptor function in vitro. J Neural Transm (Vienna). 2007;114:1143–6.

[194] Rung JP, Rung E, Helgeson L, Johansson AM, Svensson K, Carlsson A, and Carlsson ML. Effects of (-)-OSU6162 and ACR16 on motor activity in rats, indicating a unique mechanism of dopaminergic stabilization. J Neural Transm (Vienna). 2008;115:899–908.

[195] Sonesson C, Lin CH, Hansson L, Waters N, Svensson K, Carlsson A, Smith MW, and Wikstrom H. Substituted (S)-phenylpiperidines and rigid congeners as preferential dopamine autoreceptor antagonists: synthesis and structure-activity relationships. J Med Chem. 1994;37:2735–53.

[196] Steensland P, Fredriksson I, Holst S, Feltmann K, Franck J, Schilstrom B, and Carlsson A. The monoamine stabilizer (-)-OSU6162 attenuates voluntary ethanol intake and

ethanol-induced dopamine output in nucleus accumbens. Biol Psychiatry. 2012; 72:823-31

[197] Khemiri L, Steensland P, Guterstam J, Beck O, Carlsson A, Franck J, and Jayaram-Lindstrom N. The effects of the monoamine stabilizer (-)-OSU6162 on craving in alcohol dependent individuals: a human laboratory study. Eur Neuropsychopharmacol. 2015;25:2240–51.

[198] Johansson B, Carlsson A, Carlsson ML, Karlsson M, Nilsson MK, Nordquist-Brandt E, and Ronnback L. Placebo-controlled cross-over study of the monoaminergic stabiliser (-)-OSU6162 in mental fatigue following stroke or traumatic brain injury. Acta Neuropsychiatr. 2012;24:266–74.

[199] Kloberg A, Constantinescu R, Nilsson MK, Carlsson ML, Carlsson A, Wahlstrom J, and Haghighi S. Tolerability and efficacy of the monoaminergic stabilizer (-)-OSU6162 (PNU-96391A) in Huntington's disease: a double-blind cross-over study. Acta Neuropsychiatr. 2014;26:298–306.

[200] Lido HH, Ericson M, Marston H, and Soderpalm B. A role for accumbal glycine receptors in modulation of dopamine release by the glycine transporter-1 inhibitor org25935. Front Psychiatry. 2011;2:8.

[201] Lido HH, Stomberg R, Fagerberg A, Ericson M, and Soderpalm B. The glycine reuptake inhibitor org 25935 interacts with basal and ethanol-induced dopamine release in rat nucleus accumbens. Alcohol Clin Exp Res. 2009;33:1151–7.

[202] Molander A, Lido HH, Lof E, Ericson M, and Soderpalm B. The glycine reuptake inhibitor Org 25935 decreases ethanol intake and preference in male wistar rats. Alcohol Alcohol. 2007;42:11–8.

[203] Vengeliene V, Leonardi-Essmann F, Sommer WH, Marston HM, and Spanagel R. Glycine transporter-1 blockade leads to persistently reduced relapse-like alcohol drinking in rats. Biol Psychiatry. 2010;68:704–11.

[204] Larsson A and Engel JA. Neurochemical and behavioral studies on ethanol and nicotine interactions. Neurosci Biobehav Rev. 2004;27:713–720.

[205] Steensland P, Simms JA, Holgate J, Richards JK, and Bartlett SE. Varenicline, an alpha4beta2 nicotinic acetylcholine receptor partial agonist, selectively decreases ethanol consumption and seeking. Proc Natl Acad Sci USA. 2007;104:12518–23.

[206] Ericson M, Lof E, Stomberg R, and Soderpalm B. The smoking cessation medication varenicline attenuates alcohol and nicotine interactions in the rat mesolimbic dopamine system. J Pharmacol Exp Ther. 2009;329:225–30.

[207] de Bejczy A, Nations KR, Szegedi A, Schoemaker J, Ruwe F, and Soderpalm B. Efficacy and safety of the glycine transporter-1 inhibitor org 25935 for the prevention of relapse in alcohol-dependent patients: a randomized, double-blind, placebo-controlled trial. Alcohol Clin Exp Res. 2014;38:2427–35.

[208] Fucito LM, Toll BA, Wu R, Romano DM, Tek E, and O'Malley SS. A preliminary investigation of varenicline for heavy drinking smokers. Psychopharmacology (Berl). 2011;215:655–63.

[209] McKee SA, Harrison EL, O'Malley SS, Krishnan-Sarin S, Shi J, Tetrault JM, Picciotto MR, Petrakis IL, Estevez N, and Balchunas E. Varenicline reduces alcohol self-administration in heavy-drinking smokers. Biol Psychiatry. 2009;66:185–90.

[210] Mitchell JM, Teague CH, Kayser AS, Bartlett SE, and Fields HL. Varenicline decreases alcohol consumption in heavy-drinking smokers. Psychopharmacology (Berl). 2012;223:299–306.

[211] Litten RZ, Ryan ML, Fertig JB, Falk DE, Johnson B, Dunn KE, Green AI, Pettinati HM, Ciraulo DA, Sarid-Segal O, Kampman K, Brunette MF, Strain EC, Tiouririne NA, Ransom J, Scott C, and Stout R. A double-blind, placebo-controlled trial assessing the efficacy of varenicline tartrate for alcohol dependence. J Addict Med. 2013;7:277-86.

[212] de Bejczy A, Lof E, Walther L, Guterstam J, Hammarberg A, Asanovska G, Franck J, Isaksson A, and Soderpalm B. Varenicline for treatment of alcohol dependence: a randomized, placebo-controlled trial. Alcohol Clin Exp Res. 2015;39:2189–99.

[213] Schacht JP, Anton RF, Randall PK, Li X, Henderson S, and Myrick H. Varenicline effects on drinking, craving and neural reward processing among non-treatment-seeking alcohol-dependent individuals. Psychopharmacology (Berl). 2014;231:3799–807.

[214] Walther L, de Bejczy A, Lof E, Hansson T, Andersson A, Guterstam J, Hammarberg A, Asanovska G, Franck J, Soderpalm B, and Isaksson A. Phosphatidylethanol is superior to carbohydrate-deficient transferrin and gamma-glutamyltransferase as an alcohol marker and is a reliable estimate of alcohol consumption level. Alcohol Clin Exp Res. 2015;39:2200–8.

Chapter 5

Contribution of Noradrenaline, Serotonin, and the Basolateral Amygdala to Alcohol Addiction: Implications for Novel Pharmacotherapies for AUDs

Omkar L. Patkar, Arnauld Belmer and
Selena E. Bartlett

Additional information is available at the end of the chapter

http://dx.doi.org/10.5772/62843

Abstract

Alcohol use disorders (AUDs) constitute one of the 10 leading causes of preventable deaths worldwide. To date, there are only a few Food and Drug Administration (FDA)-approved medications for AUDs, all of which are only moderately effective. The development of improved and effective strategies for the management of AUDs is greatly needed. This review focuses on understanding the neurobiological basis of alcohol addiction with a special emphasis on the role of serotonin (5-hydroxytryptamine, 5-HT) and noradrenaline (NE) in AUDs and sheds light on their complex interplay in the basolateral amygdala (BLA)—a brain region widely implicated in addiction. There is a significant evidence to support the role of the amygdala in stress-induced negative emotional states resulting from withdrawal from alcohol; in fact, it has been hypothesized that this leads to craving and relapse. Dysregulation of 5-HT and NE signaling in the BLA have been proposed to alter affective behavior, memory consolidation, and most importantly increase the propensity for addiction to alcohol and other common drugs of abuse. Improving deficits in 5-HT and NE receptor signaling may provide ideal targets for the treatment of AUDs.

Keywords: Addiction, alcohol use disorders, noradrenaline, serotonin, basolateral amygdala

1. Introduction

1.1 Alcohol addiction: one drink too many

Alcohol dependence or alcohol abuse, now collectively known as alcohol use disorders (AUDs), causes significant loss of productivity, health concerns, emotional instability, career-oriented failures, and socioeconomic problems [1]. It is estimated that AUDs amount to 3.8% of global deaths and 4.6% of disability-adjusted life years [2]. *The Diagnostic and Statistical Manual of Mental Disorders*, 4th edition (DSM-IV-TR), defines AUDs on the persistence of dependence symptoms like tolerance, withdrawal, increased amounts of alcohol consumed over time, ineffective efforts to reduce use, interference with personal or professional life, significant amount of time spent obtaining, using, and recovering from alcohol or continued use of alcohol despite harmful consequences [3]. The U.S. National Institute of Alcohol Abuse and Alcoholism (NIAAA) defined men who consume more than 14 drinks per week and women having more than 11 drinks per week belong to the "At Risk" category of alcohol consumers.

1.2 Neurobiology of alcohol addiction: a vicious cycle

Alcohol addiction like any other drug addiction is a chronic relapsing disorder characterized by compulsive alcohol use and alcohol-seeking behavior [4, 5]. The neurobiology of alcohol addiction is increasingly complex; however, for the purpose of simplicity, it can be delineated in three stages. The first phase of this cycle is the *Binge and intoxication stage* [5]. During this phase, reward areas of the brain involving the mesocorticolimbic system like the dorsal striatum and nucleus accumbens (NAc) are activated, which results in pleasurable and rewarding feelings [5, 6]. Dopamine is a key neurotransmitter involved in this stage [7–9]. The positive reinforcement is triggered by the pleasurable effects of alcohol where the user wants "more" to experience the hedonic effects. This is then followed by the *Withdrawal stage* [5]. During this phase, brain regions that are associated with negative feelings and emotions are activated, such as the amygdala and bed nucleus of stria terminalis (BNST) [4, 5]. Chronic withdrawal-induced stress blunts the activity of the stress–response system and sensitizes extrahypothalamic structures of the extended amygdala [6, 10]. This stage marks a critical phase in the addiction cycle where alcohol use is primarily motivated by the desire to avoid negative feelings of stress, dysphoria, and negative emotional states of alcohol withdrawal. The third phase is the *Preoccupation and anticipation stage* [5]. During this phase, brain regions like the frontal cortex and hippocampus [11] that respond to previously paired alcohol cues and contexts are activated, intensifying alcohol-seeking behavior [12, 13]. Since the frontal cortex is involved in decision-making and higher executive functions, alcohol-induced neuroadaptations of the frontal cortex [14] impair higher cognitive and decision-making processes, increasing the rate of relapse in alcoholics.

Over time, as this cycle is repeated, alcohol-induced neuroadaptations in the reward circuitry, stress–response pathway, and brain regions involved in higher cognitive functions facilitate the transition from nondependent to dependent alcohol consumption. These maladaptive neuromodulations contribute to sensitization, tolerance, craving, and relapse to alcohol-seeking [4]. For instance, alcohol-induced plasticity in glutamatergic signaling in the NAc may contribute to behavioral sensitization to the effects of alcohol [15], while changes in the synaptic properties of NAc-medium spiny neurons contribute to relapse during withdrawal [16]. Furthermore, chronic alcohol modulates presynaptic and postsynaptic functions on glutamate neurons in the basolateral amygdala (BLA) [17]. Finally, alcohol impairs communication between the amygdala and prefrontal cortex to disrupt cognitive and emotional responses that lead to altered affective states that further contribute to the development of alcohol dependence [18, 19].

1.3. Pharmacotherapy: available treatment options for AUDs

Bill Wilson and Bob Smith took early steps toward alcohol remediation in 1935 with the introduction of Alcoholic Anonymous (AA) [20, 21]. This 12-step approach toward rehabilitation was built on the premise of acceptance of individual helplessness during addiction to alcohol and other drugs of abuse [22]. This method was adopted by the "Minnesota model of addiction treatment" in a 28-day rehabilitation setting [23]. Parallel efforts to treat alcoholism by understanding the nature and cause of alcohol dependence were gaining momentum, which led to the foundation of the National Institute of Alcohol Abuse and Alcoholism (NIAAA) in 1970 [24].

Since then, several approaches to understand and treat alcoholism were designed that took into consideration individual differences and susceptibility to AUDs. Cognitive behavioral therapy or motivational therapy was adopted as the first line of treatment to match the needs of the addict to help recuperate in a 12-week therapy session called "Project MATCH" [25]. This project was successful in rehabilitation of patients that did not have any psychiatric conditions. The next step was to combine behavioral and pharmacotherapy in the treatment of alcoholism called "Project COMBINE" [26]. This study evaluated the efficacy of available pharmacotherapies, namely acamprosate and naltrexone, in conjunction with or without medical assistance and with or without cognitive–behavioral therapy [27].

Acamprosate (Campral™), the calcium salt of N-acetyl homotaurine, suppresses alcohol consumption and relapse [28, 29]. Early reports delineating the mechanism of action of acamprosate were unclear [30]; however, recent studies have shown that acamprosate works through the calcium ion in its molecular structure [31]. This was supported with improved results in patients that showed an increase in plasma calcium levels following acamprosate treatment [31]. Acamprosate has been shown to have a good safety and a tolerability profile and is highly effective in maintenance of abstinence in patients who are abstinent at treatment initiation [32].

In addition to acamprosate, the mu-opioid receptor antagonist, naltrexone (Re Via™), was found effective as a treatment for alcohol consumption and relapse [33]. However, studies have shown that naltrexone is ineffective in achieving abstinence in alcoholic subjects; instead it is more effective to reduce consumption [34, 35]. Also, recent research demonstrated that it acts more specifically for a cohort with single nucleotide polymorphism (SNP) in exon 1 of the mu-opioid receptor gene (*OPRM1*) [36] limiting broader efficacy. Nevertheless, naltrexone reduces alcohol consumption through a dopaminergic/opioidergic reinforcement system, causing increased sedation and less arousal in patients consuming alcohol [35]. Both these drugs were successful in reducing drinking in combination with behavioral therapy, as highlighted by the COMBINE project [37].

In addition to acamprosate and naltrexone, disulfiram (Antabuse®) was approved as a therapeutic treatment for alcoholism. The anti-alcohol addiction properties of disulfiram were serendipitously discovered, when a Danish physician Jacobsen accidentally ingested alcohol over disulfiram and experienced its unpleasant and nauseous effects [38, 39]. Disulfiram inhibits the enzyme aldehyde dehydrogenase (ALDH), which results in the accumulation of acetaldehyde on alcohol ingestion [40]. This toxic metabolite produces aversive symptoms, such as flushing, nausea, and vomiting, and a desire to avoid this reaction encourages abstinence [41]. Disulfiram also inhibits dopamine-β-hydroxylase (DBH), the enzyme required to synthesize noradrenaline (NE). It reduces NE concentrations and elevates dopamine (DA) concentrations to facilitate normal DA functioning [40, 41], a pharmacotherapeutic feature of the drug that makes it an excellent treatment option even for cocaine addicts.

In addition to this, our lab has investigated the role of neuronal nicotinic acetylcholine receptors in alcohol addiction and came up with varenicline (Champix™) as a treatment option for AUDs [42, 43]. Varenicline was found to be more efficacious in heavy-drinking smokers because of the comorbid nature of both the types of addiction involving the recruitment of nicotinic acetylcholine receptors. Varenicline is now in its third stage of clinical trial as a treatment option for AUDs [44, 45].

1.4. Shortcomings of available treatment options for AUDs: need for better pharmaceutical alternatives

Acamprosate, naltrexone, and disulfiram are the only available medications for alcoholism approved by the Food and Drug Administration (FDA), while nalmefene (Selincro™), an opioid receptor antagonist having a similar mechanism of action to naltrexone [46], is approved as a medication for alcohol abstinence in Europe [47]. Most of these drugs treat one aspect of alcoholism at best without significantly altering other parameters of alcohol addiction.

Drugs like acamprosate reduce consumption and are effective in motivating abstinence for a certain period of time. However, acamprosate does not significantly affect abstinence-induced rebound consumption of alcohol [48]. Also, despite achieving an aversion for alcohol, the likelihood of the addict returning to drinking with increased tolerance cannot be assured. A case study also indicated the development of Parkinson's-like syndrome with acamprosate use [49].

Although naltrexone was shown to be very effective with and without cognitive behavioral therapy, noncompliance with maintenance of drug regimen was shown to limit efficacy [50]. About 37% patients were reported to discontinue naltrexone therapy by 12 weeks and 80% by 6 months [50]. It is possible that some of the severe complications involved with naltrexone use, that is, renal failure and hepatitis, may have contributed to its early discontinuation [51]. Furthermore, the efficacy of naltrexone appears to be related to alcohol abusers having the mu-opioid SNP [36].

All the above drugs work best when combined with an individual's motivation to quit drinking. Disulfiram works on this principle as it deters the positive reinforcing effects of alcohol and masks them with aversive and negative feelings stimulated by the action of the drug post-alcohol consumption [52]. As a result, this drug is effective for alcoholics with a goal to achieve complete abstinence, but has limited efficacy for alcoholics without these goals. Noncompliance is one of the biggest challenges in the use of disulfiram, illustrated by the 20% compliance measure in the largest controlled trial to date [53]. Also, disulfiram is contraindicated in patients with cardiac disease and on rare occasions may cause severe liver damage [54].

Despite the availability of these pharmacotherapies and behavioral therapy, AUDs are widely prevalent. As illustrated by COMBINE, no single medication or treatment strategy is effective in every case or in every person [37]. A detailed investigation of other neurobiological factors that play a role in alcohol dependence is needed as are further strategies to treat alcoholism.

The remainder of this chapter highlights the role of serotonin (5-hydroxytryptamine, 5-HT), NE, and BLA in alcohol addiction with a view to improve current treatment strategies for AUDs.

2. NE and serotonin: role in alcohol dependence

Prolonged alcohol exposure causes maladaptive changes in regions of the extended amygdala that cause sensitization to negative emotional states and reinforcement of addictive behaviors during withdrawal. These neuroadaptations alter the activity of important neurotransmitters particularly involved in stress. Such changes are well documented for increasing the activity of the stress neurotransmitter corticotrophin-releasing factor (CRF) in rodent models of alcohol dependence [4]. Additionally, changes in the function and signaling of other neurotransmitters including 5-HT [55–57] and NE [55–61] have also been implicated in the development of alcohol addiction.

NE and 5-HT play a crucial role in regulating mood, emotions, and importantly, behavioral adaptations to stress that include addictive phenotypes [57, 60]. As these neurochemicals widely innervate the reward system [62–66] and extrahypothalamic regions involving the amygdala [67–71], these are prime candidates to influence alcohol and even other drug-seeking behaviors.

Dysregulation of the 5-HT pathway is implicated in AUDs and other affective states like depression and anxiety disorders [57, 72, 73]. Recent studies have demonstrated an increase in the immunoreactivity of tryptophan hydroxylase (TRH)—the rate-limiting step in 5-HT synthesis, in the dorsal raphe nuclei (DRN) of alcohol-dependent victims of depression and suicide compared to normal psychiatric controls [74]. Such disruptions in brain serotonin levels in these individuals have widespread implications in the role of 5-HT to regulate emotional and behavioral vulnerability to alcohol and other drugs of abuse. Alcohol increases 5-HT levels in the ventral tegmental area (VTA), NAc, and amygdala [75]. These brain regions play a pivotal role in processing of information from emotional and rewarding stimuli. Chronic alcohol abuse alters the activity of these brain areas, resulting in changes in motivational and goal-directed behaviors, which further drive alcohol-seeking behavior [76, 77]. For instance, studies have shown that behavioral sensitization to alcohol is mediated by accumbal 5-HT_{2C} receptors [76], and blockade of 5-HT_3 receptors especially in the VTA attenuates alcohol consumption [77]. The 5-HT receptors, 5-HT_{1A}, 5-HT_{1B}, 5-HT_{2A}, and 5-HT_{2C}, [78–80] have been widely implicated in alcohol consumption in animal models with new evidence also implicating 5-HT_3 and 5-HT_6 receptors in alcohol addiction [81, 82].

NE has been shown to play a significant role in negative emotional states which contribute to alcohol consumption [60, 83, 84]. Acute alcohol decreases [85], while chronic alcohol and withdrawal increases the activity of neurons in the locus coeruleus (LC), a region that provides the majority of NE in the brain [86]. Activation of the α2-adrenergic autoreceptors has been shown to attenuate the overall negative effects of withdrawal [87], and blocking α1-adrenergic receptors (ARs) using prazosin reduced alcohol consumption in dependent rats [88] and human alcoholics [89]. Likewise, treatment with the β-AR antagonist, propranolol, reduced drinking in dependent rats [60]. Evidence also suggests that β-ARs may also contribute in mediating the anxiolytic effects of alcohol [58].

Furthermore, CRF is a regulating factor in the activation of the hypothalamus–pituitary–adrenal (HPA) axis to stress [90–94]. Chronic alcohol consumption affects CRF signaling in the central nucleus of amygdala (CeA) and BNST, as evidenced by alterations in CRF transmission during withdrawal [95]. Interestingly, NE and 5-HT have been shown to interact with the neurotransmitter CRF in neuroanatomical sites like the LC, DRN, CeA, and BNST [96–100] to influence addictive behaviors. For instance, yohimbine, a pharmacological agent used to promote stress in rats, has effects on NE, 5-HT, and CRF signaling to potentiate alcohol drinking and reinstatement [101, 102], suggesting possible mutual regulatory roles of these neurotransmitters in alcohol dependence and relapse. This was further evidenced by CRF antagonism in the DRN to attenuate yohimbine-induced alcohol-seeking behavior in rats [100]. Also, CRF and NE antagonism has been shown to be effective in reducing stress-induced reinstatement in human alcoholics [88, 103].

3. The BLA: role in alcohol addiction

The amygdaloid complex is made up 13 distinct nuclei which are divided in three groups: the deep or basolateral group, the superficial or cortical-like group, and the centromedial group [104]. These nuclei have been proposed to be located in such a way to maximize the amygdala's connections with other limbic, cortical, and subcortical regions of the brain to help facilitate its function in emotional processing, learning, and fear memory [105–107]. The basolateral amygdalar complex, comprising of lateral amygdala (LA), basal and basomedial nuclei [108, 109] controls behavioral expressions like emotional arousal, fear, and stress that are linked to traumatic incidents, stressful environmental stimuli, or pharmacological stressors, and consolidates them as memories [70]. The BLA communicates through excitatory efferents to

http://dx.doi.org/10.5772/62843

the prefrontal cortex and structures of the limbic system involving the hippocampus, NAc, dorsomedial striatum (DMS), and BNST [110–114], while it receives feedback from these structures through glutamatergic afferents [115, 116], majority of which converge with the cortical inputs [114] running toward the BLA.

The role of the BLA in fear, memory consolidation, and emotional learning along with its contribution in associative learning for appetitive conditioning is well documented [70, 105, 117, 118]. Since the BLA can impart incentive salience to a previously neutral stimulus in response to a motivational or a goal-directed task [119], recent efforts have now focused on the role of the BLA in drug-seeking, including cocaine [120], morphine [121], and alcohol [122–124].

Alcohol has been shown to increase neuronal activity and glucose utilization in the BLA [125]. Additionally, long-term alcohol exposure alters glutamate transmission in the BLA [126] and NAc [127], which is implicated in increased alcohol self-administration in rodents [128]. Furthermore, alcohol-induced withdrawal stress increases presynaptic glutamatergic function in thalamic afferents to the BLA that may explain the increased emotional dysregulation during withdrawal [129]. It has also been shown that altered neuropeptide S function in the BLA following long-term alcohol exposure may contribute to relapse [130]. Furthermore, a recent study has shown that IL-1 receptor signaling in the BLA contributes to binge-like alcohol consumption in mice [131].

There is growing body of evidence that supports the role of the BLA in conditioned–cued relapse [132] and context-induced reinstatement [133] for alcohol and a variety of other drugs [134–137]. It was shown that the BLA may play a significant role in cue-induced alcohol reinstatement [138], following exposure to previously alcohol-paired environmental cues [123]. Research has also shown that BLA–glutamatergic signaling attributes salience to conditioned cues that are related to alcohol-seeking [132], while the opioidergic system of the BLA may play a role in context-induced alcohol-seeking [140]. Indeed, since the BLA extensively communicates with the NAc, alcohol withdrawal-induced changes in glutamatergic function in the BLA get perpetuated in structures of the reward system that may contribute to craving and relapse [141].

It is well documented that repeated and chronic stress leads to adverse behavioral outcomes, and many studies support the reinforcing effects of chronic stress in drug addiction in animal models [86, 142–144]. Stress alters the morphology of BLA principal cells and impairs fear extinction memory [145] that may have implications in the development of affective disorders like PTSD and depression. It has been shown that the BLA modulates chronic stress-induced learning and memory deficits in the hippocampus, suggesting that dysregulation of BLA–hippocampal signaling may affect memory storage, retrieval, and extinction of fear memory that may contribute to emotional disorders and drug dependence [146]. Furthermore, early life stress causes increased excitability of pyramidal cells in the BLA [147], while chronic restraint stress in adolescent and adult rats increases BLA activity [148]. Increased BLA excitability has been positively correlated with increased anxiety and increased alcohol-seeking behavior [141, 147, 149, 150].

Long-term exposure to alcohol simulates chronic stress-like conditions [130] that have a profound effect on fear memory consolidation [151]. Alcohol withdrawal-induced stress has been shown to increase conditioned fear [152] and impair extinction of fear memory [153]. A recent study also showed that repeated alcohol exposures enhance retrieval of previously consolidated fear memories and augments activity in BLA and other brain regions involved in fear memory retrieval [154].

4. Role of 5-HT and NE in the BLA in alcohol addiction

There is significant evidence that supports the role of NE and 5-HT in drug dependence and alcohol addiction [87, 155–157]. Moreover, the BLA which is highly implicated in dependence to alcohol-seeking [17, 123, 131, 132] is densely innervated by these neurotransmitters [58, 71, 158, 159]. Since chronic alcohol exposure causes neuroadaptations that affect the signaling and receptor subtypes of these neurotransmitters, dysregulation of NE and 5-HT transmission in the BLA may lead to a constellation of aversive outcomes including altered consolidation of alcohol-related memories, anxiety disorders, and eventually higher rates of relapse [132, 138].

NE plays a vital role in facilitating the function of the BLA in fear memory consolidation [70]. It has been shown that intra-BLA infusions of β-AR agonists enhance retention of inhibitory avoidance [160], while β-AR antagonists block fear memory enhancement [69]. Also, α_1-AR activation in the BLA enhances fear memory consolidation through an interaction with β-ARs [161]. This evidence suggests that noradrenergic receptors strongly contribute to BLA function. It is possible that alteration in NE activity in the BLA may lead to altered memory consolidation and stress-coping mechanism that may enhance alcohol-seeking and relapse [162]. Indeed, antagonism of α_1-ARs reduced dependence-induced increase in alcohol consumption in rats [88]. Furthermore, recent evidence supports the role of β-ARs in alcohol-induced enhancement of GABA synapses in the BLA, suggesting a possible noradrenergic mechanism mediating the anxiolytic effects of alcohol [58] (**Figure 1**). This was further evidenced by intra-BLA infusions of a β_3-AR agonist that enhanced inhibitory GABA signaling on BLA pyramidal cells to reduce anxiety-like and alcohol-seeking behavior [163]. Furthermore, the neuroadaptive changes associated with chronic alcohol consumption including desensitization of β-ARs in the BLA have been shown to modulate its activity [164] (**Figure 1**).

In contrast to excitatory dopaminergic/glutamatergic signaling in the BLA that increases its activity, serotonergic transmission in the BLA is inhibitory [165]. The serotonergic innervations on principal glutamate cells in the BLA decrease the overall excitatory activity of these cells [166] through 5-HT_{1A} receptors [167] and modulate BLA output (**Figure 2**). This is supported by a recent study where depletion of serotonin in the BLA increased glutamate receptor density and fear-potentiated startle in mice, indicating that serotonergic inhibition regulates excitatory signaling in the BLA to modulate affective behaviors like anxiety [68].

Chronic alcohol-induced neuroadaptations change 5-HT receptor expression and function in the brain [168] that alters the regulatory control of serotonin over BLA principal cells. Loss of inhibition on BLA principal neurons increases BLA output, increasing anxiety [169, 170] and other symptoms of withdrawal. In support of this, chronic alcohol or withdrawal stress increases the expression of 5-HT_{1A} autoreceptors in the raphe nucleus [168] which causes a reduction in 5-HT levels in the BLA. This increases BLA activity, which contributes to anxiety-like behaviors following withdrawal from chronic alcohol (**Figure 2**). Furthermore, 5-$HT_{2A/2C}$ receptors have been suggested to potentiate inhibitory GABAergic tone on principal BLA glutamatergic cells to decrease excitability [67]. Chronic alcohol causes adaptive changes that lower the expression levels of these receptors, reducing inhibition over BLA principal neurons [67]. This augments BLA output and increases the possibility of anxiety-induced relapse following a period of chronic alcohol exposure [141] (**Figure 2**). In addition to this,

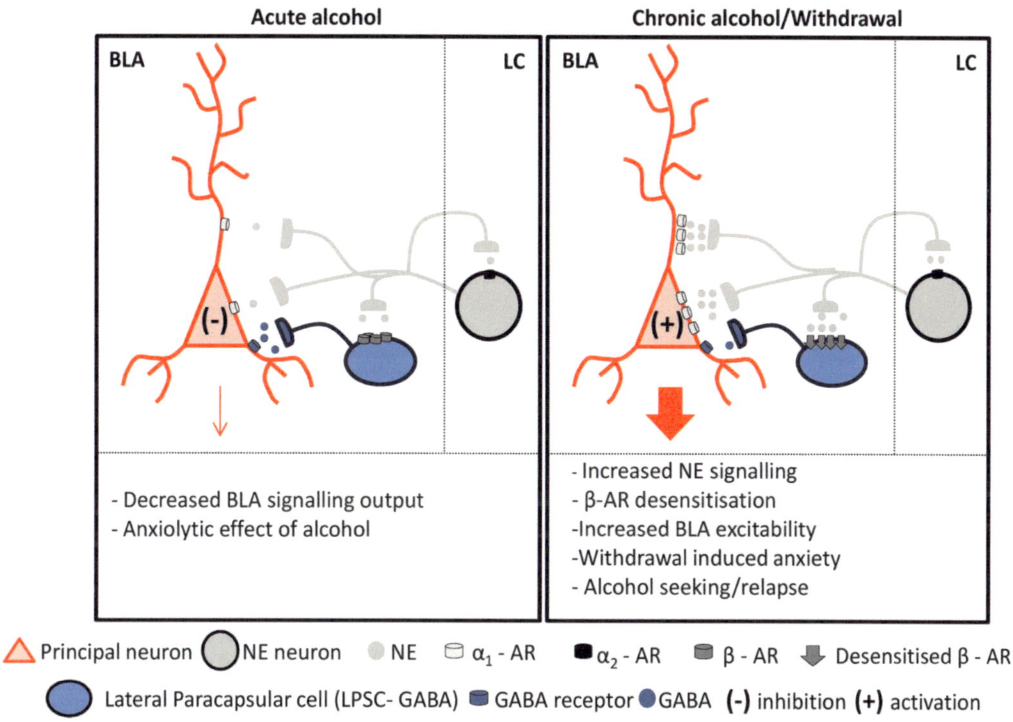

Figure 1. Changes in NE signaling and BLA output following acute and chronic alcohol exposure or withdrawal. Acute alcohol decreases NE signaling in the BLA, which is regulated by a feedback loop through presynaptic α_2-adrenergic autoreceptors expressed on NE fibers in the LC. Decreased BLA-NE levels decrease the excitation of BLA principal cells through postsynaptic α_1-ARs. Acute alcohol further enhances the inhibition of BLA principal cells by NE-mediated enhancement of GABA synapses through β-ARs expressed on GABAergic LPSCs. The net result of this inhibition is decreased BLA principal neuron excitability and BLA activity which has been suggested to reduce anxiety and may explain the anxiolytic effect of acute alcohol. Chronic alcohol/withdrawal increases NE levels that enhance α_1-AR mediated excitation of BLA principal cells. Chronic ethanol has been shown to desensitize β-ARs in the brain which leads to a reduction in NE's effects on GABA-LPSCs causing a decrease in the inhibitory tone over BLA principal cells, increasing excitability. This increases the net excitability of BLA principal cells and increases BLA activity causing anxiety during withdrawal and may contribute to alcohol-seeking and relapse.

chronic alcohol-induced neuroadaptations in other receptor subtypes like the GABA-A receptors facilitate the anxiolytic effects of alcohol [171]. Increasing the activity of 5-HT on GABA-A receptors on BLA principal cells may contribute in reducing withdrawal-induced anxiety and alcohol-seeking.

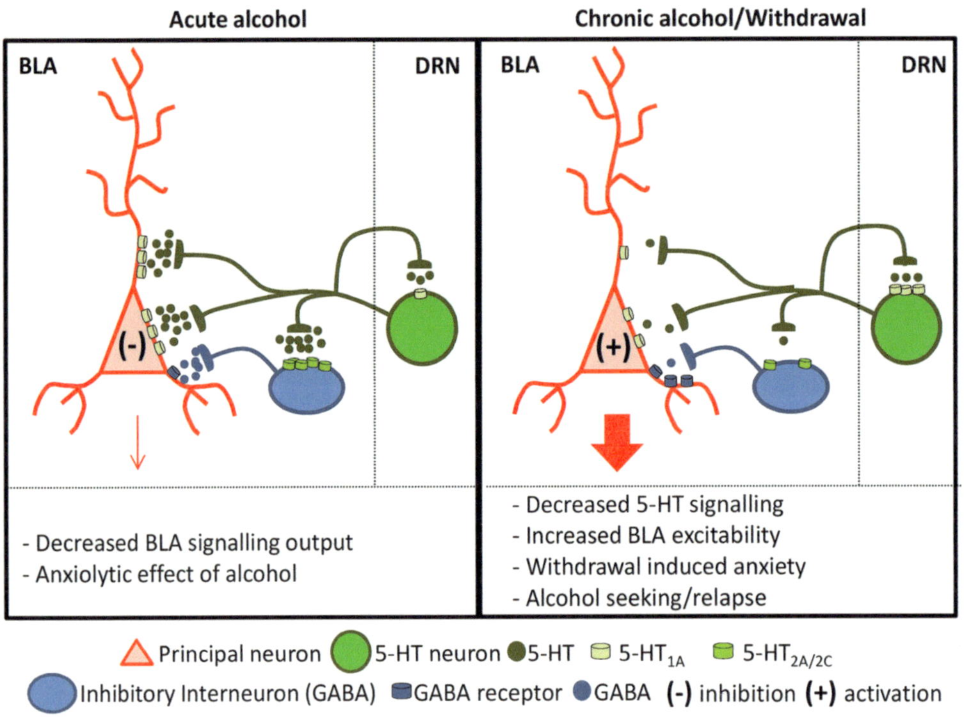

Figure 2. Changes in 5-HT signaling and BLA output following acute and chronic alcohol exposure or withdrawal. Acute alcohol increases 5-HT release in the BLA which is regulated by a feedback loop through 5-HT_{1A} autoreceptors expressed on 5-HT neurons in the DRN. Increased BLA-5-HT levels enhance the inhibition of BLA activity through postsynaptic 5-HT_{1A} receptors expressed on principal neurons. Increased 5-HT signaling also activates 5-$HT_{2A/2C}$ receptors expressed on GABAergic interneurons in the BLA that further increase the inhibition on BLA principal cells through increased GABAergic tone. The net result of this inhibition is decreased BLA principal neuron excitability and BLA activity, which has been shown to reduce anxiety and may explain the anxiolytic effect of acute alcohol. Chronic alcohol/withdrawal increases the expression of 5-HT_{1A} autoreceptors in the DRN which decreases 5-HT levels in the BLA. This reduces 5-HT_{1A}-mediated inhibition on BLA principal cells. Chronic alcohol-induced withdrawal downregulates the expression of 5-$HT_{2A/2C}$ receptors on GABAergic interneurons to further decrease the inhibitory GABA tone on BLA principal cells, increasing excitability. Chronic alcohol also upregulates GABA receptors on principal cells. This results in a net increase in BLA activity causing anxiety that may contribute to alcohol-seeking and relapse.

Furthermore, cross-modulation of synaptic transmission in the BLA by 5-$HT_{1A/1B}$ receptors and β-ARs dictates BLA output [159] that may affect behavioral outcomes like stress, anxiety, and drug dependence. In support of this, we have shown that pindolol, a drug having dual pharmacological activity on 5-$HT_{1A/1B}$ receptors and β_1/β_2 ARs, decreases alcohol consumption in mice following long-term alcohol exposure. Our electrophysiological experiments also indicate that the BLA may mediate the effects of pindolol on alcohol consumption [172].

http://dx.doi.org/10.5772/62843

5. Conclusion

Research in the past few decades has significantly increased our understanding of the neurobiological basis of alcohol dependence. Recent research has targeted pathways that mediate more than just the reinforcing properties of alcohol. However, despite these concerted efforts, effective pharmacological interventions for the management of AUDs remain elusive.

Chronic alcohol consumption causes maladaptive changes in brain regions like the extended amygdala that cause sensitization to negative emotional states of withdrawal. These changes disrupt the signaling of many neurotransmitters including those involved in stress. Dysregulation of NE and 5-HT signaling has been widely implicated in the development of affective disorders and alcohol addiction. Specifically, NE and/or 5-HT impairments in the BLA, a region involved in stress, emotional processing, and reward-seeking have been suggested to play a major role in the development of alcohol dependence (**Figures 1** and **2**).

In addition to the growing evidence in animal models of alcohol addiction, pharmacological compounds that target NE and 5-HT receptors have also shown promise as potential treatment strategies for AUDs in human patients [173, 174]. Noradrenergic compounds like propranolol [175, 176] and atenolol [174] have been shown to attenuate alcohol-seeking behavior and reduce craving in human alcoholics. Similarly, serotonergic compounds like buspirone show efficacy to reduce anxiety-induced consumption in alcoholics [177, 178]. Moreover, our research indicates that pindolol, the FDA-approved antihypertensive drug having activity on both 5-HT and NE receptors, may have a similar mechanism of action to more effectively reduce alcohol consumption following chronic intake [172].

Since the BLA plays a vital role in affective disorders and stress-induced maladaptive behavioral conditioning, drugs that selectively modulate NE and 5-HT signaling in the BLA offer great promise in the treatment of AUDs. With the increasing need for improved pharmacotherapeutic strategies for the management of AUDs combined with the modest efficacy of current treatments, putative compounds that target 5-HT and NE receptors may prove useful for the development of more effective treatment strategies for alcohol dependence.

Acknowledgements

This work was supported by funding from grants from the Australian Research Council and National Health and Medical Research Council to S.E.B. We thank Dr. Paul Klenowski and Ms Joan Holgate in providing their valuable suggestions to this manuscript.

Financial disclosures

All the authors who have participated in this study report no biomedical financial interests or potential conflicts of interest.

Author's contributions

All authors have been involved in the preparation and have approved the submitted manuscript. Omkar Patkar was the lead author and responsible for conducting the literature review and writing the manuscript. Arnauld Belmer assisted in writing and editing the manuscript. As the senior author, Selena Bartlett supervised Omkar Patkar's work, reviewed, and edited the manuscript.

Author details

Omkar L. Patkar[1,2], Arnauld Belmer[1,2] and Selena E. Bartlett[1,2*]

*Address all correspondence to: selena.bartlett@qut.edu.au

1 Translational Research Institute, Queensland University of Technology, Brisbane, Australia

2 Institute of Health and Biomedical Innovation (IHBI), Queensland University of Technology, Brisbane, Australia

References

[1] Gnanavel S, Robert RS. Diagnostic and Statistical Manual of Mental Disorders, fifth edition, and the impact of events scale—revised. Chest. 2013;144(6):1974.

[2] Rehm J, Mathers C, Popova S, Thavorncharoensap M, Teerawattananon Y, Patra J. Global burden of disease and injury and economic cost attributable to alcohol use and alcohol-use disorders. The Lancet. 2009;373(9682):2223–33.

[3] Trull TJ, Verges A, Wood PK, Jahng S, Sher KJ. The structure of Diagnostic and Statistical Manual of Mental Disorders (4th edition, text revision) personality disorder symptoms in a large national sample. Personal Disorders. 2012;3(4):355–69.

[4] Gilpin NW, Koob GF. Neurobiology of alcohol dependence: focus on motivational mechanisms. Alcohol Research & Health: The Journal of the National Institute on Alcohol Abuse and Alcoholism. 2008;31(3):185–95.

[5] Koob GF, Volkow ND. Neurocircuitry of addiction. Neuropsychopharmacology: Official Publication of the American College of Neuropsychopharmacology. 2010;35(1): 217–38.

[6] Koob GF. A role for brain stress systems in addiction. Neuron. 2008;59(1):11–34.

[7] Harris RA, Brodie MS, Dunwiddie TV. Possible substrates of ethanol reinforcement: GABA and dopamine. Annals of the New York Academy of Sciences. 1992;654:61–9.

[8] Yorgason JT, Ferris MJ, Steffensen SC, Jones SR. Frequency-dependent effects of ethanol on dopamine release in the nucleus accumbens. Alcoholism: Clinical and Experimental Research. 2014;38(2):438–47.

[9] Young KA, Gobrogge KL, Wang Z. The role of mesocorticolimbic dopamine in regulating interactions between drugs of abuse and social behavior. Neuroscience & Biobehavioral Reviews. 2011;35(3):498–515.

[10] Zorrilla, E.P., M.L. Logrip, and G.F. Koob, *Corticotropin releasing factor: a key role in the neurobiology of addiction*. Front Neuroendocrinol, 2014. 35(2): p. 234-44.

[11] Kalivas PW, O'Brien C. Drug addiction as a pathology of staged neuroplasticity. Neuropsychopharmacology: Official Publication of the American College of Neuropsychopharmacology. 2008;33(1):166–80.

[12] Baimel C, Bartlett SE, Chiou L-C, Lawrence AJ, Muschamp JW, Patkar O, Tung L-W, Borgland SL. Orexin/hypocretin role in reward: implications for opioid and other addictions. British Journal of Pharmacology. 2015;172(2):334–48.

[13] Abernathy K, chandler lJ, Woodward JJ. Alcohol and the prefrontal cortex. International Review of Neurobiology. 2010;91:289–320.

[14] Bechara A, Dolan S, Denburg N, Hindes A, Anderson SW, Nathan PE. Decision-making deficits, linked to a dysfunctional ventromedial prefrontal cortex, revealed in alcohol and stimulant abusers. Neuropsychologia. 2001;39(4):376–89.

[15] Abrahao KP, Ariwodola OJ, Butler TR, Rau AR, Skelly MJ, Carter E, Alexander NP, McCool BA, Souza-Formigoni MLO, Weiner JL. Locomotor sensitization to ethanol impairs NMDA receptor-dependent synaptic plasticity in the nucleus accumbens and increases ethanol self-administration. The Journal of Neuroscience: The Official Journal of the Society for Neuroscience. 2013;33(11):4834–42.

[16] Marty VN, Spigelman I. Effects of alcohol on the membrane excitability and synaptic transmission of medium spiny neurons in the nucleus accumbens. Alcohol (Fayetteville, NY). 2012;46(4):317–27.

[17] Lack AK, Diaz MR, Chappell A, DuBois DW, McCool BA. Chronic ethanol and withdrawal differentially modulate pre- and postsynaptic function at glutamatergic synapses in rat basolateral amygdala. Journal of Neurophysiology. 2007;98(6):3185–96.

[18] Stephens DN, Duka T. Cognitive and emotional consequences of binge drinking: role of amygdala and prefrontal cortex. Philosophical Transactions of the Royal Society B: Biological Sciences. 2008;363(1507):3169–79.

[19] Pleil KE, Lowery-Gionta EG, Crowley NA, Li C, Marcinkiewcz CA, Rose JH, McCall NM, Maldonado-Devincci AM, Morrow AL, Jones SR, Kash TL. Effects of chronic ethanol exposure on neuronal function in the prefrontal cortex and extended amygdala. Neuropharmacology. 2015;99:735–49.

[20] Krentzman AR, Farkas KJ, Townsend AL. Spirituality, religiousness, and alcoholism treatment outcomes: a comparison between black and white participants. Alcoholism Treatment Quarterly. 2010;28(2):128–50.

[21] Tonigan JS, Rynes KN, McCrady BS. Spirituality as a change mechanism in 12-step programs: a replication, extension, and refinement. Substance Use & Misuse. 2013;48(12):1161–73.

[22] Bogenschutz MP, Rice SL, Tonigan JS, Vogel HS, Nowinski J, Hume D, Arenella PB. 12-Step facilitation for the dually diagnosed: a randomized clinical trial. Journal of Substance Abuse Treatment. 2014;46(4):403–11.

[23] Anderson DJ, McGovern JP, DuPont RL. The origins of the Minnesota model of addiction treatment – a first person account. Journal of Addictive Diseases. 1999;18(1): 107–14.

[24] Huebner RB, Kantor LW. Advances in alcoholism treatment. Alcohol Research & Health: The Journal of the National Institute on Alcohol Abuse and Alcoholism. 2011;33(4):295–9.

[25] Project MATCH secondary a priori hypotheses. Project MATCH Research Group. Addiction. 1997;92(12):1671–98.

[26] Gueorguieva R, Wu R, Donovan D, Rounsaville BJ, Couper D, Krystal JH, O'Malley SS. Naltrexone and combined behavioral intervention effects on trajectories of drinking in the COMBINE study. Drug and Alcohol Dependence. 2010;107(2–3):221–9.

[27] Kranzler HR, Kirk J. Efficacy of naltrexone and acamprosate for alcoholism treatment: a meta-analysis. Alcoholism: Clinical and Experimental Research. 2001;25(9):1335–41.

[28] Acamprosate. Drugs in R&D. 2002;3(1):13–8.

[29] Acamprosate campral for alcoholism. Medical Letter on Drugs and Therapeutics. 2005;47(1199):1–3.

[30] De Witte P, Littleton J, Parot P, Koob G. Neuroprotective and abstinence-promoting effects of acamprosate: elucidating the mechanism of action. CNS Drugs. 2005;19(6): 517–37.

[31] Spanagel R, Vengeliene V, Jandeleit B, Fischer W-N, Grindstaff K, Zhang X, Gallop MA, Krstew EV, Lawrence AJ, Kiefer F. Acamprosate produces its anti-relapse effects via calcium. Neuropsychopharmacology: Official Publication of the American College of Neuropsychopharmacology. 2014;39(4):783–91.

[32] Yahn SL, Watterson LR, Olive MF. Safety and efficacy of acamprosate for the treatment of alcohol dependence. Substance Abuse: Research and Treatment. 2013;7:1–12.

[33] Hoque MM, Hossain KJ, Kamal MM, Akhtaruzzaman M. Naltrexone in drug addiction: significance in the prevention of relapse. Mymensingh Medical Journal. 2009;18(1 Suppl):S56–65.

[34] Del Re AC, Maisel N, Blodgett J, Finney J. The declining efficacy of naltrexone pharmacotherapy for alcohol use disorders over time: a multivariate meta-analysis. Alcoholism: Clinical and Experimental Research. 2013;37(6):1064–8.

[35] Chen A, Morgenstern J, Davis CM, Kuerbis AN, Covault J, Kranzler HR. Variation in Mu-Opioid Receptor Gene (OPRM1) as a moderator of naltrexone treatment to reduce heavy drinking in a high functioning cohort. Journal of Drug & Alcohol Dependence. 2013;1(1):101.

[36] Oslin DW, Berrettini W, Kranzler HR, Pettinati H, Gelernter J, Volpicelli JR, O'Brien CP. A functional polymorphism of the mu-opioid receptor gene is associated with naltrexone response in alcohol-dependent patients. Neuropsychopharmacology: Official Publication of the American College of Neuropsychopharmacology. 2003;28(8): 1546–52.

[37] Anton RF, O'Malley SS, Ciraulo DA, Cisler RA, Couper D, Donovan DM, Gastfriend DR, Hosking JD, Johnson BA, LoCastro JS, Longabaugh R, Mason BJ, Mattson ME, Miller WR, Pettinati HM, Randall CL, Swift R, Weiss RD, Williams LD, Zweben A, Group CSR. Combined pharmacotherapies and behavioral interventions for alcohol dependence: the COMBINE study: a randomized controlled trial. JAMA. 2006;295(17): 2003–17.

[38] Hald J, Jacobsen E. A drug sensitizing the organism to ethyl alcohol. The Lancet. 1948;2(6539):1001–4.

[39] Krampe H, Ehrenreich H. Supervised disulfiram as adjunct to psychotherapy in alcoholism treatment. Current Pharmaceutical Design. 2010;16(19):2076–90.

[40] Kalra G, De Sousa A, Shrivastava A. Disulfiram in the management of alcohol dependence: a comprehensive clinical review. Open Journal of Psychiatry. 2014;4:43.

[41] Schroeder JP, Cooper DA, Schank JR, Lyle MA, Gaval-Cruz M, Ogbonmwan YE, Pozdeyev N, Freeman KG, Iuvone PM, Edwards GL, Holmes PV, Weinshenker D. Disulfiram attenuates drug-primed reinstatement of cocaine seeking via inhibition of dopamine beta-hydroxylase. Neuropsychopharmacology: Official Publication of the American College of Neuropsychopharmacology. 2010;35(12):2440–9.

[42] Bito-Onon JJ, Simms JA, Chatterjee S, Holgate J, Bartlett SE. Varenicline, a partial agonist at neuronal nicotinic acetylcholine receptors, reduces nicotine-induced increases in 20% ethanol operant self-administration in Sprague–Dawley rats. Addiction Biology. 2011;16(3):440–9.

[43] Steensland P, Simms JA, Holgate J, Richards JK, Bartlett SE. Varenicline, an alpha4beta2 nicotinic acetylcholine receptor partial agonist, selectively decreases ethanol consumption and seeking. Proceedings of the National Academy of Sciences of the United States of America. 2007;104(30):12518–23.

[44] Mitchell JM, Teague CH, Kayser AS, Bartlett SE, Fields HL. Varenicline decreases alcohol consumption in heavy-drinking smokers. Psychopharmacology. 2012;223(3): 299–306.

[45] Litten RZ, Ryan ML, Fertig JB, Falk DE, Johnson B, Dunn KE, Green AI, Pettinati HM, Ciraulo DA, Sarid-Segal O, Kampman K, Brunette MF, Strain EC, Tiouririne NA, Ransom J, Scott C, Stout R. A double-blind, placebo-controlled trial assessing the efficacy of varenicline tartrate for alcohol dependence. Journal of Addiction Medicine. 2013;7(4):277–86.

[46] Osborn MD, Lowery JJ, Skorput AGJ, Giuvelis D, Bilsky EJ. In vivo characterization of the opioid antagonist nalmefene in mice. Life Sciences. 2010;86(15–16):624–30.

[47] Robin C. Alcohol use disorder: pathophysiology, effects, and pharmacologic options for treatment. 2014;5:1–12.

[48] Mann K, Lemenager T, Hoffmann S, Reinhard I, Hermann D, Batra A, Berner M, Wodarz N, Heinz A, Smolka MN, Zimmermann US, Wellek S, Kiefer F, Anton RF, Team PS. Results of a double-blind, placebo-controlled pharmacotherapy trial in alcoholism conducted in Germany and comparison with the US COMBINE study. Addiction Biology. 2013;18(6):937–46.

[49] Sidana AK, Mangla D. Unusual side effects with acamprosate. Indian Journal of Psychiatry. 2007;49(2):143.

[50] Hulse GK. Improving clinical outcomes for naltrexone as a management of problem alcohol use. British Journal of Clinical Pharmacology. 2013;76(5):632–41.

[51] Waal H, Christophersen AS, Frogopsahl G, Olsen LH, Morland J. [Naltrexone implants – a pilot project]. Tidsskr Nor Laegeforen. 2003;123(12):1660–1.

[52] Weiss RD. Pharmacotherapy of alcohol dependence: how and when to use disulfiram and naltrexone. Current Psychiatry. 2002;1(1):51–60.

[53] Fuller RK, Branchey L, Brightwell DR, Derman RM, Emrick CD, Iber FL, James KE, Lacoursiere RB, Lee KK, Lowenstam I, et al. Disulfiram treatment of alcoholism. A Veterans Administration cooperative study. JAMA. 1986;256(11):1449–55.

[54] Fuller RK, Gordis E. Does disulfiram have a role in alcoholism treatment today? Addiction. 2004;99(1):21–4.

[55] Gorelick DA. Serotonin uptake blockers and the treatment of alcoholism. Recent Developments in Alcoholism: An Official Publication of the American Medical Society on Alcoholism, the Research Society on Alcoholism, and the National Council on Alcoholism. 1989;7:267–81.

[56] George FR. Pharmacotherapy in alcoholism treatment: integrating and understanding the use of serotonin reuptake inhibitors. Alcohol and Alcoholism (Oxford, Oxfordshire) Supplement. 1994;2:537–43.

[57] Gallant D. The serotonin system and alcoholism: basic research and clinical problems. Alcoholism: Clinical and Experimental Research. 1993;17(6):1345.

[58] Silberman Y, Ariwodola OJ, Weiner JL. beta1-adrenoceptor activation is required for ethanol enhancement of lateral paracapsular GABAergic synapses in the rat basolateral amygdala. The Journal of Pharmacology and Experimental Therapeutics. 2012;343(2):451–9.

[59] Petrakis IL, Ralevski E, Desai N, Trevisan L, Gueorguieva R, Rounsaville B, Krystal JH. Noradrenergic vs serotonergic antidepressant with or without naltrexone for veterans with PTSD and comorbid alcohol dependence. Neuropsychopharmacology: Official Publication of the American College of Neuropsychopharmacology. 2012;37(4): 996–1004.

[60] Gilpin NW, Koob GF. Effects of beta-adrenoceptor antagonists on alcohol drinking by alcohol-dependent rats. Psychopharmacology. 2010;212(3):431–9.

[61] Fahlke C, Berggren U, Berglund KJ, Zetterberg H, Blennow K, Engel JA, Balldin J. Neuroendocrine assessment of serotonergic, dopaminergic, and noradrenergic functions in alcohol-dependent individuals. Alcoholism: Clinical and Experimental Research. 2012;36(1):97–103.

[62] Ossewaarde L, Verkes RJ, Hermans EJ, Kooijman SC, Urner M, Tendolkar I, van Wingen GA, Fernandez G. Two-week administration of the combined serotonin-noradrenaline reuptake inhibitor duloxetine augments functioning of mesolimbic incentive processing circuits. Biological Psychiatry. 2011;70(6):568–74.

[63] Orejarena MJ, Lanfumey L, Maldonado R, Robledo P. Involvement of 5-HT2A receptors in MDMA reinforcement and cue-induced reinstatement of MDMA-seeking behaviour. International Journal of Neuropsychopharmacology. 2011;14(7):927–40.

[64] Gomez-Milanes I, Almela P, Garcia-Carmona JA, Garcia-Gutierrez MS, Aracil-Fernandez A, Manzanares J, Milanes Maquilon MV, Laorden ML. Accumbal dopamine, noradrenaline and serotonin activity after naloxone-conditioned place aversion in morphine-dependent mice. Neurochemistry International. 2012;61(3):433–40.

[65] Fallon S, Shearman E, Sershen H, Lajtha A. Food reward-induced neurotransmitter changes in cognitive brain regions. Neurochemical Research. 2007;32(10):1772–82.

[66] Dzirasa K, Phillips HW, Sotnikova TD, Salahpour A, Kumar S, Gainetdinov RR, Caron MG, Nicolelis MA. Noradrenergic control of cortico-striato-thalamic and mesolimbic cross-structural synchrony. The Journal of Neuroscience: The Official Journal of the Society for Neuroscience. 2010;30(18):6387–97.

[67] McCool BA, Christian DT, Fetzer JA, Chappell AM. Lateral/basolateral amygdala serotonin type-2 receptors modulate operant self-administration of a sweetened ethanol solution via inhibition of principal neuron activity. Frontiers in Integrative Neuroscience. 2014;8:5.

[68] Tran L, Lasher BK, Young KA, Keele NB. Depletion of serotonin in the basolateral amygdala elevates glutamate receptors and facilitates fear-potentiated startle. Translational Psychiatry. 2013;3:e298.

[69] Roozendaal B, Nguyen BT, Power AE, McGaugh JL. Basolateral amygdala noradrenergic influence enables enhancement of memory consolidation induced by hippocampal glucocorticoid receptor activation. Proceedings of the National Academy of Sciences of the United States of America. 1999;96(20):11642–7.

[70] Pare D. Role of the basolateral amygdala in memory consolidation. Progress in Neurobiology. 2003;70(5):409–20.

[71] Zhang J, Muller JF, McDonald AJ. Noradrenergic innervation of pyramidal cells in the rat basolateral amygdala. Neuroscience. 2013;228:395–408.

[72] Commons KG, Connolley KR, Valentino RJ. A neurochemically distinct dorsal raphe-limbic circuit with a potential role in affective disorders. Neuropsychopharmacology: Official Publication of the American College of Neuropsychopharmacology. 2003;28(2): 206–15.

[73] Le AD, Harding S, Juzytsch W, Fletcher PJ, Shaham Y. The role of corticotropin-releasing factor in the median raphe nucleus in relapse to alcohol. The Journal of Neuroscience: The Official Journal of the Society for Neuroscience. 2002;22(18):7844–9.

[74] Bonkale WL, Turecki G, Austin MC. Increased tryptophan hydroxylase immunoreactivity in the dorsal raphe nucleus of alcohol-dependent, depressed suicide subjects is restricted to the dorsal subnucleus. Synapse. 2006;60(1):81–5.

[75] Ketcherside A, Mathews I, Filbey F. The serotonin link between alcohol use and 25 affective disorders. Journal of Addiction and Prevention. 2013;1(2).3p. n/a-n/a.

[76] Andrade AL, Abrahao KP, Goeldner FO, Souza-Formigoni ML. Administration of the 5-HT2C receptor antagonist SB-242084 into the nucleus accumbens blocks the expression of ethanol-induced behavioral sensitization in Albino Swiss mice. Neuroscience. 2011;189:178–86.

[77] Ding ZM, Oster SM, Hauser SR, Toalston JE, Bell RL, McBride WJ, Rodd ZA. Synergistic self-administration of ethanol and cocaine directly into the posterior ventral tegmental area: involvement of serotonin-3 receptors. The Journal of Pharmacology and Experimental Therapeutics. 2012;340(1):202–9.

[78] Burnett EJ, Grant KA, Davenport AT, Hemby SE, Friedman DP. The effects of chronic ethanol self-administration on hippocampal 5-HT $_{1A}$ receptors in monkeys. Drug and Alcohol Dependence. 2014;136:135–142.

[79] Kasper JM. Characterization of the effects of novel 5-HT2C receptor agonists on neurotransmission and voluntary alcohol consumption in rats. Thesis, University of Florida; 2013.

[80] Sari Y. Role of 5-hydroxytryptamine 1B (5-HT1B) receptors in the regulation of ethanol intake in rodents. Journal of Psychopharmacology. 2013;27(1):3–12.

[81] Yang, J. and M.D. Li, *Association and Interaction Analyses of 5-HT3 Receptor and Serotonin Transporter Genes with Alcohol, Cocaine, and Nicotine Dependence Using the SAGE Data*. Human genetics, 2014. 133(7): p. 905-918. .

[82] De Bruin N, McCreary A, Van Loevezijn A, De Vries T, Venhorst J, Van Drimmelen M, Kruse C. A novel highly selective 5-HT $_6$ receptor antagonist attenuates ethanol and nicotine seeking but does not affect inhibitory response control in Wistar rats. Behavioural Brain Research. 2013;236:157–65.

[83] Smith RJ, Aston-Jones G. Noradrenergic transmission in the extended amygdala: role in increased drug-seeking and relapse during protracted drug abstinence. Brain Structure and Function. 2008;213(1–2):43–61.

[84] Becker HC. Effects of alcohol dependence and withdrawal on stress responsiveness and alcohol consumption. Alcohol Research. 2012;34(4):448–58.

[85] Howes LG, Reid JL. Changes in plasma free 3,4-dihydroxyphenylethylene glycol and noradrenaline levels after acute alcohol administration. Clinical Science. 1985;69(4): 423–8.

[86] Higley AE, Koob GF, Mason BJ. Treatment of alcohol dependence with drug antagonists of the stress response. Alcohol Research. 2012;34(4):516–21.

[87] Le AD, Harding S, Juzytsch W, Funk D, Shaham Y. Role of alpha-2 adrenoceptors in stress-induced reinstatement of alcohol seeking and alcohol self-administration in rats. Psychopharmacology. 2005;179(2):366–73.

[88] Walker BM, Rasmussen DD, Raskind MA, Koob GF. alpha1-noradrenergic receptor antagonism blocks dependence-induced increases in responding for ethanol. Alcohol. 2008;42(2):91–7.

[89] Simpson TL, Saxon AJ, Meredith CW, Malte CA, McBride B, Ferguson LC, Gross CA, Hart KL, Raskind M. A pilot trial of the alpha-1 adrenergic antagonist, prazosin, for alcohol dependence. Alcoholism: Clinical and Experimental Research. 2009;33(2):255–63.

[90] Walsh JJ, Friedman AK, Sun H, Heller EA, Ku SM, Juarez B, Burnham VL, Mazei-Robison MS, Ferguson D, Golden SA, Koo JW, Chaudhury D, Christoffel DJ, Pomeranz L, Friedman JM, Russo SJ, Nestler EJ, Han MH. Stress and CRF gate neural activation of BDNF in the mesolimbic reward pathway. Nature Neuroscience. 2014;17(1):27–9.

[91] Philbert J, Pichat P, Palme R, Belzung C, Griebel G. The CRF(1) receptor antagonist SSR125543 attenuates long-term cognitive deficit induced by acute inescapable stress in mice, independently from the hypothalamic pituitary adrenal axis. Pharmacology, Biochemistry, and Behavior. 2012;102(3):415–22.

[92] Lemos JC, Wanat MJ, Smith JS, Reyes BA, Hollon NG, Van Bockstaele EJ, Chavkin C, Phillips PE. Severe stress switches CRF action in the nucleus accumbens from appetitive to aversive. Nature. 2012;490(7420):402–6.

[93] Huang MM, Overstreet DH, Knapp DJ, Angel R, Wills TA, Navarro M, Rivier J, Vale W, Breese GR. Corticotropin-releasing factor (CRF) sensitization of ethanol withdrawal-induced anxiety-like behavior is brain site specific and mediated by CRF-1 receptors: relation to stress-induced sensitization. The Journal of Pharmacology and Experimental Therapeutics. 2010;332(1):298–307.

[94] Hauger RL, Risbrough V, Oakley RH, Olivares-Reyes JA, Dautzenberg FM. Role of CRF receptor signaling in stress vulnerability, anxiety, and depression. Annals of the New York Academy of Sciences. 2009;1179:120–43.

[95] Koob G, Kreek MJ. Stress, dysregulation of drug reward pathways, and the transition to drug dependence. American Journal of Psychiatry. 2007;164(8):1149–59.

[96] Hammack SE, Guo JD, Hazra R, Dabrowska J, Myers KM, Rainnie DG. The response of neurons in the bed nucleus of the stria terminalis to serotonin: implications for anxiety. Progress in Neuro-Psychopharmacology & Biological Psychiatry. 2009;33(8): 1309–20.

[97] Wenzel JM, Cotten SW, Dominguez HM, Lane JE, Shelton K, Su ZI, Ettenberg A. Noradrenergic beta-receptor antagonism within the central nucleus of the amygdala or bed nucleus of the stria terminalis attenuates the negative/anxiogenic effects of cocaine. The Journal of Neuroscience: The Official Journal of the Society for Neuroscience. 2014;34(10):3467–74.

[98] Flavin SA, Winder DG. Noradrenergic control of the bed nucleus of the stria terminalis in stress and reward. Neuropharmacology. 2013;70:324–30.

[99] Leri F, Flores J, Rodaros D, Stewart J. Blockade of stress-induced but not cocaine-induced reinstatement by infusion of noradrenergic antagonists into the bed nucleus of the stria terminalis or the central nucleus of the amygdala. The Journal of Neuroscience: The Official Journal of the Society for Neuroscience. 2002;22(13):5713–8.

[100] Le AD, Funk D, Coen K, Li Z, Shaham Y. Role of corticotropin-releasing factor in the median raphe nucleus in yohimbine-induced reinstatement of alcohol seeking in rats. Addiction Biology. 2013;18(3):448–51.

[101] Dzung Le A, Funk D, Harding S, Juzytsch W, Fletcher PJ. The role of noradrenaline and 5-hydroxytryptamine in yohimbine-induced increases in alcohol-seeking in rats. Psychopharmacology. 2009;204(3):477–88.

[102] Marinelli PW, Funk D, Juzytsch W, Harding S, Rice KC, Shaham Y, Le A. The CRF1 receptor antagonist antalarmin attenuates yohimbine-induced increases in operant alcohol self-administration and reinstatement of alcohol seeking in rats. Psychopharmacology. 2007;195(3):345–55.

[103] Funk CK, Koob GF. A CRF(2) agonist administered into the central nucleus of the amygdala decreases ethanol self-administration in ethanol-dependent rats. Brain Research. 2007;1155:172–8.

[104] Krettek JE, Price JL. A description of the amygdaloid complex in the rat and cat with observations on intra-amygdaloid axonal connections. The Journal of Comparative Neurology. 1978;178(2):255–79.

[105] Davis M, Rainnie D, Cassell M. Neurotransmission in the rat amygdala related to fear and anxiety. Trends in Neurosciences. 1994;17(5):208–14.

[106] Cardinal RN, Parkinson JA, Hall J, Everitt BJ. Emotion and motivation: the role of the amygdala, ventral striatum, and prefrontal cortex. Neuroscience & Biobehavioral Reviews. 2002;26(3):321–52.

[107] Cahill L, Weinberger NM, Roozendaal B, McGaugh JL. Is the amygdala a locus of "conditioned fear"? Some questions and caveats. Neuron. 1999;23(2):227–8.

[108] Johnston JB. Further contributions to the study of the evolution of the forebrain. The Journal of Comparative Neurology. 1923;35(5):337–481.

[109] Roozendaal B, McEwen BS, Chattarji S. Stress, memory and the amygdala. Nature Reviews Neuroscience. 2009;10(6):423–33.

[110] Paré D, Smith Y, Paré JF. Intra-amygdaloid projections of the basolateral and basomedial nuclei in the cat: phaseolus vulgaris-leucoagglutinin anterograde tracing at the light and electron microscopic level. Neuroscience. 1995;69(2):567–83.

[111] Dong H-W, Petrovich GD, Swanson LW. Topography of projections from amygdala to bed nuclei of the stria terminalis. Brain Research Reviews. 2001;38(1–2):192–246.

[112] Petrovich GD, Canteras NS, Swanson LW. Combinatorial amygdalar inputs to hippocampal domains and hypothalamic behavior systems. Brain Research Reviews. 2001;38(1–2):247–89.

[113] McDonald AJ. Topographical organization of amygdaloid projections to the caudatoputamen, nucleus accumbens, and related striatal-like areas of the rat brain. Neuroscience. 1991;44(1):15–33.

[114] Ray JP, Price JL. The organization of the thalamocortical connections of the mediodorsal thalamic nucleus in the rat, related to the ventral forebrain–prefrontal cortex topography. The Journal of Comparative Neurology. 1992;323(2):167–97.

[115] Ottersen OP, Fischer BO, Rinvik E, Storm-Mathisen J. Putative amino acid transmitters in the amygdala. Advances in Experimental Medicine and Biology. 1986;203:53–66.

[116] Amaral D, Insausti R. Retrograde transport of D-[3H]-aspartate injected into the monkey amygdaloid complex. Experimental Brain Research. 1992;88(2):375–88.

[117] Killcross S, Robbins TW, Everitt BJ. Different types of fear-conditioned behaviour mediated by separate nuclei within amygdala. Nature. 1997;388(6640):377–80.

[118] Nomura M, Izaki Y, Takita M, Tanaka J, Hori K. Extracellular level of basolateral amygdalar dopamine responding to reversal of appetitive-conditioned discrimination in young and old rats. Brain Research. 2004;1018(2):241–6.

[119] Ramirez DR, Savage LM. Differential involvement of the basolateral amygdala, orbitofrontal cortex, and nucleus accumbens core in the acquisition and use of reward expectancies. Behavioral Neuroscience. 2007;121(5):896–906.

[120] Meil WM, See RE. Lesions of the basolateral amygdala abolish the ability of drug associated cues to reinstate responding during withdrawal from self-administered cocaine. Behavioural Brain Research. 1997;87(2):139–48.

[121] Valizadegan F, Oryan S, Nasehi M, Zarrindast MR. Interaction between morphine and noradrenergic system of basolateral amygdala on anxiety and memory in the elevated plus-maze test based on a test-retest paradigm. Archives of Iranian Medicine. 2013;16(5):281–7.

[122] Varodayan, F.P., et al., *Chronic alcohol exposure disrupts CB1 regulation of GABAergic transmission in the rat basolateral amygdala*. Addiction Biology, 2016: p. n/a-n/a.In press.

[123] Sciascia JM, Reese RM, Janak PH, Chaudhri N. Alcohol-seeking triggered by discrete pavlovian cues is invigorated by alcohol contexts and mediated by glutamate signaling in the basolateral amygdala. Neuropsychopharmacology: Official Publication of the American College of Neuropsychopharmacology. 2015;40(12):2801–12.

[124] Gass JT, Sinclair CM, Cleva RM, Widholm JJ, Olive MF. Alcohol-seeking behavior is associated with increased glutamate transmission in basolateral amygdala and nucleus accumbens as measured by glutamate-oxidase-coated biosensors. Addiction Biology. 2011;16(2):215–28.

[125] Porrino LJ, Williams-Hemby L, Whitlow C, Bowen C, Samson HH. Metabolic mapping of the effects of oral alcohol self-administration in rats. Alcoholism: Clinical and Experimental Research. 1998;22(1):176–82.

[126] Läck AK, Diaz MR, Chappell A, DuBois DW, McCool BA. Chronic ethanol and withdrawal differentially modulate pre- and post-synaptic function at glutamatergic synapses in rat basolateral amygdala. Journal of Neurophysiology. 2007;98(6):3185–96.

[127] Rassnick S, Pulvirenti L, Koob GF. Oral ethanol self-administration in rats is reduced by the administration of dopamine and glutamate receptor antagonists into the nucleus accumbens. Psychopharmacology. 1992;109(1):92–8.

[128] Hyytia P, Kiianmaa K. Suppression of ethanol responding by centrally administered CTOP and naltrindole in AA and Wistar rats. Alcoholism: Clinical and Experimental Research. 2001;25(1):25–33.

[129] Christian DT, Alexander NJ, Diaz MR, McCool BA. Thalamic glutamatergic afferents into the rat basolateral amygdala exhibit increased presynaptic glutamate function following withdrawal from chronic intermittent ethanol. Neuropharmacology. 2013;65:134–42.

[130] Enquist J, Ferwerda M, Madhavan A, Hok D, Whistler JL. Chronic ethanol potentiates the effect of neuropeptide s in the basolateral amygdala and shows increased anxiolytic and anti-depressive effects. Neuropsychopharmacology: Official Publication of the American College of Neuropsychopharmacology. 2012;37(11):2436–45.

[131] Marshall SA, Casachahua JD, Rinker JA, Blose AK, Lysle DT, Thiele TE. IL-1 receptor signaling in the basolateral amygdala modulates binge-like ethanol consumption in male C57BL/6J mice. Brain, Behavior, and Immunity. 2016;51:258–67.

[132] Sinclair CM, Cleva RM, Hood LE, Olive MF, Gass JT. mGluR5 receptors in the basolateral amygdala and nucleus accumbens regulate cue-induced reinstatement of ethanol-seeking behavior. Pharmacology, Biochemistry, and Behavior. 2012;101(3): 329–35.

[133] Chaudhri N, Woods CA, Sahuque LL, Gill TM, Janak PH. Unilateral inactivation of the basolateral amygdala attenuates context-induced renewal of pavlovian-conditioned alcohol-seeking. The European Journal of Neuroscience. 2013;38(5):2751–61.

[134] McLaughlin J, See RE. Selective inactivation of the dorsomedial prefrontal cortex and the basolateral amygdala attenuates conditioned-cued reinstatement of extinguished cocaine-seeking behavior in rats. Psychopharmacology. 2003;168(1–2):57–65.

[135] Fuchs RA, Feltenstein MW, See RE. The role of the basolateral amygdala in stimulus-reward memory and extinction memory consolidation and in subsequent conditioned cued reinstatement of cocaine seeking. The European Journal of Neuroscience. 2006;23(10):2809–13.

[136] Di Ciano P, Everitt BJ. Direct interactions between the basolateral amygdala and nucleus accumbens core underlie cocaine-seeking behavior by rats. The Journal of Neuroscience: The Official Journal of the Society for Neuroscience. 2004;24(32):7167–73.

[137] Alderson HL, Robbins TW, Everitt BJ. The effects of excitotoxic lesions of the basolateral amygdala on the acquisition of heroin-seeking behaviour in rats. Psychopharmacology. 2000;153(1):111–9.

[138] Radwanska K, Wrobel E, Korkosz A, Rogowski A, Kostowski W, Bienkowski P, Kaczmarek L. Alcohol relapse induced by discrete cues activates components of AP-1 transcription factor and ERK pathway in the rat basolateral and central amygdala. Neuropsychopharmacology: Official Publication of the American College of Neuropsychopharmacology. 2008;33(8):1835–46.

[139] Wilden J, Hauser S, Deehanjr G, Ding Z-M, Truitt W, Mcbride W, Rodd Z. The basolateral amygdala is a critical structure for environmental cue augmentation of EtOH-seeking. 2012.

[140] Marinelli PW, Funk D, Juzytsch W, Le AD. Opioid receptors in the basolateral amygdala but not dorsal hippocampus mediate context-induced alcohol seeking. Behavioural Brain Research. 2010;211(1):58–63.

[141] Gass JT, Sinclair CM, Cleva RM, Widholm JJ, Olive MF. Alcohol-seeking behavior is associated with increased glutamate transmission in basolateral amygdala and nucleus accumbens as measured by glutamate-oxidase-coated biosensors. Addiction Biology. 2011;16(2):215–28.

[142] Silberman Y, Matthews RT, Winder DG. A corticotropin releasing factor pathway for ethanol regulation of the ventral tegmental area in the bed nucleus of the stria terminalis. The Journal of Neuroscience: The Official Journal of the Society for Neuroscience. 2013;33(3):950–60.

[143] Simms JA, Haass-Koffler CL, Bito-Onon J, Li R, Bartlett SE. Mifepristone in the central nucleus of the amygdala reduces yohimbine stress-induced reinstatement of ethanol-seeking. Neuropsychopharmacology: Official Publication of the American College of Neuropsychopharmacology. 2012;37(4):906–18.

[144] Valdez GR, Sabino V, Koob GF. Increased anxiety-like behavior and ethanol self-administration in dependent rats: reversal via corticotropin-releasing factor-2 receptor activation. Alcoholism: Clinical and Experimental Research. 2004;28(6):865–72.

[145] Maroun M, Ioannides PJ, Bergman KL, Kavushansky A, Holmes A, Wellman CL. Fear extinction deficits following acute stress associate with increased spine density and dendritic retraction in basolateral amygdala neurons. The European Journal of Neuroscience. 2013;38(4):2611–20.

[146] Rei D, Mason X, Seo J, Gräff J, Rudenko A, Wang J, Rueda R, Siegert S, Cho S, Canter RG, Mungenast AE, Deisseroth K, Tsai L-H. Basolateral amygdala bidirectionally modulates stress-induced hippocampal learning and memory deficits through a p25/Cdk5-dependent pathway. Proceedings of the National Academy of Sciences of the United States of America. 2015;112(23):7291–6.

[147] Rau AR, Chappell AM, Butler TR, Ariwodola OJ, Weiner JL. Increased basolateral amygdala pyramidal cell excitability may contribute to the anxiogenic phenotype induced by chronic early-life stress. The Journal of Neuroscience: The Official Journal of the Society for Neuroscience. 2015;35(26):9730–40.

[148] Zhang W, Rosenkranz JA. Repeated restraint stress increases basolateral amygdala neuronal activity in an age-dependent manner. Neuroscience. 2012;226:459–74.

[149] Silberman Y, Bajo M, Chappell AM, Christian DT, Cruz M, Diaz MR, Kash T, Lack AK, Messing RO, Siggins GR, Winder D, Roberto M, McCool BA, Weiner JL. Neurobiolog-

ical mechanisms contributing to alcohol–stress–anxiety interactions. Alcohol. 2009;43(7):509–19.

[150] Baculis BC, Diaz MR, Valenzuela CF. Third trimester-equivalent ethanol exposure increases anxiety-like behavior and glutamatergic transmission in the basolateral amygdala. Pharmacology, Biochemistry, and Behavior. 2015;137:78–85.

[151] Weitemier AZ, Ryabinin AE. Alcohol-induced memory impairment in trace fear conditioning: a hippocampus-specific effect. Hippocampus. 2003;13(3):305–15.

[152] Bertotto ME, Bustos SG, Molina VA, Martijena ID. Influence of ethanol withdrawal on fear memory: effect of d-cycloserine. Neuroscience. 2006;142(4):979–90.

[153] Holmes A, Fitzgerald PJ, MacPherson KP, DeBrouse L, Colacicco G, Flynn SM, Masneuf S, Pleil KE, Li C, Marcinkiewcz CA, Kash TL, Gunduz-Cinar O, Camp M. Chronic alcohol remodels prefrontal neurons and disrupts NMDAR-mediated fear extinction encoding. Nature neuroscience. 2012;15(10):1359–61.

[154] Quinones-Laracuente K, Hernandez-Rodriguez MY, Bravo-Rivera C, Melendez RI, Quirk GJ. The effect of repeated exposure to ethanol on pre-existing fear memories in rats. Psychopharmacology. 2015;232(19):3615–22.

[155] Le AD, Funk D, Juzytsch W, Coen K, Navarre BM, Cifani C, Shaham Y. Effect of prazosin and guanfacine on stress-induced reinstatement of alcohol and food seeking in rats. Psychopharmacology. 2011;218(1):89–99.

[156] Marcinkiewcz, C.A., *Serotonergic Systems In The Pathophysiology Of Ethanol Dependence: Relevance To Clinical Alcoholism*. ACS Chem Neurosci, 2015. 6(7): p. 1026-39.

[157] McBride WJ, Guan XM, Chernet E, Lumeng L, Li TK. Regional serotonin1A receptors in the CNS of alcohol-preferring and -nonpreferring rats. Pharmacology, Biochemistry, and Behavior. 1994;49(1):7–12.

[158] Muller JF, Mascagni F, McDonald AJ. Serotonin-immunoreactive axon terminals innervate pyramidal cells and interneurons in the rat basolateral amygdala. The Journal of Comparative Neurology. 2007;505(3):314–35.

[159] Wang SJ, Cheng LL, Gean PW. Cross-modulation of synaptic plasticity by beta-adrenergic and 5-HT1A receptors in the rat basolateral amygdala. The Journal of Neuroscience: The Official Journal of the Society for Neuroscience. 1999;19(2):570–7.

[160] Barbara Ferry and Gina L. Quirarte (2012). Role of Norepinephrine in Modulating Inhibitory Avoidance Memory Storage: Critical Involvement of the Basolateral Amygdala, The Amygdala - A Discrete Multitasking Manager, Dr. Barbara Ferry (Ed.), InTech, DOI: 10.5772/53246. Available from: http://www.intechopen.com/books/the-amygdala-a-discrete-multitasking-manager/role-of-norepinephrine-in-modulating-inhibitory-avoidance-memory-storage-critical-involvement-of-the.

[161] Ferry B, Roozendaal B, McGaugh JL. Basolateral amygdala noradrenergic influences on memory storage are mediated by an interaction between β- and α1-adrenoceptors. Journal of Neuroscience. 1999;19(12):5119–23.

[162] Barak S, Liu F, Hamida SB, Yowell QV, Neasta J, Kharazia V, Janak PH, Ron D. Disruption of alcohol-related memories by mTORC1 inhibition prevents relapse. Nature Neuroscience. 2013;16(8):1111–7.

[163] Butler TR, Chappell AM, Weiner JL. Effect of beta3 adrenoceptor activation in the basolateral amygdala on ethanol seeking behaviors. Psychopharmacology. 2014;231(1): 293–303.

[164] Hoffman PL, Valverius P, Kwast M, Tabakoff B. Comparison of the effects of ethanol on beta-adrenergic receptors in heart and brain. Alcohol and Alcoholism (Oxford, Oxfordshire) Supplement. 1987;1:749–54.

[165] Rainnie DG. Serotonergic modulation of neurotransmission in the rat basolateral amygdala. Journal of Neurophysiology. 1999;82(1):69–85.

[166] Cheng LL, Wang SJ, Gean PW. Serotonin depresses excitatory synaptic transmission and depolarization-evoked Ca^{2+} influx in rat basolateral amygdala via 5-HT1A receptors. The European Journal of Neuroscience. 1998;10(6):2163–72.

[167] de Andrade Strauss CV, Vicente MA, Zangrossi Jr H. Activation of 5-HT1A receptors in the rat basolateral amygdala induces both anxiolytic and antipanic-like effects. Behavioural Brain Research. 2013;246:103–10.

[168] Nevo I, Langlois X, Laporte AM, Kleven M, Koek W, Lima L, Maudhuit C, Martres MP, Hamon M. Chronic alcoholization alters the expression of 5-HT1A and 5-HT1B receptor subtypes in rat brain. The European Journal of Pharmacology. 1995;281(3):229–39.

[169] Christianson JP, Ragole T, Amat J, Greenwood BN, Strong PV, Paul ED, Fleshner M, Watkins LR, Maier SF. 5-Hydroxytryptamine 2C receptors in the basolateral amygdala are involved in the expression of anxiety after uncontrollable traumatic stress. Biological Psychiatry. 2010;67(4):339–45.

[170] Gonzalez LE, Andrews N, File SE. 5-HT1A and benzodiazepine receptors in the basolateral amygdala modulate anxiety in the social interaction test, but not in the elevated plus-maze. Brain Research. 1996;732(1–2):145–53.

[171] McCool BA, Frye GD, Pulido MD, Botting SK. Effects of chronic ethanol consumption on rat GABA(A) and strychnine-sensitive glycine receptors expressed by lateral/ basolateral amygdala neurons. Brain Research. 2003;963(1–2):165–77.

[172] Patkar, O.L., et al., *The antihypertensive drug pindolol attenuates long-term but not short-term binge-like ethanol consumption in mice.* Addiction Biology, 2016: p. n/a-n/a. In press. 2016.

[173] Kraus ML, Gottlieb LD, Horwitz RI, Anscher M. Randomized clinical trial of atenolol in patients with alcohol withdrawal. The New England Journal of Medicine. 1985;313(15):905–9.

[174] Horwitz RI, Gottlieb LD, Kraus ML. The efficacy of atenolol in the outpatient management of the alcohol withdrawal syndrome. Results of a randomized clinical trial. Archives of Internal Medicine. 1989;149(5):1089–93.

[175] Johnsson G, Regardh CG. Clinical pharmacokinetics of beta-adrenoreceptor blocking drugs. Clinical Pharmacokinetics. 1976;1(4):233–63.

[176] Carlsson C, Johansson T. The psychological effects of propranolol in the abstinence phase of chronic alcoholics. The British Journal of Psychiatry: The Journal of Mental Science. 1971;119(553):605–6.

[177] Malcolm R, Anton RF, Randall CL, Johnston A, Brady K, Thevos A. A placebo-controlled trial of buspirone in anxious inpatient alcoholics. Alcoholism: Clinical and Experimental Research. 1992;16(6):1007–13.

[178] Kranzler HR, Burleson JA, Del Boca FK, Babor TF, Korner P, Brown J, Bohn MJ. Buspirone treatment of anxious alcoholics. A placebo-controlled trial. Archives of General Psychiatry. 1994;51(9):720–31.

Chapter 6

Substance Abuse Therapeutics

John Andrew Mills

Additional information is available at the end of the chapter

http://dx.doi.org/10.5772/64264

Abstract

This chapter provides a broad overview of therapies for substance abuse. These therapies are understood in the context of the history of drug use in the United States and factors that influenced the expansion and regulation of substance use. This is followed by a discussion of how the complexity of these factors was associated with difficulties in understanding substance misuse and created challenges to the creation of effective treatment systems. The chapter reviews the moral and disease models of addiction before discussing the diagnosis of substance-related disorders. The chapter describes major treatment approaches and their efficacy.

Keywords: Substance abuse, Treatment

1. Introduction

This chapter will provide a brief overview of the history of substance abuse therapeutics and survey of approaches to the treatment of substance use disorders. To fit the history of, and approaches to, substance abuse therapeutics into a chapter of this type, great simplification is required; at the same time, the entire enterprise bears much resemblance to the well-worn parable of the group of blind men attempting to describe an elephant. The elephant parable illustrates beautifully that reasonable people may disagree vigorously about the essence of something by virtue of how they encounter it. This array of views has been likened to metaphors [1], but the significance of each metaphor has profound implications. So, while the parable of the men and the elephant *does* highlight the potential validity of differing perspectives on substance use, the parable *does not* do enough to consider the implications and consequences of substance abuse. Community and professional responses to substance use have reflected the untold conflict and enormous consequences that have still not yielded widely agreed upon responses to the destructive effects of substance use. The vast social issues include, but are certainly not limited to moral, legal, ethical, economic, political, sociological, and psychological considerations. So, it is virtually impossible to be exhaustive in one's review of these issues, and this chapter will focus only on the highlights of treatment of substance use conditions.

Modern data indicate that substance use and misuse continue to be widespread [2]. For 2014, nearly 140 million people over the age of 12 used alcohol, more than 60 million reported some binge drinking, and more than 16 million people reported heavy binge drinking in the United States. Estimates for the use of illicit drugs overall appear to be overshadowed by data pertaining specifically to marijuana use. More than 22 million people reported use of marijuana, nearly 67 million reported use of tobacco, and more than 4 million persons reported misuse of prescription medication. Perhaps of greater concern than the reported patterns of use overall is the reported 17 million people whose self-reported use is consistent with a diagnosis of an alcohol use disorder and more than 21 million people whose self-reported use is consistent with a diagnosis of a substance use disorder. Clearly, misuse of psychoactive substances remains a significant problem.

2. Early roots of treatment in the United States

The treatment of substance-related problems in the United States came from the intersection of various forces in the middle of the nineteenth century. Patterns of alcohol and other substance use, social reform movements, regulatory efforts, and the dynamics of professional guilds all combined to shape the beginning of attempts to intervene with these problems. Both the Europeans on the North American continent and the Africans who were brought as slaves were users of alcohol, but the Native Americans were mostly *not* users of alcohol. Cultural factors were significant and patterns of usage and resulting problems, including the catastrophic effect of alcohol on Native American tribes [3]. As colonization progressed, public drunkenness may have been the most significant problem that was explicitly identified [4]. Benjamin Rush (1746–1913) was an influential writer on a number of subjects, having been a member of the Continental Congress, a signer of the Declaration of Independence, and notable hospital reformer of the eighteenth century. Rush's work was rich with descriptions of alcohol use as a progressive *medical* condition that required abstinence as a method of invention. Until the influence of his writings, alcohol had previously been seen as a moral problem or a manifestation of mental illness [4].

2.1. Temperance

The American temperance movement emerged as alcohol-related problems became more salient. As one might discern from the name of the organizations ("Temperance"), the initial goals were to promote moderate use. However, the goals of the temperance movement changed to a perspective that emphasized abstinence [5]. While modern abusers of substances must battle for recovery in the context of a variety of possible interventions, substance abusers in the nineteenth century had far fewer alternatives. There is evidence that these persons turned to a variety of social change movements and were met with various attitudes. For example, the political attitudes of temperance movement participants could sometimes be confused with other political stances (e.g., slavery). Thus, factors that were associated with the rise and fall of various social movements were also critical to attempts to establish programs to assist substance users (primarily alcoholics at that time).

2.2. Institutional treatment

Because of the difficulties associated with substance misuse, attempts have been made to provide shelter for persons who needed some form of assistance. These efforts to provide residential care have been referenced in writings as long as 5000 years ago [6]. By the early 1800s in the United States, the physical effects of alcohol were becoming clearer, and there was a significant increase in the number of institutions that emphasized the treatment of alcohol and other addictions [7].

Just as the public response to substance abuse was a product of complex forces, complex forces were also significant to treating institutions. Economic forces, primitive clinical methods, conflict within the field, and problems associated with individual behavior all contributed to a decline in the institutional treatment movement. It was clear by the mid-1800s that the search was on for more effective approaches to treating addictions. Not surprisingly, miracle cures were suggested in the context of entrepreneurialism. Innumerable chemical preparations and marketing techniques were seen [8]. The first "inebriate asylum" was called for by Dr. Samuel B. Woodward, whose efforts led to the establishment of the first real institutional treatment in the form of the New York State Inebriate Asylum, established in 1864. The first facility for women was the Martha Washington Home in Chicago that was established in 1867. Further progression in institutional care as part of the moral treatment that Dr. Woodward espoused was slow to grow.

2.3. The increase in legal controls

The sentiment of many Americans seemed to have been critical of the non-medical use of any drug, including alcohol and tobacco. From colonial times through the Civil War, these attitudes were associated with abstentionist outcries against alcohol and tobacco and calls for regulation. The regulation of substance use has been increasingly relevant to treatment since the proliferation of public regulations in the early 1900s. However, the energy expended to stem the availability and use of psychoactive substances has met with controversy. The specific consequences of both direct and indirect action included the intention to eliminate use, pressure to make the price of substances rise, and efforts to reduce social costs of use [9]. History has been clear that race, ethnicity, and social class have been highly tied to efforts to control substance use and that legal controls frequently represented bigotry and oppression that served the aims of dominant groups.

The path to regulation began with registration and taxation mandates. The first significant step in this regard was the Pure Food and Drug Act of 1906. At time in which there had been decades of proliferation of substances and their combination in Patent Medications, the Pure Food and

Drug Act established the requirement that medications with opiates and other drugs must provide a list of ingredients. This made opium and cocaine were early casualties of regulation attempts [10].

The Harrison Narcotic Act was passed in 1914 by the United States government. The original intention of the bill was to place a special tax on opium and coca, but the effect was to eliminate legal opiates. Alcohol and tobacco were also soon to be subject to growing legal pressure. Tobacco was not traditionally used in the form of modern cigarettes, but tobacco habits were fostered by the development of modern cigarettes, leading to large increases in tobacco use between 1900 and 1910.

The battle over alcohol was even to be more visible and controversial. Andrew Volstead of Minnesota saw his name attached to the Eighteenth Amendment to the United States Constitution. The result of the "Volstead Act" (H.R. 6810) was that from 1920 until 1933, and the manufacture, sale, and consumption of alcohol were prohibited in the United States. The failure of prohibition leads to the Twentieth Amendment that repealed federal prohibition in 1933. The states gradually repealed their own legislation ending with Mississippi in 1966.

As one alternative to the futility of broad prohibition, legally mandated treatment for substance abusers is now widely practiced [11], and legally mandated treatment is seen as a sensible approach for persons whose criminal offense is substance related. The intention is to direct the convicted individual to a system in which treatment is a more central focus then would be expected in a traditional correctional context. Critics of the approach question the propriety and efficacy of this strategy.

2.4. Spiritual traditions and intervention

Another common perspective on treatment of substance-related problems emerged from spiritual traditions. Spiritual traditions provided the foundation for a variety of approaches to substance-related problems. Some of this influence has been direct and some indirect. For example, a movement as broad as the American temperance movement was substantially derived from the evangelical movement. The Benjamin Rush speculated that religion by itself could "carry the day" with substance abusers [12]. The early view that religious experiences were an important path to recovery was bolstered by the perspectives of some early mental health professionals. Some professionals in health care were skeptical of religious approaches and others opined that religious approaches were only good for certain patients. Even within psychology, there were advocates for spiritually based intervention. The prominent work of George Cutton's *The Psychology of Alcoholism* (1907) and the broad work of the pragmatist William James (non-practicing M.D. and Harvard psychologist) went far to legitimize the spiritual view. James was well known because of the variety of his contributions related to psychology. James operationalized the center of religious conversion as anti-Christian by referring to it as "the hot place in a person's consciousness ... The habitual center of one's personal energy ([13], p. 196)." Despite knowing that reports of religious conversion experiences would be met with skepticism in a professional community of materialists, James felt that the results or specific components of spiritual interventions should be considered independent of the underlying assumptions of a particular spiritual perspective. The continued significance of the spiritual contribution to substance abuse therapeutics is reflected in a number of contemporary realities. The United States Congress passed a measure in 1996 that allowed states to contract with faith-based programs in substance abuse treatment. This led to an increase in emphasis on such programs and associated research into the effectiveness of such approaches [14, 15]. Typically, such programs include Bible study, church services, spiritually based therapy, in addition to a strict regimen of activities. There are continued efforts to clarify the precise nature of treatment that is based on Christian principles [16].

3. Models of misuse and methods of treatment

3.1. The diversification of substances

Many types of substances have been used throughout history for a host of purposes. Early North American settlers used a variety of preparations for a variety of medicinal and recreational purposes. Until the late 1800s, it was easy for opponents of substance use to locate their targets. Many substances began as legitimate medications and became used outside the clinic. Despite the widespread use of a variety of substances, it was not until the Controlled Substance Act of 1970 that anti-substance law began to keep up with the great variety of substances that are used. The proliferation and diversification of substance use, the variety of substance pharmacologic action, the impact of route of administration, and the host of socio-cultural factors have all been significant in the development of effective treatment methods [17].

Tobacco was first introduced to Europeans by Native Americans. Sailors adopted tobacco, both smoking the leaf and chewing it and brought tobacco home to Europe. By the time of the Civil War, alcohol and tobacco were established and clearly the most common American substances associated with problematic use.

Marijuana use has a long and complex history. Varied types of cannabis existed long before its appearance in the United States. Cannabis sativa was available in the early days of the new world, first appearing in South America in the 1500s [16]. Varieties of cannabis were both a medicinal/recreational substance and a critical crop for the American colonies in the 1700s. Hemp was grown for its fiber, and it was a major export for farmers as well as a source of rope and sail material. In the 1800s, hemp plantations thrived in Staten Island, New York, as well as in Mississippi, Georgia, California, South Carolina, and Nebraska [17].

At the same time that Hemp was so commercially and strategically significant, cannabis sativa was becoming better known. Cannabis was known to have been used for thousands of years in China, and "marijuana" became a widely accepted medication in the nineteenth century. Limited non-medical use of cannabis began to appear and the allegedly scandalous behavior of cannabis users was a featured item in the popular press in the early decades of the 1900s [17]. Publicity associated with anti-cannabis sentiments demonized the substance and patterns of its use and manifest subtle themes of bigotry against Mexican people.

Opium was a new entry to the American scene in the 1800s. Railroad laborers from China brought their opium smoking habit with them as they were hired by railroad magnates as less expensive labor than Americans. The connection between opium and the displacement of American workers was not to be forgotten and became a part of legislation that emerged later. However, the use of opium was not regulated by the mid-1800s, so opium and its extractions were readily available. For medical purposes, morphine had been derived from opium in the early 1800s and became an ingredient in some patent medicines (discussed below) in the United States. A vibrant patent medicine industry developed in the United States, with widespread marketing and distribution of a many products that contained large quantities of opium. These "medicines" claimed to cure just about anything, but they were really a vehicle for opium at an inexpensive price [17]. Perhaps, the most commercially dramatic development among the opioids was heroin. The Bayer Company first marketed heroin in 1898 as an (allegedly) addiction-free pain medication as well as a curative for abuse of other opioids.

Cocaine has a long history that first appeared in accounts of the chewing of coca leaves by the native populations of South America [17]. By 1844, cocaine had been isolated in pure form, though little use of it was made until later in the century. In the late 1870s, cocaine was used for the treatment of alcoholism and morphine addiction. In the 1880s, Sigmund Freud became aware of the use of cocaine to sustain Bavarian soldiers and started to experiment himself. He published his exuberance quickly, but he came to see cocaine as more problematic than he originally reported. Other distinguished medical professionals saw cocaine's beneficial potential. William Stewart Halstead found the mood enhancing and anesthetic properties of cocaine in the mid-1880s.

Amphetamines were first created in the laboratory in 1887, but it took 40 years for clinical applications to be realized. Military physicians used these stimulants for various purposes in the combat theater as well as in clinics. Illicit use increased in the military in the 1950s [17], and the use was also seen in truck drivers and students for a variety of medical conditions.

By the 1870s, Native Americans had begun ritual use of peyote, as had the Aztecs before them. For the Comanches, Cheyennes, Arapahoes, and other tribes, peyote rituals were a completely religious practice, requiring total abstinence from alcohol. Among these tribes, alcohol was considered to be a substance of considerable abuse. White land speculators sought to have peyote outlawed as a way to join with Christian missionaries and secure the Indian land. Much like other pursuits of criminalization of substances, there was a powerful motive that was different than the overt motivation [17].

As existing medications took more complex and pure forms, there was an increase in the promotion of "patent medicines." These preparations were promoted with great vigor, so had creative names and claims of effectiveness that were more associated with marketing than clinical effect. These preparations that were not actually patented were produced in England and began to appear in the colonies in the 1700s. The production of patent medications grew independently in the United States in the nineteenth century and was available through a wide range of vendors. Alcohol, cocaine, and morphine were common ingredients [18, 19]. These products included Laudanum (an alcohol preparation that originally included all of the opium alkaloids), Vin Mariani (a wine with coca leaves), and Coca-Cola (with cocaine as an ingredient).

In 1943, Dr. Albert Hofmann discovered what came to be a popular and widely used hallucinogen, lysergic acid diethylamide (LSD). Working with the fungus ergot to isolate components for pharmaceuticals, he accidentally ingested a small amount of the substance and had what has been described as the "first acid trip." Despite his careful account of the experience in a professional publication [20], his serendipitous discovery has been widely repeated and distorted. Hofmann went on to do further research in several areas and was persistent throughout his career in his criticisms of public claims of the great dangers of LSD.

3.2. Expanding treatment in the early twentieth century

Before the Second World War, there were relatively few treatment alternatives for a person in trouble with substance use. Concerned persons and some healthcare professionals complained about the limited treatment options, but most addiction treatment centered on the management of withdrawal symptoms (now known as detoxification). The result of the lack of treatment was increased the expansion of where addicts would seek mood-altering substances. The lack of treatment and expanding drug seeking combined with advancing criminalization led to the evolution of a new category of criminal. In addition, the United States Public Health Service became involved in the problem of addiction in the 1920s. State facilities for psychiatric patients and prisons were being overcrowded because of the arrests following the Harrison Narcotic Act [17]. In 1929, the Porter Act was passed, allocating funds to develop to rehabilitation facilities. The first results of this legislation were the new facilities in Lexington, Kentucky (1935) and Forth Worth Texas (1938). Treatment consisted primarily of withdrawal, convalescence, and rehabilitation. Outcome studies yielded disappointing results.

Three groups were critical to the development of what has become known as the "modern alcoholism movement." The Research Council on Problems of Alcohol, the Yale Center of Alcohol Studies, and the National Committee for Education on Alcoholism combined to promote a host of initiatives aimed at promoting treatment [21]. Following the Second World War, there was increasing understanding about substance abuse disorders and the need to organize public health efforts. The "disease model" (discussed below) was instrumental in promoting significant discussions about substance-related problems. Most treatment still occurred in general hospitals, state psychiatric hospitals, and private sanitariums. It is also significant that freestanding treatment programs began to appear. Many of the early freestanding programs became well known because of the unique ways in which they were developed. What came to be important to all of the treatment efforts that began to emerge was the nature of each facility's connection to alcoholics anonymous.

3.3. Alcoholics and narcotics anonymous

Alcoholics anonymous was established in 1935, and the eponymously named book of the central tenets of AA was published in 1939. AA is based on 12 "steps" that are central to the process of recovery and are considered to be indispensable to success. These steps are part of a program that is codified in the "Big Book" and is very specific about being effective for 75% of the participants [21]. With an avowed spiritual foundation (e.g., Step 2: "Came to believe that a Power greater than ourselves could restore us to sanity" and Step 5: "Admitted to God, to ourselves, and to another human being the exact nature of our wrongs"), AA developed a strong following and claimed considerable success. When AA was established, the treatment industry and the understanding of addiction could reasonably describe as being in its infancy. Despite claims made in the Big Book, the efficacy of AA is very difficult to submit to rigorous empirical evaluation due to the structure and procedures of the organization [22].

As noted above, the range of substances used and the associated problems expanded in the early twentieth century. Efforts to assist users of substances other than alcohol gradually expanded. By the mid-1940s, AA's co-founder Bill Wilson discussed the possibility of a group for a drug addicts that was separate from AA.

The first realization of Wilson's idea was called NARCO; it first appeared in 1947 and met weekly at the United States Public Health Service's treatment center in the Lexington, Kentucky federal prison. By the end of the 1940s, a NARCO member started a short-lived group called "Narcotics Anonymous" in the New York Prison System. By 1953, Narcotics Anonymous was clearly established in California [17]. Early members, many of whom were from AA, worked out the 12 Traditions for the new organization. Within a year, the first NA publication was printed, called the "Little Brown Book." There was controversy in AA and NA regarding Bill Wilson's experimentation with LSD. While he experimented under the supervision of a psychiatrist and a psychologist, the use of another drug (in addition to alcohol) was seen as antithetical to the letter and spirit of "Anonymous" teachings.

AA continues to foster a spiritual foundation and works to alter the thinking of alcoholics through "spiritual awakening." Studies of the effectiveness of AA have not produced clear results. AA is supported primarily by voluntary donations, and meetings are held in a vast array of facilities, including prisons, treatment facilities, hospitals, and churches. AA groups are available in most towns in the United States. Despite the relative paucity of efficacy studies, AA has been recognized by professional groups [21]. In addition, despite initial scorn by much of the medical profession, the American Medical Society recommended use of such self-help groups in 1979.

3.4. The moral and disease models

3.4.1. The moral model

Modern medical views of substance misuse claim to view the problem as a medical, rather than moral, problem. This appears to refrain from giving serious consideration to morality or values as the foundation for the problem. However, there is considerable evidence, in public opinion and its reflection in political discourse and the law, that substance misuse continues to be viewed as a moral problem. Consistent with current views, there is extensive history of morality as a dominant component of the views of substance abuse by many [23]. The moral view was, in part, a part of an absence of other useful perspectives. However, there is also substantial evidence for social control exerted from class and culture-related factors [24, 25]. Social groups who were so oriented would promote public campaigns in which misinformation and inflammatory information were promoted related to the types of substances used, the nature of substance use, and other conduct associated with substance use. Substance use and certainly misuse was proclaimed to be a manifestation of misplaced values and lack of moral standing. Today, criminal penalty remains a dominant approach to substance-related problems, despite considerable evidence that argues against the practical value of such an approach. Some elements of faith-related perspectives, while offering assistance to some users, continue to communicate judgment of these problems.

3.4.2. The disease model

One of the most significant developments in the intellectual representation of substance use disorders was the "Disease Model" of addiction. The first major proponent of this approach was Morton Jellenik [26]. Jellinek had witnessed the massive failure of the Volstead Act to stem the use of alcohol and began to write from the Yale Summer School of Alcohol Studies. The Disease model posits that certain individuals are vulnerable to substance use disorders as a result of (inferred) neurochemical dysfunction. This "disease" is characterized by, in part, an inability to control/inhibit behavior, loss of control, a failure to recognize the syndrome in one's self, and predictable decline. The disease model also suggests that the substance abuse vulnerability can/does occur independent of other problems and is chronic. Thus, the enlightened practitioner refrains from judgment of the abuser, and problems with substance use should be permitted to mitigate criminal punishment when crimes are committed [27]. The disease model is not always described in the same way, and it may be seen as having evolved since its first description. For example, despite the focus on factors internal to the substance abuser in the disease model, [28] characterized the disease model as being "multidimensional" and including psychological and sociocultural factors.

The later diversification of the disease model has done little to mute its detractors. Major objections to the disease model appear to be linked to the basic assumptions of any disease-related approach. For example, Wallace [29] called for a move beyond the disease model in the context of Native North Americans, suggesting that the disease model is particularly toxic in its neglect of context and culture in evaluating and intervening with substance-related problems. Feminist theorists have highlighted the construction of gender in the context of research and treatment approaches in general [30]. A behaviorist approach has also made cogent arguments against the disease model [31].

Recognizing the actual physical destruction that is a possible result of substance use, some behaviorists argue that a disease model is not needed at all for there to be adequate rationale for effective treatment. Consistent with general behavioral principles, the behavioral approach finds it more useful and even humane to view the problematic use of substances is a by-product of the interaction between unique features of virtual and reinforcement contingencies within their environment. That is, what is rewarding about the context in which a person has learned to use the substance? The behaviorist perspective also gives careful consideration to the nature of motivation, since the nature of motivation, or drive states, is critical to the reward value of environmental features.

3.5. Diagnosis of the substance-related disorders

The history of psychology and psychiatry includes a legacy of efforts to develop the most elegant and powerful nosology of disorders of psychological adaptation. There is evidence of attempts to categorize disorders as far back as the ancients, but increased focus emerged around 1900 and has accelerated since. The first comprehensive modern work was the Diagnostic and Statistical Manual (DSM) in 1952 [32]. Given that psychoanalysis still enjoyed hegemony in the clinical world of the late 1940s, the original DSM was relatively brief and grounded in clinical lore and psychoanalytic theory. The DSM subsequently evolved from a primarily psychoanalytic work to an atheoretical compendium that is designed to reflect the highest levels of clinical and empirical science. By the time of DSM-II (1968 [33]), the role of theory was substantially reduced and increasing specificity in diagnostic criteria was realized.

The introduction of the Diagnostic and Statistical Manual of Mental Disorders (Fifth edition: DSM-V [34]) brought revisions to previous diagnostic criteria in the DSM tradition. Most recently, the DSM-IV [35] used two main categories of substance misuse conditions, substance abuse and substance dependence. The DSM-IV criteria were considered to be inadequately descriptive of what was seen clinically, and the new criteria are claimed to be a substantial improvement. These two categories from DSM-IV were combined into one disorder in DSM-V that is diagnosed in conjunction with a rating from mild to severe. This also eliminates the "substance dependence" category, which was widely seen as easily confused with "addiction." While using the same underlying criteria, each substance is indicated as a distinct use disorder, including alcohol, cannabis, hallucinogens, inhalants, opioids, sedatives, hypnotics or anxiolytics, stimulants, and tobacco. Caffeine-related syndromes are not included.

It is important to review the DSM-V criteria for substance use disorder. It is important to bear in mind that each of these eleven criteria may be manifest in different ways and will be influenced heavily by the pharmacology of the specific substance. For each of the substances, the following are the eleven possible symptoms:

1. Taking the substance in larger amounts and for longer than intended
2. Wanting to cut down or quit but not being able to do it
3. Spending a lot of time obtaining the substance
4. Craving or a strong desire to use the substance
5. Repeatedly unable to carry out major obligations at work, school, or home due to substance use
6. Continued use despite persistent or recurring social or interpersonal problems caused or made worse by substance use
7. Stopping or reducing important social, occupational, or recreational activities due to substance use
8. Recurrent use of substance in physically hazardous situations

9. Consistent use of opioids despite acknowledgment of persistent or recurrent physical or psychological difficulties from using substance

10. *Tolerance as defined by either a need for markedly increased amounts to achieve intoxication or desired effect or markedly diminished effect with continued use of the same amount (does not apply for diminished effect when used appropriately under medical supervision).

11. *Withdrawal manifesting as either characteristic syndrome or the substance is used to avoid withdrawal (does not apply when used appropriately under medical supervision).

The DSM-V section with substance-related disorders includes gambling, which was not in the same section as substances in prior versions of DSM. The task force members for the substance and other addictive disorders section gathered findings that suggest that gambling disorder is similar in a number of respects to substance-related disorders. It is also thought that this development will make the accessing of treatment more likely. Other disorders that may be considered relevant (e.g., Internet, social media) have not yet been seen as having the empirical support needed for inclusion in this section.

4. Treatment approaches

There have been a staggering number of treatment approaches substance-related problems over the centuries [17]. It is virtually impossible to organize and categorize all treatment approaches, and the intersection of treatment method and type of professional further complicates the picture. The difficulties of professional domains and perspectives are further exacerbated by the relative lack of evidence for the effectiveness for different interventions [36]. In fact, there is some evidence to suggest that the specific treatment approach or technique is not as important to outcome as are factors associated with intervention relationships such as empathy [37]. Garner [38] issued a clear call for greater methodological rigor in studies of treatment efficacy to ensure development of treatment approaches that are grounded in empirical support. Recent suggestions have begun to clarify how this research might be conducted. DuPont et al. [39] suggested that addiction should be considered separate from other forms of health care because of the complexity and need for better kinds of research. In addition, they highlighted the high level of investment required in successful treatment, the variety of substances associated with disorders, and the varieties of organizational structures present in the treatment community. They also highlighted the severity, complexity, and chronicity of these disorders as important guideposts for the development of outcome measures. In light of the complexity of the treatment factors just noted, the final section of this chapter will highlight a few of the major treatment perspectives.

4.1. Detoxification

The critical role of detoxification in substance abuse treatment has continued since its central place in nineteenth century treatment. Because of a relative lack of knowledge about the exact impact of substance use, addictive processes, and treatment, there was obvious emphasis detoxification as an essential step in recovery. In addition, there was considerable emphasis on physical dependence as a central element of addiction. So, work with a patient began with simply clearing the body of the toxic substances, often with inpatient medical supervision and sometimes medications such as benzodiazepines. Today, detoxification is not technically considered to be actual treatment for a substance use disorder, though it is widely seen as a fundamental first step for treatment. However, contemporary perspectives on treatment manifest great variability in the rate of movement from detoxification to longer forms of intervention. The relative merits of gradual versus sudden withdrawal quickly became a matter of intense dispute in the medical community [1,42–44]. Modern research has identified factors that make detoxification a more effective part of a treatment system in which approximately one-fifth of annual admissions include detoxification [40]. The availability of intervention beyond detoxification is greatly influenced by healthcare economics. Despite efforts associated with the Affordable Care Act, many persons with substance use disorders are uninsured or underinsured. It is clear that finances are associated with the quality of intervention as well as limitations on the quantity and nature of service modalities. The Wellstone and Domenici move in 2008 to bring parity to mental health care did attempt to reduce barriers to treatment utilization, reduce financial burdens, and decrease stigma, though the success of those efforts is a matter of debate [41].

4.2. Harm reduction

"Harm reduction" is a relatively recent approach that functions in contrast to abstinence-only models. There have been several major contributors who have influenced this approach, though their assumptions and strategies are similar (in particular [1, 42–44]. With a pragmatic perspective that is theoretically inclusive, the harm reduction approach considers psychoactive substance use to be a part of the human experience and works to minimize damage resulting from use. The harm reduction approach, like many other approaches, considers substance use (and misuse) to be a complex result of many forces and maintains the view that there are constructive and destructive ways to use many substances. Without minimizing the real destruction from use, this perspective emphasizes the participation of substance users in reducing harm as well as the great significance of poverty, class, racism, social isolation, past trauma, sex-based discrimination and other social inequalities as vulnerability factors. With this broad emphasis, intervention is associated with the unique realities of the person who is struggling with substances and predetermined treatments are not embraced. Proponents of harm reduction thus characterize it as a public health alternative to moral, criminal, or disease models. From this point of view, it is appropriate to adopt a "whatever it takes" perspective on intervention with persons who abuse substances.

Peele, in particular, supports harm reduction and speaks in contrast to the AA tradition, promoting natural solutions in the context of careful goal-setting and the making of personal meaning in recovery. His writing includes specific arguments about the perils of the disease model. Peele argues that addicts are not different from other people in respects other than the addiction. In addition, Peele disputes a number of long-standing assumptions of the AA

http://dx.doi.org/10.5772/64264

tradition. He does not agree that recovery depends on forces outside the individual or that substance abusers are unable to control themselves in any situation. Since Jellenik's seminal contributions to the disease model, "addiction" has been perceived as a predictable, progressive, and fatal disease. Peele argues that this is not the standard progression through which an addict must inexorably pass, and recovery does not consist of a lifelong conscription to absence and twelve-step methods. In fact, Peele argues that the pessimism and determinism that are intrinsic to the disease model actually contribute to the likelihood of relapse and continued harm.

Some harm reduction techniques include methadone maintenance, which serves as a safer alternative to heroin use because of the longer half-life of methadone and the safer route of administration. Other approaches may include over the counter medications or even care in maintaining hydration with club drugs [45]. Needle exchange programs have been a highly visible and controversial approach to harm reduction that targets the high levels of risk associated with sharing intravenous drug administration supplies [46].

The harm reduction approach has been bolstered by the addition of mindfulness techniques [47]. Grounded in Buddhist tradition, mindfulness is considered to be the cultivation of awareness in the present moment. Mindfulness practices have been integrated into many of the therapeutic approaches since it began to appear in Western teachings in the 1950s. Mindfulness began to appear into the scientific literature associated with substance abuse treatment relatively recently [48].

4.3. Relapse prevention

"Relapse" refers to a return of problem behavior following an interval during which an individual has been relatively problem free. The study of relapse has been motivated by the prevalence of relapse, by attempts to bolster treatment effectiveness as well as to understand the persistence of substance-related problems. The practice of relapse prevention is an eclectic blend of a variety of approaches that have mixed empirical support. Many of these approaches are rooted in clinician beliefs and experience as well as guidance from recovering users. For example, "booster sessions" may follow the termination of regular treatment contact. Relapse prevention strategies are likely to be a part of a final phase of treatment and attempts to solidify relapse prevention may be a routine protocol during a termination phase. Recovering users are called upon to identify high risk situations and develop a range of robust coping mechanisms. Similar to this evaluation of the environment, persons in the treatment are encouraged to identify warning signs within him or herself as well as overall factors of vulnerability that may increase the risk of relapse. Attempts to generalize training experiences that are cultivated in treatment include exercises to bring lessons from treatment to real-life situations.

4.4. Interpersonal therapies

Since the inception of psychoanalysis in the late 1800s, the *relationship* between a would-be healer and a suffering person has been considered to be critical to the success of interventions. As the understanding of the fundamental conditions of therapeutic relationships advanced in the twentieth century, so did empirical support for the essential quality of certain therapeutic conditions. Interpersonal therapies were not initially designed for substance abusing persons, and the psychopharmacology of substances was recognized early in the history of psychotherapy as a complicating factor in treatment. Freud's exaltation of and subsequent struggle with cocaine is a well-known example of this uncomfortable reality. Early psychoanalytic theories of substance misuse were provocative and controversial [49–52]. In general, however, themes emerged that suggested that substance use problems developed in association with the person's inability to meet their inner needs in more adaptive ways [53].

Interpersonal approaches to substance use disorders are optimized when recognizing and incorporating psychopharmacological and substance use realities. In addition to the realities of substance misuse, patients are encouraged to confront issues that emerge in the absence of the substances. For example, a recovering user may be encouraged to grieve the "lost friend" of the substance. Shame is frequently identified and challenged as a factor in the inevitable frustration of needs. Defense mechanisms, originally couched in psychoanalytic language as negative factors, became seen as essential elements of psychic life and forces which need to be improved and not eliminated. For persons who use substances in problematic ways, defense mechanisms are identified as adaptive or maladaptive and modified accordingly. In general, the enhancement of self-expression and the relative satisfaction associated with human connections are bolstered in this approach.

4.5. Cognitive behavior therapy

Cognitive behavior therapy (CBT) may reasonably consider one of the dominant perspectives in mental health and substance abuse therapeutics today [54]. CBT is a blend of behavior therapy (BT) and cognitive therapy (CT). BT was originally introduced as an attempt to apply laboratory-based behaviorism to human change processes. BT was, in part, a reaction to psychoanalysis that was seen as pessimistic, deterministic, and nearly impossible to investigate empirically. An example of a behavioral approach to substance abuse therapeutics is contingency management (CM[55, 56]). CM uses the principles of operant conditioning and provides established reinforcers for drug abstinence or other objective measures of drug abstinence. The rewards may be a coupon for goods and services, a verbal reward, or small monetary tokens. This approach includes escalating rewards with rules for resetting the reward when there has been a relapse. Another example of a behavioral approach illustrates the role of contingencies on task participation (in contrast to abstinence as in the previous example). Spohr et al. [57] reported the results of behavioral approach in which rewards were established related to participation in probation and treatment of tasks.

Cognitive therapy has a broad history, in as much as there is evidence of some of the central tenets of the approach in the writings of the ancients [54]. While there are an increasing number of variants, cognitive therapy addresses thinking patterns that contribute to problems in adaptation.

Another approach that some consider to be within the cognitive behavioral tradition is dialectical behavior therapy (DBT [58]). DBT is an empirically supported therapy approach that was designed originally to assist persons who are struggling with symptoms of borderline personality disorder. Since its original development, it has been adapted for the treatment of substance use disorders [59]. DBT prioritizes risky behaviors (self-injury) and then works directly with substance use issues. Next, the approach attends to effects of substance use, such as legal jeopardy and vocational difficulties. Finally, DBT builds skills for broad psychological adaptation and relapse prevention.

4.6. Contributions from contemporary pharmacology and neuroscience

With the rise of neuroscience and a deeper understanding of cognitive processes, contemporary neuroscience has begun to offer evidence holds some promise of informing clinical efforts. It has been suggested [60] that mechanisms associated with motivation and control elements of addictive processes are better illuminated by advances in the neurocognitive laboratory than prior models. In particular, attentional bias, reward processing, and cognitive control are important areas of research that are soon to make direct contributions to treatment. These findings are consistent with early findings related in impulse control that indicate that impulse control problems is a likely culprit in at least the exacerbation if not a cause of substance abuse problems [61]. EEG study has suggested that patterns of substance misuse may be associated with detectable deflections in brain activity as assessed via quantitative electroencephalography (qEEG) methods [62]. The decade of the 2000s reflected increased interest in the role of executive function in a number of human problems in adaptation including substance abuse patterns. An essential element of executive function is the capacity to postpone, prevent, and/or arrest a behavioral response to permit time for the development of more constructive paths of behavior [63].

Some facets of substance misuse phenomena are being treated with repetitive transcranial magnetic stimulation (rTMS [64]). This non-invasive method uses an electromagnetic field that changes rapidly and induces electrical currents in the brain. rTMS has been found to have promising effects on some aspects of addiction-related cognitions. While there is continued investigation into the exact mechanism of effect of rTMS, craving has been seen as an area of patient difficulty that responds to rTMS [65].

The role of dopamine represents another avenue of research/treatment progress. While the direct treatment implications are not clear, it is important to note that the emerging work in physiology indicates that substance abuse and disinhibition are different [66]. Prominent striatal dopamine has an important influence on externalizing proneness (disinhibition) and on reward-based decision-making. Using eyeblink rate as estimator of dopamine level associated with disinhibition, investigators have found that dopamine is more strongly associated how much an individual "wants" (motivation) to learn about making decisions associated with tangible rewards. This orientation to learning about decision-making is then accompanied by working with an individual's broader substance use patterns that are associated with learning of action-reward contingencies [67].

For a number of reasons consistent with the approaches just noted, psychotropic medications have been used with some success to reduce vulnerabilities associated with substance misuse syndromes. Medication-assisted treatment (MAT) uses medications that can reduce cravings (agonists or partial agonists), interfere with the pleasurable sensations that come from use (antagonists), or create negative feelings with a substance is taken. Methadone, buprenorphine (opioid partial agonist-antagonist), and naltrexone (antagonist) have been used for opioid addiction. Antabuse has been used for alcohol since tire manufacturers noticed that workers could not drink alcohol after the vapors of the precursor of antabuse was inhaled during the vulcanization of rubber [17]. In the wake of problems associated with methadone maintenance, buprenorphine has become an effective alternative in reducing withdrawal symptoms and cravings associated with opioid dependence. For nicotine, there are three FDA-approved approaches to nicotine replacement. The FDA first approved nicotine gum (approved in 1984 and available over the counter in 1996) and the transdermal nicotine patch (approved in 1992 and over the counter in 1996) for smoking cessation. Finally, nicotine sprays (1996) and inhalers (1998) were approved for dispensing by prescription. Other psychotropic medications have been used in an off-label fashion to reduce depression and anxiety associated with recovery.

4.7. Motivational interviewing

Motivational interviewing (MI) is defined by its originators as a directive, client-centered counseling style for eliciting behavior change by helping clients to explore and resolve ambivalence [68]. The developers of MI affirm that MI is primarily a style of relating to service recipients rather than a specific set of techniques [69]. The originators of MI explicitly described borrowing many ideas from the interpersonal therapy tradition, and MI has become a "Gold Standard" for intervention. MI concepts include a focus on the capacities of the client, maintaining positive communication, an emphasis on resolving change-related ambivalence, and appreciating the variability in change readiness. In addition, empathy is emphasized and therapeutic resistance is a force with which one collaborates, and client inconsistencies are challenged. Further, MI emphasizes engagement with clients in empathic and collaborative communication, attention to established behavior change goals, and the initiation of change planning when the client is ready. There is a growing body of empirical work that supports the efficacy of MI for substance abuse disorders [70, 71].

Despite the fact that MI is touted primarily as a style of relating to patients, literature that followed its introduction highlighted specific techniques. These techniques were not forwarded as specifically essential to the approach but rather were considered to be naturally emerging and optimal examples of how the perspective might appear in practice.

4.8. Efficacy of treatment approaches

As has been discussed, various treatment approaches have developed for the treatment of substance-related disorders. In the interest of brevity, **Table 1** is presented with references pertaining to the nature of the treatment approaches and their efficacy. There are some important observations that are worth noting beyond the specifics of the table. Evidence continues to accumulate for the effectiveness of a variety of treatment approaches as well as the distinct cost advantage that treatment has over incarceration [72]. There is a continued call for "translational research" that takes findings from the laboratory and cultivates enhanced clinical practice [73]. New methods of assessing efficacy have been proposed that are more ecologically valid than traditional outcome studies, particularly emphasizing longer periods of follow-up [74].

	References	Notes
Evidence-based approach	[77]	Argues for more specific targets in treatment and reviews difficulties in empirical support for empirically supported treatments
	[78]	Examines issues associated with the development and use of evidence-based treatment research
Detoxification	[40]	An evaluation of the factors that are associated with successful detox completion
	[79]	Examined the impact of medically assisted detoxification on subsequent outcomes
Harm reduction	[80]	Reviews approaches to and perspectives on the harm reduction approach
	[81]	Evaluation of syringe dispensing machines and public impact – example of harm reduction strategy
Relapse prevention	[82]	Reviews three main approaches to pharmacological intervention for relapse prevention
	[83]	Review of the effectiveness of relapse prevention with substance abuse disorders
Interpersonal therapies	[84]	Description of practical elements of family therapy approaches to substance abuse treatment
	[85]	Review of six articles that considered creative writing as a facilitator of the interpersonal therapy process
	[86]	Considers a broad array of approaches to improving the life of a substance abuser, including expressive therapy, art therapy, spiritual intervention, etc.
	[87]	Brief discussion of elements of interpersonal intervention with substance abusers
	[37]	A discussion of relationship factors in treatment of substance use disorders
Cognitive behavioral and behavioral therapy	[88]	Examined the impact of adding a trauma component to group-based cognitive behavioral therapy
	[57]	Outcome study of electronic reminders of goals for group of drug-involved offenders.
	[89]	Review of the effectiveness of mindfulness interventions with substance use disorders
	[55]	Evaluation of a contingency management program to reduce substance use

	References	Notes
Medication assisted and physiologic therapy	[90]	Report of a review of studies of transcranial magnetic stimulation on addiction
	[62]	A review outcome studies of the effectiveness of EEG Biofeedback for treatment of substance use disorder
	[65]	Evaluated the use of transcranial magnetic stimulation on smoking cue-induced craving
	[91]	Evaluated the use of selective serotonin reuptake inhibitors for substance use disorders.
Motivational interviewing (MI)	[92]	Discusses the combination of MI with cognitive behavioral technique
	[93]	Considered the connection between therapist attitude toward MI and impact on client interpersonal functioning
Drug court	[94]	Evaluated drug courts as a promoter of "turning points" for offenders in areas of self-esteem, relationship, educational development, employment
	[95]	Examination of the value of compulsory treatment of addiction in Australia and the United States
Alcoholics anonymous	[96]	Considers the value of the "therapeutic alliance" that develops in AA as a significant curative factor
	[97]	Examines the effectiveness of AA in a research method that reduces previous method problems. Support for the effectiveness of AA is reported.

Table 1. Representative literature of efficacy and application of treatment approaches.

5. Conclusion

The history of use of mood-altering substances is complex and controversial. For centuries, the conflict between the benefits of varied substances and the massive societal costs of the misuse of substances has been confused by political and economic motivations for action related to substance users. A contemporary response to the complexity and cost of substance-related disorders is the development of the drug court. The first drug court was created in Florida in 1989 [75] as there was growing awareness of the widespread presence of substance abusing offenders in the criminal justice system. As testimony to the appeal of the drug court concept, one may note that National institute of Justice reported that there were more than 3400 drug courts in the United States by the middle of 2014. Drug court programs consider an individual's unique patterns of use and associated consequences with a graduated series of rewards for the attainment of target behaviors. Early evidence suggests that drug courts are associated with lower recidivism [76]. Drug court may reflect the type of approach that fits the

http://dx.doi.org/10.5772/64264

complex and destructive influence of substance misuse. Drug court is a program that offers many services to legally mandated individuals, and it represents an intersection between several models of addiction, most notably the moral and medical models. Following a legal adjudication, a treatment and follow-up plan is created that involves the judgment and leverage intrinsic to the criminal justice system. Thus, the moral dimension of drug court serves as the "teeth" for the accountability built into the program. At the same time, the nature of the substance use problem is assessed and diagnosed by treatment facilities that work in concert with the court. Treatment is based on the prevailing diagnostic system (DSM, ICD) that reflects the specific diagnostic criteria and decision rules that characterize the medical model. With this combination of perspectives, the drug court concept may represent the interdisciplinary future of substance abuse therapeutics.

Author details

John Andrew Mills

Address all correspondence to: jamills@iup.edu

Indiana University of Pennsylvania, Indiana, Pennsylvania, USA

References

[1] Marlatt, G.A. (1998). Basic principles and strategies of harm reductions. In G. Alan Marlatt (Ed.) *Harm Reduction: Pragmatic strategies for managing high risk behaviors.* (pp. 49–66). New York: Guilford Press.

[2] Center for Behavioral Health Statistics and Quality (2015). *Behavioral health trends in the United States: Results from the 2014 National Survey on Drug Use and Health* (HHS Publication No. SMA 15-4927, NSDUH Series H-50). Retrieved from http://www.samhsa.gov/data/

[3] Mancall, P. (1995). *Deadly Medicine: Indians and Alcohol in Early America.* Ithaca, New York: Cornell University Press.

[4] Bynum, W. (1968). Chronic alcoholism in the first half of the 19th century. *Bulletin of the History of Medicine*, 42, 160–185.

[5] Dorchester, D. (1984). *The Liquor Problem in all Ages.* New York: Phillips and Hunt.

[6] Crothers, T.D. (1912). A review of the history and literature of inebriety, the first journal and its work to present. *Journal of Inebriety*, 33, 139–151.

[7] Jaffe, A. (1978). Addiction performing the present age: scientific and social responses to drug dependence in the United States, 1870–1930.

[8] Mason, L. (1903). Patent and proprietary medicines is the cause of the alcoholic and opium habit or other forms of narcomania: with some suggestions else to have the evil may be remedied. *Quarterly Journal of Inebriety*, 25, 1–13.

[9] Weissman, J.C. (1979). Drug control principles: instrumentalism and symbolism. *Journal of Psychedelic Drugs*, 11, 203–210.

[10] Terry, C.E., Pellens, M. (1928). *The Opium Problem*. New York: Committee on Drug Addictions, Bureau of Social Hygiene.

[11] Stevens., A., Berto, D., Heckmann, W., Kerschl, V., Oeuvray, K., Ooyen, M., Uchtenhagen, A. (2005). Quasi-compulsory treatment of drug dependent offenders: an international literature review. *Substance Use & Misuse*, 40, 269–283.

[12] Tyler, A. (1944). *Freedom's Ferment*. New York: Harper & Row.

[13] James, W. (1902/1985). *The Varieties of Religious Experience*. New York: Penguin Books.

[14] Grettenberger, S.E., Bartkowski, J.P., Smith, S.R. (2006). Evaluating the effectiveness of faith-based welfare agencies: Methodological challenges and possibilities. *Journal of Religion and Spirituality in Social Work*, 25, 223–240.

[15] Windsor, L.C., Shorley, C. (2010). Spiritual change in drug treatment: utility of the Christian Inventory of Spirituality, *Substance Abuse*, 31, 136–145.

[16] Neff, J.A., Shorkey, C.T., Windsor, L. (2006). Contrasting faith-based and traditional substance abuse treatment programs. *Journal of Substance Abuse Treatment*, 30, 49–61.

[17] Brecher, E.M. (1972). *Licit and Illicit Drugs; The Consumers Union Report on Narcotics, Stimulants, Depressants, Inhalants, Hallucinogens, and Marijuana—Including Caffeine*. NY: Little, Brown and Co.

[18] Cook, J.G. (1976). *Remedies and Rackets. The Truth About Patent Medicines Today*. New York: Arno Press.

[19] Hechtlinger, A. (1974). *A Great Patent Medicine Era; Or, Without Benefit of Doctor*. New York: Galahad Books.

[20] Hofmann, A. (1979). How LSD originated. *Journal of Psychedelic Drugs*, 11, 53–60.

[21] White, W. (2014). *Slaying the Dragon: The History of Addiction Treatment and Recovery in America (2nd ed)*. Illinois: Chestnut Health Systems

[22] Vetulani, J. (2001). Drug addiction. Part I. Psychoactive substances in the past and presence. *Polish Journal of Pharmacology*, 53, 201–214.

[23] Glaser, G. (2015). The false gospel of alcoholics anonymous. *The Atlantic*, 315(3), 50–60.

[24] Peele, S. (1987). A moral vision of addiction: how people's values determine whether they become and remain addicts. *Journal of Drug Issues*, 17, 187–215.

[25] Berridge, V., Edwards, G. (1981). *Opium and the People: Opiate Use in Nineteenth Century England*. London: Allen Lane.

[26] Harding, G. (1986). Constructive addiction as a moral failing. *Sociology of Health & Illness*, 8, 75–85.

[27] Jellinek, E.M. (1942). *Alcohol Addiction and Chronic Alcoholism*. New Haven: Yale University Press.

[28] Mills, W.R. (1993). Alcoholism: toward a better disease model. *Psychology of Addictive Behaviors*, 7, 129–136.

[29] Wallace, J. (1990). The new disease model of alcoholism. *Addiction medicine and the primary care physician. Addiction Medicine [Special Issue]. Western Journal of Medicine*, 152, 502–505.

[30] Thatcher, R. (2004). Fighting Firewater Fictions: Moving Beyond the Disease Model of Alcoholism in First Nations. Toronto: University of Toronto Press.; Peralta, R.L., Jauk, D. (2011). A brief feminist review and critique of the Sociology of Alcohol-use and substance-abuse treatment approaches, *Sociology Compass*, 5, 882–897.

[31] Heather, N. (1992). Why alcoholism is not a disease. *The Medical Journal of Australia*, 156, 212–215.

[32] American Psychiatric Association (1952). *Diagnostic and Statistical Manual of Mental Disorders* (1st ed.). Arlington: Author.

[33] American Psychiatric Association (1968). *Diagnostic and Statistical Manual of Mental Disorders* (2nd ed.). Arlington: Author.

[34] American Psychiatric Association (2013). *Diagnostic and Statistical Manual of Mental Disorders* (5th ed.). Washington, DC: Author.

[35] American Psychiatric Association (2000). *Diagnostic and Statistical Manual of Mental Disorders* (4th ed., text rev.). Arlington: Author.

[36] Cleary, M., Hunt, G.E., Matheson, Walter, G. (2009). Psychosocial treatments for people with co-occurring severe mental illness and substance misuse: systematic review. *Journal of Advanced Nursing*, 65, 238–258.

[37] Miller, W.R., Moyers, T.B. (2014). The forest and the trees: relational and specific factors in addiction treatment. *Addiction*, 110, 401–413.

[38] Garner, B.R. (2009). Research on the diffusion of evidence-based treatments within substance abuse treatment: a systematic review. *Journal of Substance Abuse Treatment*, 36, 376–399.

[39] DuPont, R.L., Compton, W.M., McLellan, A.T. (2015). Editorial. Five-year recovery: a new standard for assessing effectiveness of substance use disorder treatment. *Journal of Substance Abuse Treatment*, 58, 1–5.

[40] Timko, C., Below, M., Schultz, N.R., Brief, D., Cucciare, M.A. (2015). Patient and program factors that bridge the detoxification-treatment gap: a structured evidence review. *Journal of Substance Abuse Treatment*, 52, 31–39.

[41] Stewart, M.T., Horgan, C.M. (2011). Health services and financing of treatment. *Alcohol Research and Health*, 33, 389–394.

[42] Peele, S. (1975/2014). *Love and Addiction*. Watertown: Broadrow Publications.

[43] Peele, S., Brodsky, A. (1992). *The Truth about Addiction and Recovery*. New York: Simon & Shuster.

[44] Peele, S., Thompson, I. (2015). *Recover!: An Empowering Program to Help You Stop Thinking like an Addict and Reclaim Your Life*. Boston: Lifelong Books.

[45] Akram, G., Galt, M. (2009). A profile of harm-reduction practices and co-use of illicit and licit drugs in users of dance drugs. *Drugs: Education, Prevention, and Policy*, 6, 215–225. doi:10.1080/09687639997188.

[46] Ksobiech, K. (2004). Assessing and improving needle exchange programs: gaps and problems in the literature. *Harm Reduction Journal, 1*. doi:10.1186/1477-7517-1-4.

[47] Bayles, C. (2014). Using mindfulness in a harm reduction approach to substance abuse treatment. A literature review. *International Journal of Behavioral Consultation and Therapy*, 9(2), 22–25.

[48] Bowen, S., Chawla, N., Collins, S.E., Witkiewitz, K., Hsu, S., Grow, J., Marlatt, A. (2009). Mindfulness-based relapse prevention for substance use disorders: a pilot efficacy trial. *Substance Abuse,* 30. doi:10.1080/08897070903250084.

[49] Abraham, K. (1979). The psychological relations between sexuality and alcoholism. *In Selected Papers on Psychoanalysis* (pp. 80–90). NY: Brunner/Mazel (original work published in 1908).

[50] Jung, C.G. (1973). *C.G. Jung*: Letters, Vol. 11, 1951–1961 (pp. 623–625). Princeton: Princeton University Press.

[51] Petrie, A. (1978). *Individuality in Pain and Suffering* (2nd ed.). Chicago: University of Chicago Press.

[52] Witkin, J.A., Karp, S.A., Goodnough, D.D. (1959). Dependence in alcoholics. *Quarterly Journal of Studies on Alcohol*, 20, 493–504.

[53] Fenichel, O. (1945). The Psychoanalytic Therapist of Neurosis. New York: Norton.

[54] Thoma, N., Pilecki, B., McKay, D. (2015). Contemporary cognitive behavior therapy: a review of theory, history, and evidence. *Psychodynamic Psychiatry*, 43, 523–462.

[55] Benishek, L.A., Dugosh, K.L., Kirby, K.C., Matejkowski, J., Clements, N.T., Seymour, B.L., Festinger, D.S. (2014). Prize-based contingency management for the treatment of substance abusers: a meta-analysis. *Addiction*, 109, 1426–1436. doi:10.1111/add.12589.

[56] Burch, A.E., Morasco, B.J., Petry, N.M. (2015). Patients undergoing substance abuse treatment and receiving financial assistance for physical disability respond well to contingency management treatment. *Journal of Substance Abuse Treatment*, 58, 67–71.

[57] Spohr, S.A., Taxman, F.S., Walters, S.T. (2015). The relationship between electronic goal reminders and subsequent drug use and treatment initiation in a criminal justice setting. *Addictive Behaviors*, 51, 51–56.

[58] Linehan, M.M. (2015). DBT *Skills Training Manual (2nd ed)*. New York: Guilford.

[59] Neacsiu, A.D., Linehan, M.M. (2014). Borderline personality disorder. In Barlow, D.H. (ed.), *Clinical Handbook of Psychological Disorders* (pp. 394–461) (5th ed.), New York: Guilford Press.

[60] Franken, I.H.A., van de Wetering, B.J.M. (2015). Bridging the gap between the neurocognitive lab and the addiction clinic. *Addictive Behaviors*, 44, 108–114.

[61] Bechara, A., Damasio, H. (2002). Decision-making and addiction (part I): impaired activation of somatic states in substance dependent individuals when pondering decisions with negative future consequences. *Neuropsychologia*, 40, 1675–1689.

[62] Sokhadze, T.M., Cannon, R.L., Trudeau, D.L. (2008). EEG biofeedback as a treatment for substance use disorders: review, rating of efficiency, and recommendations for further research. *Applied Psychophysiology and Biofeedback*, 33, 1–28.

[63] Barkley, R.A. (1997). Behavioral inhibition, sustained attention, and executive functions: constructing the unifying theory of ADHD, *Psychological Bulletin*, 121, 65–94.

[64] Herremans, S.C., Van Schuerbeek, P., De Raedt, R., Matthys, F., Buyl, R., De Mey, J., Baeken, C. (2015). The impact of accelerated right prefrontal high-frequency repetitive transcranial magnetic stimulation (rTMS) on cue-reactivity: an fMRI study on craving in recently detoxified alcohol-dependent patients. PLoS One 10 (8): e0136182. doi:10.1371/journal.pone.0136182.

[65] Flores-Leal, M., Sacristán-Rock, E., Jiménez-Ángeles, L., Leehan, J.A. (2016). Primed low frequency transcranial magnetic stimulation effects on smoking cue-induced craving. *Revista Mexicana de Ingeniería Biomédica*, 37, 39–48.

[66] Finn, P.R., Rickert, M.E., Miller, M.A., Lucas, J., Bogg, T., Bobova., L., Cantrell, H. (2009). Reduced cognitive ability in alcohol dependence: examining the role of covarying-externalizing psychopathology. *Journal of Abnormal Psychology*, 118, 100–116.

[67] Byrne, K.A., Patrick, C.J., Worthy, D.A. (2015). Striatal dopamine, externalizing proneness, and substance abuse: effects on wanting and learning during reward-based decision making. *Clinical Psychological Science*, 1–15. doi:10.1177/2167702615618163.

[68] Rollnick, S., Miller, W.R. (1995). What is motivational interviewing? *Behavioral and Cognitive Psychotherapy*, 23, 325–334.

[69] Hettema, J., Steele, J., Miller, W.R. (2005). Motivational interviewing. *Annual Review of Clinical Psychology*, 1, 91–111.

[70] Lundall, B., Kunz, C., Brownell, C., Tollefson, D., Burke, B. (2010). A meta-analysis of motivational interviewing: twenty-five years of empirical students. *Research on Social Work Practice*, 20, 137–160.

[71] Shorey, R.C., Martino, S., Lamb, K.E., LaRowe, S.D., Santa Ana, E.J. (2015). Change talk and relatedness in group motivational interviewing: a pilot study. *Journal of Substance Abuse Treatment*, 51, 75–81.

[72] Mignon, S.I. (2015). *Substance Abuse Treatment: Options, Challenges, and Effectiveness.* New York: Springer Publishing.

[73] Woolf, S.H. (2008). The meaning of translational research and why it matters. *Journal of the American Medical Association*, 299, 211–213.

[74] DuPont, R.L., Compton, W.M., McLellan, A.T. (2015). Five-year recovery: a new standard for assessing effectiveness of substance use disorder treatment. *Journal of Substance Use Treatment*, 58, 1–5.

[75] Fulkerson, A. (2009). The drug treatment court as a form of restorative justice. *Contemporary Justice Review*, 12, 253–267.

[76] Shaffer, D.K. (2011). Looking inside the black box of drug courts: a meta-analytic review. *Justice Quarterly*, 28, 493–521.

[77] Magill, M., Longabaugh, R. (2012). Efficacy combined with specific ingredients: a new direction for empirically supported addiction treatment. *Addiction*, 108, 874–881 doi: 10.1111/add.12013.

[78] Miller W.R., Zweben, J., Johnson, W.R. (2005). Evidence-based treatment: why, what, where, when, and how? *Journal of Substance Abuse Treatment*, 29, 267–276.

[79] Merkx, M.J.M., Schippers, G.M., Koeter, M.W., de Wildt, W.A.J., Vedel, E., Goudriaan, A.E., dan den Brink, W. (2014). Treatment outcome of alcohol use disorder outpatients with or without medically assisted detoxification. *Journal of Studies on Alcohol and Drugs*, 75, 993–998.

[80] Kelly, S. (2014). Contingencies of the will: uses of harm reduction and the disease model of addiction among health care practitioners. Health: *An interdisciplinary Journal for the Social Study of Health, Illness and Medicine*, 19(5), 507–522.

[81] Duplessy, C, Reynaud, E.G. (2014). Long-term survey of a syringe dispensing machine needle exchange program: answering pubic concerns. *Harm Reduction Journal*, 11, doi:10.1186/1477-7517-11-16.

[82] Chithiramohan, A., George, S. (2015). Pharmacological interventions for alcohol relapse prevention. *Internet Journal of Medical Update*, 10(2), 41–45. doi: 10.4314/ijmu.v10i2.7.

[83] Witkiewitz, K., Marlatt, G.A. (2004). Relapse prevention for alcohol and drug problems. That was Zen, This is Tao. *American Psychologist*, 59 (4), 224–235.

[84] Kaslow, N.J., Broth, M.R., Smith, C.O., Collins, M.H. (2012). Family-based interventions for child and adolescent disorders. *Journal of marital and Family therapy*, 38, 82–100.

[85] Snead, B., Pakstis, D., Evans, B., Nelson, R. (2015). The use of creative writing interventions in substance abuse treatment. *Therapeutic Recreation Journal*, 44 (3), 179–182.

[86] Adedoyn, C., Burns, N., Jackson, H.M., Franklin, S. (2014). Revisiting holistic interventions in substance abuse treatment, *Journal of Human Behavior in the Social Environment*, 24, 538–546.

[87] Lorman, W.J. (2015). Psychotherapy in addictions treatment. *Journal of Addictions Nursing*, 26, 99–100.

[88] Haller, M., Norman, S.B., Cummins, K., Trim, R.S., Xu, X., Ruifeng, C., Allard, C.B., Brown, S.A., Tate, S.R. (2016). Integrated congitive behavioral therapy versus cognitive processing therapy for adults with depression, substance use disorder, and trauma. *Journal of Substance Abuse Treatment*, 62, 38–48.

[89] Chiesa, A., Serretti, A. (2014). Are mindfulness-based interventions effective for substance use disorders? A systematic review of the evidence. *Substance Use and Misuse*, 49, 492–512.

[90] Gorelick, D.A., Zangen, A., George, M.S. (2014). Transcranial magnetic stimulation in the treatment of substance addiction. *Annals of the New York Academy of Sciences*, 1327, 79–93. doi:10.111/nyas.12479.

[91] Zhou, X., Qin, B., Del Giovane, C., Pan, J., Gentile, S., Liu, Y., Lan, X., Yu, J., Xie, P. (2014). Efficacy and tolerability of antidepressants in the treatment of adolescents and young adults with depression and substance use disorders: a systematic review and meta-analysis. *Addiction, 110, 38–48. doi:10.1111/add.12698.*

[92] Cooper, L. (2012). Combined motivational interviewing and cognitive-behavioral therapy with older adult drug and alcohol abusers. *Health and Social Work*, 37(3), 173–179. doi:10.1093/hsw/hls023.

[93] Saarnio, P. (2011). Therapist's preference on motivational interviewing and its relationship to interpersonal functioning and personality traits. *Counselling Psychology Quarterly*, 24 (3), 171–180.

[94] Messer, S., Patten, R., Candela, K. (2016). Drug courts and the facilitation of turning points: an expansion of life course theory. *Contemporary Drug Problems*, 43, 6–24.

[95] Hall, W., Farrell, M., Carter, A. (2014). Compulsory treatment of addiction in the patient's best interests: more rigorous evaluations are essential. *Drug and Alcohol Review*, 33, 268–271.

[96] Kelly, J.F., Green, M.C., Bergman, B.C. (2016). Recovery benefits of the "therapeutic alliance" among 12-step mutual-help organization attendees and their sponsors. *Drug and Alcohol Dependence*, 162, 64–71. doi:10.1016/j.drugalcdep.2016.02.028.

[97] Humphreys, K., Blodgett, J.C., Wagner, T.H. (2014). Estimating the efficacy of alcoholics anonymous without self-selection bias: an instrumental variables re-analysis of randomized clinical trials. *Alcoholism: Clinical and Experimental Research*, 38, 2688–2694. doi:10.1111/acer.12557.

Chapter 7

Dual Diagnosis Patients First Admitted to a Psychiatric Ward for Acute Psychiatric Patients: 2-Year Period 2003–2004 versus 2013–2014

Carla Gramaglia, Ada Lombardi, Annalisa Rossi,
Alessandro Feggi, Fabrizio Bert,
Roberta Siliquini and Patrizia Zeppegno

Additional information is available at the end of the chapter

http://dx.doi.org/10.5772/63102

Abstract

Dual diagnosis (DD) is the coexistence of severe mental illness (SMI) and substance use disorder (SUD). The increase of DD observed in recent years has important implications for mental health services organization. The aim of this study is to assess the prevalence and features of DD over a decade, comparing the periods 2003–2004 and 2013–2014. We performed a retrospective study retrieving sociodemographic and clinical data from the medical records of patients at their first admission to the Psychiatric Ward of University Hospital "Maggiore della Carità" in Novara, Italy. Patients with SMI and comorbid SUD (SMI-SUD) and patients with SMI without comorbidity (SMI) were compared in the two periods, 2003–2004 versus 2013–2014. SMI-SUD patients in both 2-year periods were more likely to be male, younger, unemployed, living with parents (or alone, for the 2013–2014 period) rather than with a family of their own, and single (or divorced, in 2003–2004). The 2003–2004 patients were more frequently diagnosed with a personality disorder, whereas the 2013–2014 patients had mixed diagnoses. We have found differences in the possible predictors of substance abuse in the two periods as well: in both periods, male gender was associated with an increased risk of DD, whereas age >61 years was associated with decreased risk. Only in the first period (2003–2004) was having a university degree associated with a decreased risk of DD, whereas the diagnosis of a personality disorder was associated with an increased risk of DD; on the contrary, in the second period (2013–2014), living in a protective environment was associated with a decreased risk of DD. The identification of changes in the prevalence of first admission DD patients and their clinical and sociodemographic features may help to highlight an evolving pattern of substance use and to identify possible risk factors that may be the target of prevention and treatment approaches.

Keywords: dual diagnosis, first admission, inpatients, substance use disorder, addiction

1. Introduction

1.1. Addiction

The pathway that leads to addiction is characterized by specific steps: the initiation of substance use, the established use, and, finally, the development of addiction. Several factors are involved in this process, including genetic and environmental ones. The availability of the substance may play a role in each stage in the development of addiction, whereas the accessibility of a substance seems relatively more important in the initiation of substance use [1]. Evidence from family, adoption, and twin studies converges on the relevance of genetic factors in the development of addiction according to a complex model of inheritance and clinical and genetic heterogeneity [2–10]. The role of genetic, sociocultural, biological, and other factors, including drug availability, peer influence, social support, and type and psychoactive properties of the drug, varies across the lifespan and in different stages of the addiction process. Briefly, it seems that environmental factors (such as peer influences and family environment) have a stronger effect on exposure and initial pattern of use, whereas genetic factors play a major role in the transition from regular use to the development of addiction [11,12]. Moreover, it should not be overlooked that genetic factors underlying addiction may overlap to various degrees with those underlying other psychiatric disorders. For instance, studies focusing on the role of the COMT gene polymorphism in the genetic predisposition to mental disorders [including severe mental illness (SMI), such as schizophrenia, bipolar disorder, obsessive-compulsive disorder, anorexia nervosa, and attention-deficit hyperactivity disorder] have found that the same polymorphism may be involved in the pathogenesis of addiction and substance use disorder (SUD). Probably COMT increases susceptibility to mental disorders in general, whereas other genetic or environmental factors may influence the development of specific disorders, including SUD [13].

1.2. Dual diagnosis (DD)

The World Health Organization defines DD as the co-occurrence, in the same person, of a severe mental health condition (SMI) with a drug abuse or dependence disorder (SUD).

In 1993, First and Gladis [14] proposed to classify DD patients as follows: (1) main psychiatric disorder and secondary drug dependence, (2) main SUD and secondary psychiatric disorder, and (3) main psychiatric disorder and drug dependence. Discriminating among these three options may be particularly challenging in clinical settings, where it can be hard to understand whether it is the SMI that induced drug consumption or the drug consumption that induced or worsened the SMI.

http://dx.doi.org/10.5772/63102

Consistent with the first class proposed by First and Gladis (psychiatric disorder first and subsequent drug dependence), the study of the psychological attitudes in addiction disorders has lead to the self-medication hypothesis (SMH) proposed by Khantzian [15]. The SMH primarily derives from clinical observations and posits substance dependence as a compensatory means to modulate emotions and aimed at self-soothing in response to distressing psychological states. According to this hypothesis, drugs would become addicting because of their power to alleviate, counteract, or modulate psychological suffering; there would also be a considerable degree of specificity in a person's choice of drugs because of unique psychological and physiological effects [15]. Hence, emotional states and distress, as well as expectancy of positive affective modifications, would be associated with substance use or relapse in people with SUD [16]. The SMH has received a variable empirical support, particularly as far as drug specificity is concerned [17]. The choice of type of drug according to the SMH is sometimes counterintuitive. For instance, while DD bipolar patients seem to use substances to maintain a euphoric state or soothe a depressive suffering, depressed patients, who might be expected to choose stimulants as well, often turn to depressants such as alcohol. Schizophrenic patients are often strongly nicotine addicted, and their heavy smoking may be an attempt to alleviate cognitive deficits and to reduce extrapyramidal side effects induced by antipsychotic medication, through the effect of nicotine on dopaminergic activity [18]. Briefly, the choice of a particular type of substance could depend on the symptoms that patients wish to relieve, as well as on substance availability, and on patients' basic personality traits [19]. Moreover, clinical experience in the last years has highlighted clear and ongoing changes in the choice of type of drug [from heroin and lysergic acid diethylamide (LSD) to the current so-called "smart drugs", vegetable or synthetic origin compounds with psychoactive effects that are not yet considered illegal]. For instance, changes in the prevalence of commonly used substances in people with DD have been discussed in two studies that estimated the prevalence of SUD in patients with SMI in Philadelphia [20,21]. These studies found a shift from cannabis being the most commonly used drug to cocaine and associated changes in demographic correlates. Although these data date back to more than 20 years ago, they highlight the changing pattern of SUD [22,23].

Consistent with these results, in Italy, in the last two decades, significant changes in the main drug used by patients attending addiction services have been noticed. Although the use of alcohol has remained relatively stable, there has been a significant decrease in the use of heroin and an opposite tendency regarding the use of cocaine; moreover, the use of "smart drugs" and polyabuse (i.e., the abuse of several substances simultaneously) has increased in an alarming way. The reasons underlying the use of new drugs may be different from those guiding the first heroin addicts. For instance, ecstasy has been generally chosen by adolescents and young adults for its entactogenic properties (the stimulation and enhancement of feelings of empathy, love, and presumed emotional closeness to others) [24,25].

As already suggested, personality may play a relevant role in the choice of the drug and expectations concerning the desired effect of the drug itself. The motivation leading to drug abuse may span from alleviating boredom and active search for pleasure, improvement of attention and performance, to reducing tension and decreasing mental illness symptoms.

Hence, personality traits should be assessed to improve the understanding of the complex relation between patients, drugs, and environment [26].

According to Cloninger's model [27,28], personality consists of temperament and character traits. Temperament is defined as a biological disposition reflected by relatively stable features related to mood, attitudes towards the environment, and reactivity to external and internal stimuli, including variability and intensity in emotional dispositions [29,30], whereas character is based on mechanisms that are developed through life experience. Although only a few studies have investigated personality dimensions in DD patients with the model developed by Cloninger, most of these found an association with high scores on the temperamental dimension of "novelty seeking" [31,32] as well as with high scores on "harm avoidance" [31]. According to Cloninger's descriptions of these temperament dimensions, we may expect patients with high scores on "novelty seeking" using drugs to search pleasure and to escape boredom and patients with high scores on "harm avoidance" using substances to achieve relief from tension and unpleasant or painful emotional states [33].

1.3. Epidemiology and clinical features of DD patients

Comorbidity between drug and/or alcohol dependence and a SMI is highly prevalent, and clinicians should be aware that patients asking for a psychiatric advice are likely to conceal their problems related to use and/or abuse of substances, unless specifically asked about them [34,35], possibly leading to an underestimation of DD. Recent studies report that the prevalence of DD in patients attending mental health service and substance misuse services ranges between 55% and 85% [36,37], and an association between SUD and mood and anxiety disorders has been supported by epidemiological and clinical studies [38–41]. In 2014, in the United States, among adults with a past year SUD, 39.1% had a comorbid psychiatric disorder, whereas, among adults without a past year SUD, only 16.2% had a SMI [42]. Moreover, epidemiological studies consistently describe a gender difference in DD patients as far as diagnosis is concerned; overall, DD is more common in males, and male patients usually suffer from psychotic and bipolar disorders, whereas depression and anxiety are more represented in women who, on the contrary, represent a smaller percentage of DD samples [43,44].

Many longitudinal or cross-sectional studies tried to identify recurrent and significant sociodemographic features and pattern/type of abuse typical of DD patients. The literature suggests that DD patients, compared to those with SMI but no comorbidity with SUD, are usually younger, males, with a lower level of education, often unemployed, still living with parents rather than with a family of their own, and with an overall lower social functioning [45–47]. DD is related to worst compliance to treatments, higher relapse rates and health services usage, more functional disability, and cognitive as well as psychological, physical, and social impairment [37,43,47,48]. Overall, DD patients show a poorer quality of life and reduced life expectancy [49] compared with patients with SMI or patients with SUD with no other comorbid psychiatric disorder.

The treatment of DD patients is particularly challenging because of the poor compliance and significant deterioration in social functioning that often occurs in these patients. They are more likely to suffer from comorbid medical conditions; as described above, they may experience

http://dx.doi.org/10.5772/63102

more difficulties in family relationships and troubles maintaining a stable job and financial situation; moreover, they may have legal problems related to the behavioral consequences of substance use and/or to the illegal attempts to obtain the substance. Compared to schizophrenia patients who do not use alcohol and drugs, patients with DD tend to have an earlier age of onset, more frequent and sometimes longer periods of hospitalization, more severe depressive and psychotic symptoms, more episodes of suicidal and violent behavior, more legal and financial problems, and higher mortality risk [50–56]. Likewise, bipolar patients with DD have 6.4-fold risk for violent crime compared with bipolar patients without comorbidity [57,58]. Overall, because they are less likely to adhere to their medication regimen, patients with DD also are at an increased risk of relapse and re-hospitalization [59,60]. However, even in those who do adhere to their medication, commonly abused substances can trigger or exacerbate psychiatric symptoms, eventually leading to relapse and need for inpatient treatment.

Although, in the last years, several studies have been performed about early detection and treatment of DD [59–64], there is a dearth of studies focused on the changes in the prevalence of DD in psychiatric inpatients [65]. A study about comorbidity with SUD in psychiatric inpatients performed in Spain [66] found 24.9% of inpatients having a SUD as well as another psychiatric disorder. Consistent with the literature about DD, a statistically significant predominance of men was found in the DD group together with younger age at the time of their first psychiatric admission; the most common diagnoses in this group were schizophrenia or related psychoses, although patients with SMI only had mostly affective disorders. As described above for preferred substance of abuse, the most used was alcohol followed by cannabis and cocaine.

Another interesting study assessing the trends in the incidence and demographic and clinical correlates of DD among patients whose first psychiatric hospitalization occurred between 1996 and 2010 was performed in Israel by Ponizovsky et al. in 2015 [67]. Based on the literature and their clinical experience, they hypothesized an increase of the proportion of DD among all first psychiatric hospitalizations during the study period due to the increasing prevalence of substance-related disorders in the general population, an increased vulnerability to DD on behalf of specific population groups (e.g., new immigrants) [68–70], and, lastly, higher DD rates in involuntarily hospitalized patients because they may be more likely to show episodes of suicidal and violent behavior [52] compared to voluntarily admitted patients. Over the study period, DD with drugs decreased from 1996 to 2010, whereas DD with alcohol and DD with both drugs and alcohol increased. The changing pattern of DD over time was supported as well as most findings concerning the sociodemographic features of DD patients reported in the literature. The positive predictors of DD with alcohol were male gender, previous suicide attempt, compulsory hospitalizations, and marital status. DD with alcohol was found mainly in immigrants, whereas DD with drugs was more common in the native population.

1.4. Challenges and perspectives in research

Treatment of DD patients requires a thorough understanding of both mental illness and addiction and the consequent integration of the traditional treatment approaches in both the mental health and addiction treatment fields [71].

In the research field, a complicating issue for DD studies is that they may focus on different populations: the general public, the population of subjects referring to psychiatric services, and the population of people currently treated by addiction services [72]. This diversity affecting the research field may be a concrete, challenging reality from a clinical standpoint. In Italy, this is particularly important because the standard practice for patients with comorbid psychiatric disorders and SUD is a parallel treatment. In our country, mental health and addiction facilities have different institutional cultures, etiological concepts, administrative arrangements, screening, and treatment approaches [73]. The problematic issues of such treatment approach include possible flaws in communication, collaboration, and linkage, which might significantly hinder or complicate comorbidity service delivery [74,75].

Even if it is clearly a changing and growing problem, the number of studies on DD prevalence in patients admitted to psychiatric wards in general hospitals in Italy is still scant. A recent study [76] has focused on differences in the length of stay in first-hospitalization schizophrenic patients with and without comorbid SUD and found that the first showed poorer symptom improvement and required longer stays than the latter. The flaws of communication and linkage between psychiatric and addiction services emerged from the study by Preti et al. [77], who reported that only approximately 30% of patients with SUD discharged from acute psychiatric inpatient facilities were referred to drug addiction services. Other issues that have been investigated in this field include SUD in emergency room settings [78], gender differences in DD patients [65], and attempts to understand whether SUD follows or predates the psychiatric diagnosis [79,80].

Considering these premises, the aim of our study was to describe the sociodemographic and clinical features of DD patients at their first admission to the Psychiatric Ward of University Hospital "Maggiore della Carità" in Novara, Italy. With more detail, we collected data about all patients admitted for the first time during the 2-year periods 2003–2004 and 2013–2014 to (1) assess the extent of comorbidity with drug abuse in a sample of patients at their first admission to a psychiatric ward in a general hospital in Italy; (2) investigate whether there are differences between inpatients with and without comorbid SUD, focusing on sociodemographic, clinical, and other background variables in both periods; (3) investigate the possible differences between patients with comorbid SUD in the two 2-year periods; and (4) identify the possible predictors of comorbidity with SUD and their changes over a decade.

2. Methods

We performed a retrospective study reviewing the clinical charts of patients at their first admission to the Psychiatric Ward of University Hospital "Maggiore della Carità" in Novara,

http://dx.doi.org/10.5772/63102

Italy. We assessed two 2-year periods: 2003–2004 and 2013–2014. We excluded the records of patients with a diagnosis at discharge of SUD with no comorbid psychiatric disorder. Because our interest was to focus on DD, we collected data about patients with comorbid psychiatric and SUD diagnosis (later on described as SMI-SUD) and about psychiatric patients without comorbid SUD (SMI).

The following information was retrieved from the clinical charts: (1) sociodemographic data, including age, sex, education, occupational status, living accommodation, marital status, and legal problems and (2) clinical and psychopathological history, information concerning drug use, history of self-harm (including suicidal and parasuicidal behaviors), and history of aggressive behaviors and acting out.

Psychiatric diagnoses were made during the hospital stay by experienced psychiatrists with the aid of the Structured Clinical Interview I [81] and II [82] for Axis I and Axis II disorders, respectively. According to the International Classification of Diseases [83], diagnoses were the following: schizophrenia and other psychoses, affective disorders, anxiety disorders, and personality disorders; disturbance of conduct, mental retardation, eating disorders, acute stress reaction, and adaptation reaction were grouped as "other diagnoses".

Information about the use of psychotropic drugs was collected by the treating psychiatrist during inpatient treatment, including age at first use and type of substance (alcohol, psychiatric drugs, cannabis, heroin, and cocaine; methamphetamine, ketamine, phencyclidine, LSD, butyl nitrite, amyl nitrite, and γ-hydroxybutyric acid were grouped together as "other drugs"). As for diagnosis, these data were then gathered for research purposes from clinical charts. The research project was approved by the Institutional Review Board of Università del Piemonte Orientale.

Statistical analyses were performed using STATA 11 (Stata Corp., College Station, TX, 2011). Initial descriptive statistics included the χ^2 test to evaluate the differences in proportions between groups (SMI-SUD vs SMI patients in the two periods). Then, a multivariate analysis was performed using a logistic regression to assess the potential predictors of substance abuse. The covariates included in the final model were selected using a stepwise forward selection process, with a univariate $p<0.25$ as the main criterion [84]. Results are expressed as odds ratio (OR) with 95% confidence interval (CI). A two-tailed $p<0.05$ was considered significant for all analyses.

3. Results

Patients first admitted to our psychiatric ward and matching the inclusion criteria described above were 227 in 2003–2004 and 257 in 2013–2014, respectively. The percentage of SMI-SUD patients was 25.1% in 2003–2004 and 32.7% in 2013–2014.

We divided patients in the following age categories: <18, 19–40, 41–60, and ≥61 years. In 2003–2004, SMI and SMI-SUD patients were 1.8% and 3.5% for <18 years, 42.9% and 56.1% for 19–40 years, 31.2% and 36.8% for 41–60 years, and 24.1% and 3.5% for ≥61 years, respectively. In

2013–2014, SMI and SMI-SUD patients were 2.9% and 7.1% for <18 years, 31.8% and 54.8% for 19–40 years, 38.7% and 33.3% for 41–60 years, and 26.6% and 4.8% for ≥61 years, respectively. Differences between SMI-SUD and SMI patients in age distribution were statistically significant in both 2-year periods, and patients in the SMI-SUD group were more frequently in the age category 19–40 years; moreover, in 2013–2014, this difference was found also in the age category <18 years.

Table 1 reports data about sociodemographic features in the 2003–2004 and 2013–2014 groups, further subdivided according to the presence or absence of comorbid SUD. The main statistically significant differences between SMI and SMI-SUD patients included gender, occupational status, and educational level. SMI-SUD patients compared to SMI patients were more frequently males (70.2% vs 39.4% in 2003–2004 and 70.2% vs 36.6% in 2013–2014) and unemployed (33.3% vs 15.0% in 2003–2004 and 41.3% vs 22.5% in 2013–2014) in both 2-year periods. Furthermore, in 2013–2014, a higher percentage of students (10.0% vs 6.5%) and lower educational level (junior high school; 63.0% vs 37.3%) were found in SMI-SUD patients compared to SMI.

	2003–2004 (*n* = 227)			2013–2014 (*n* = 257)		
	SMI, % (*n*)	SMI-SUD, % (*n*)	p*	SMI, % (*n*)	SMI-SUD, % (*n*)	p*
Gender			**≤0.05**			**≤0.05**
Male	39.4 (67)	70.2 (40)		36.6 (63)	70.2 (59)	
Female	60.6 (103)	29.8 (17)		63.4 (109)	29.8 (25)	
Nationality			0.209			0.334
Italian	94.1 (160)	98.3 (56)		86.7 (150)	82.1 (69)	
Foreign	5.9 (10)	1.8 (1)		13.3 (23)	17.9 (15)	
Educational level			0.179			**≤0.05**
Primary school	28.8 (49)	28.1 (16)		16.9 (28)	13.6 (11)	
Junior high school	38.2 (65)	50.9 (29)		37.3 (62)	63.0 (51)	
High school	24.7 (42)	19.3 (11)		37.9 (63)	18.5 (15)	
University degree	8.2 (14)	1.8 (1)		7.8 (13)	4.9 (4)	
Occupational status			**≤0.05**			**≤0.05**
Employed	38.1 (61)	48.1 (26)		31.4 (53)	33.7 (27)	
Unemployed	15.0 (24)	33.3 (18)		22.5 (38)	41.3 (33)	
Student	0.0 (0)	0.0 (0)		6.5 (11)	10.0 (8)	
Disabled/retired	25.6 (41)	7.4 (4)		29.6 (50)	10.0 (8)	
Other	21.3 (34)	11.1 (6)		10. 1(17)	5.0 (4)	

Table 1. Sociodemographic features of patients in 2003–2004 and 2013–2014. A comparison of the subgroups of patients, subdivided according to the presence or absence of comorbid SUD.

http://dx.doi.org/10.5772/63102

Table 2 describes the living accommodation and family features of patients in 2003–2004 and 2013–2014 and the comparison of the subgroups of patients, subdivided according to the presence or absence of comorbid SUD. The main statistically significant differences between SMI and SMI-SUD patients included living accommodation and marital status in both 2-year periods and having kids in 2013–2014. SMI-SUD patients compared to SMI patients lived more frequently with their family of origin (33.9% vs 19.2% in 2003–2004 and 33.8% vs 21.2% in 2013–2014) rather than with a family of their own, and they were more frequently single (48.2% vs 41.3% in 2003–2004 and 60.2% vs 33.5% in 2013–2014) or divorced in 2003–2004 (28.6% vs 12%). Moreover, in 2013–2014, SMI-SUD patients more frequently had no kids compared to SMI patients.

	2003–2004 (*n* = 227)			2013–2014 (*n* = 257)		
	SMI, % (*n*)	**SMI-SUD, % (*n*)**	**p***	**SMI, % (*n*)**	**SMI-SUD, % (*n*)**	**p***
Accommodation			**≤0.05**			**≤0.05**
Alone	25.8 (43)	23.2 (13)		18.6 (30)	27.3 (21)	
With parents	19.2 (32)	33.9 (19)		21.1 (34)	33.8 (26)	
Own family	49.1 (82)	28.6 (16)		49.1 (79)	29.9 (19)	
Therapeutic community	3.0 (5)	3.6 (2)		7.5 (12)	6.5 (5)	
Other	3.0 (5)	10.7 (6)		3.7 (6)	2.6 (2)	
Marital status			**≤0.05**			**≤0.05**
Married	38.3 (64)	21.4 (12)		44.1 (75)	22.9 (19)	
Single	41.3 (69)	48.2 (27)		33.5 (57)	60.2 (50)	
Widowed	8.4 (14)	1.8 (1)		6.5 (11)	3.6 (3)	
Divorced	12.0 (20)	28.6 (16)		15.9 (27)	13.2 (11)	
Siblings			0.412			0.112
No	22.9 (39)	31.6 (18)		20.0 (31)	29.9 (23)	
1	33.5 (57)	31.6 (18)		38.1 (59)	28.2 (22)	
≥2	43.5 (74)	36.8 (21)		41.9 (65)	56.4 (44)	
Children			0.277			**≤0.05**
No	47.1 (80)	50.9 (29)		35.6 (58)	63.3 (50)	
1–2	40.0 (68)	43.9 (25)		57.7 (4)	32.9 (26)	
≥3	12.9 (22)	5.3 (3)		6.8 (11)	3.8 (3)	

Table 2. Living accommodation and family features of patients in 2003–2004 and 2013–2014. A comparison of the subgroups of patients subdivided according to the presence or absence of comorbid SUD.

Family problems were reported as significantly more common by SMI-SUD patients in the years 2003–2004 than in SMI patients (21.1% vs 8.2 %, p=0.009), although no statistically significant difference was found between the two groups in the years 2013–2014 (47.9% vs 44.0%, p=0.588). Similarly, patients' parents were divorced in a significantly higher percentage of SMI-SUD patients than in SMI patients in the years 2003–2004 (7.0% vs 1.8%, p=0.047), although no significant difference was found in the two groups for this variable in the years 2013–2014 (84.2% vs 76.9%, p=0.604).

	2003–2004 (*n* = 227)			**2013–2014 (*n* = 257)**		
	SMI, % (*n*)	**SMI-SUD, % (*n*)**	**p***	**SMI, % (*n*)**	**SMI-SUD, % (*n*)**	**p***
Diagnosis			**≤0.05**			**≤0.05**
Affective disorders	24.1 (41)	10.5 (6)		17.9 (31)	4.8 (4)	
Schizophrenia/psychosis	25.3 (43)	7.0 (4)		22.5 (39)	26.2 (22)	
Personality disorders	23.5 (40)	52.6 (30)		19.1 (33)	23.8 (20)	
Anxiety disorders	7.6 (13)	0.0 (0)		30.1 (52)	22.6 (19)	
Other	19.4 (33)	29.8 (17)		10.4 (18)	22.6 (19)	
Self-injury behaviors	32.9 (56)	26.3 (15)	0.350	35.3 (60)	30.0 (24)	0.408
Acts of harm	4.7 (8)	12.3 (7)	**≤0.05**	11.8 (20)	26.3 (21)	**≤0.05**
Imprisonment	1.8 (3)	8.8 (5)	**≤0.05**	2.9 (5)	7.4 (6)	0.104

Table 3. Clinical features of patients in 2003–2004 and 2013–2014. Comparison of the subgroups of patients subdivided according to the presence or absence of comorbid SUD.

Table 3 reports the clinical and legal features of patients in 2003–2004 and 2013–2014, and the results of the comparison of the subgroups of patients, subdivided according to the presence or absence of comorbid SUD. The main statistically significant differences between SMI and SMI-SUD patients included diagnosis and acts of harm in both 2-year periods and imprisonment in 2003–2004. In 2003–2004, SMI-SUD patients compared to SMI patients were more frequently diagnosed with a personality disorder (52.6% vs 23.5%). In 2013–2014, the same difference was found, albeit less striking (23.8% vs 19.1%), together with a higher percentage of schizophrenia and psychosis in SMI-SUD patients compared to SMI patients (26.2% vs 22.5%). Acts of harm were more common in SMI-SUD patients than in SMI ones in both periods (12.3% vs 4.7% in 2003–2004 and 26.3% vs 11.8% in 2013–2014), whereas imprisonment was significantly more common in SMI-SUD patients only in 2003–2004 (8.8% vs 1.8%).

The following variables were included in the multivariate analysis: gender, nationality, educational level, occupation, marital status, living accommodation, family problems, acts of harm, imprisonment, age at admission, and diagnosis. The statistically significant results of the multivariate analysis performed to investigate the possible predictors of comorbidity with SUD are described in **Table 4**.

http://dx.doi.org/10.5772/63102

In both 2-year periods, female gender and age >61 years were associated with comorbidity with SUD with an OR <1 (adjusted OR 0.24, 95% CI 0.09–0.64, p=0.004 vs adjusted OR 0.15, 95% CI 0.06–0.39, p<0.001; adjusted OR 0.92, 95% CI 0.01–0.81, p=0.031 vs adjusted OR 0.03, 95% CI 0.01–0.31, p=0.003).

In 2003–2004, having a university degree was associated with a decreased risk of comorbid SUD (adjusted OR 0.04, 95% CI 0.01–0.64, p=0.023), whereas having a diagnosis of personality disorder was associated with an increased risk of SMI-SUD comorbidity (adjusted OR 3.51, 95% CI 1.05–11.77, p=0.042).

In 2013–2014, living in therapeutic rehabilitation center (compared to living alone) was associated with a decreased risk of SMI-SUD comorbidity (adjusted OR 0.02, 95% CI 0.01–0.41, p=0.011).

	2003–2004		**2013–2014**	
	OR (95% CI)	p	**OR (95% CI)**	p
Gender	0.24 (0.09–0.64)	**≤0.05**	0.15 (0.06–0.39)	**≤0.05**
Education level				
Primary school	Ref.	–	Ref.	–
Junior high school	0.46 (0.12–1.69)	0.239	0.63 (0.14–2.81)	0.546
High school	0.40 (0.10–1.64)	0.205	0.19 (0.04–1.03)	0.054
University degree	0.04 (0.01–0.64)	**≤0.05**	0.65 (0.08–5.02)	0.675
Accommodation status				
Alone	Ref.	–	Ref.	–
With parents	3.63 (0.92–14.27)	0.065	0.87 (0.23–3.26)	0.837
Own family	1.11 (0.17–7.14)	0.916	0.49 (0.12–1.98)	0.318
Therapeutic community	0.45 (0.04–5.84)	0.544	0.02 (0.01–0.41)	**≤0.05**
Other	5.40 (0.56–52.40)	0.146	0.63 (0.07–5.91)	0.691
Age at admission				
19–40 years old	Ref.	–	Ref.	–
<18 years old	1.39 (0.15–12.88)	0.771	0.60 (0.07–5.16)	0.644
41–60 years old	0.90 (0.30–2.74)	0.851	0.66 (0.23–1.87)	0.437
≥61 years old	0.92 (0.01–0.81)	**≤0.05**	0.03 (0.01–0.31)	**≤0.05**
Disease				
Affective disorders	Ref.	–	Ref.	–
Psychosis/schizophrenia	0.29 (0.06–1.38)	0.120	0.77 (0.16–3.68)	0.739
Personality disorders	3.51 (1.05–11.77)	**≤0.05**	2.21 (0.44–11.01)	0.334
Anxiety disorders	–	–	0.96 (0.22–4.18)	0.961

	2003–2004		2013–2014	
	OR (95% CI)	p	OR (95% CI)	p
Other	3.94 (0.99–15.69)	0.052	3.11 (0.56–17.11)	0.192

Table 4. Multivariate analysis for the assessment of potential predictors of comorbid SUD in psychiatric patients in 2003–2004 and 2013–2014.

As far as substance used is concerned, the assessment of the SMI-SUD sample in 2003–2004 and 2013–2014 highlighted a decrease of alcohol (78.9% of SMI-SUD patients in 2003–2004 vs 64.6% of SMI-SUD patients in 2013–2014) and heroin consumption (19.2% of SMI-SUD patients in 2003–2004 vs 14.6% of SMI-SUD patients in 2013–2014). Polyabuse did not seem to change after 10 years (42.1% vs 42.6%). On the contrary, we found an increase of the use of medication, cannabinoids, cocaine, and other drugs (0.05% vs 17.0%, 33.3% vs 57.3%, 28.0% vs 36.5%, and 0.05% vs 17.0%, respectively).

4. Discussion

The percentage of first admissions for SMI-SUD increased from the first to the second 2-year period considered (2003–2004 vs 2013–2014), being 25.1% and 32.7%, respectively. According to the existing literature, DD is a growing phenomenon. Studies performed in similar settings report a percentage of DD patients ranging from 24% to 51% [85,86]. In Italy, data from mental health departments and from addiction services describe a prevalence of psychiatric disorders with comorbid SUD ranging from 4% to 42%, respectively [87–91].

4.1. Sociodemographic and family features

Statistically significant differences were found in both periods between SMI and SMI-SUD patients as far as gender, age at admission, occupational status, marital status, and living accommodation are concerned. With more detail, SMI-SUD patients in both 2-year periods were more likely to be male, younger, unemployed, living with parents (or alone, for the 2013–2014 period) rather than with a family of their own, and single (or divorced, in 2003–2004). All these results are in line with similar reports from most other studies in this field. Regarding marital status and living accommodation, DD patients seem to experience relational problems in their families and have difficulties either creating or maintaining lasting relationships. Besides, comorbidity of psychiatric disorders and SUD may impact on relationships in and of itself. In a previous study [65], we found that this impact was particularly meaningful in female patients. Some differences between SMI and SMI-SUD patients were not shared between the two 2-year periods. For instance, in the 2-year period 2013–2014, SMI-SUD patients were more likely than SMI ones to have a junior high school degree rather than a high school one or a university degree and to have no kids [92]. On the contrary, family problems and parents' divorce were reported as significantly more common by SMI-SUD patients in the years 2003–2004 than in SMI patients. We may suppose an evolving pattern of substance seeking through the years; it may be that the motivation leading to addiction is shifting in most cases from relief of psychological and emotional distress to active search for pleasure and entactogenic effects. This hypothesis is consistent with the widespread changes in the choice of the main substance of abuse.

Overall, consistent with the literature [91,93], what emerges from these data is that SMI-SUD patients are more likely to have a poorer sociorelational functioning and achievement, albeit our results do not allow to discriminate which came first, whether comorbidity or a poorer performance, which are likely to be strictly intertwined.

4.2. Clinical features

In both 2-year periods examined, psychiatric diagnosis was significantly different between SMI-SUD and SMI patients. This difference is striking in 2003–2004 patients: SMI-SUD patients are more frequently affected by personality disorders and "other" diagnoses (including disturbance of conduct, mental retardation, eating disorders, acute stress reaction, and adaptation reaction), whereas, in 2013–2014, there is still a difference as far as personality disorders is concerned, albeit less striking, together with differences in "other" diagnoses and schizophrenia, which is more frequent in SMI-SUD than in SMI patients. These results are partially consistent with the existing literature [37,94–97] especially because of the under-representation of mood disorders in the SMI-SUD group of patients. On the contrary, this change in diagnosis is interesting, as it may suggest a different pattern of substance use after 10 years. It seems that schizophrenic and psychotic patients are more likely, in recent years, to use substances, but it is not clear whether this change suggests a trend towards more self-medication seeking on behalf of these patients or rather a greater potential of substances to induce long-lasting psychotic symptoms. It should be considered that the type of substances used have changed a lot over a decade; cannabinoid, ecstasy, and new drugs are studied for their potential of inducing psychosis, and in clinical settings, it is quite common to observe long-lasting, medication-resistant psychotic symptoms in young patients who have taken one of the several new synthetic drugs. Besides, these are difficult or impossible to identify and detect with standard laboratory methods.

As far as acts of harm are concerned, these were significantly more common in SMI-SUD patients than in SMI ones, in both 2-year periods, and overall, the percentage of acts of harm was higher in 2013–2014. Several studies have focused on the relation between substance abuse and aggressive behaviors; the use of substances may result in poor insight, neurocognitive impairments, hallucinations, impulsivity, as well as other emotional or physiological problems that may underlie aggressiveness. Moreover, some studies report that SMI-SUD patients are more likely to have a criminal history and legal problems than SMI ones [36]. Violent behaviors and substance abuse may be entangled because of the close relationship between drug distribution and the criminal system; moreover, the constant need of money to get the drug may lead patients to aggressive acts to obtain it [98]. Despite the almost 2-fold increase in the percentage of acts of harm from 2003–2004 to 2013–2014, only in 2003–2004 was the frequency of imprisonment significantly different in SMI-SUD and SMI patients, being higher in the first.

As far as substance used is concerned, our findings are consistent with the literature and with clinical observations, especially regarding the increased use of cannabinoids, cocaine, and "other" drugs on the one hand and the decreased consumption of heroin on the other. Surprisingly, we found polyabuse to be relatively stable even after 10 years.

4.3. Multivariate analysis

In both 2-year periods, female gender and being ≥61 years old appear to be associated with a decreased risk of SMI-SUD comorbidity. Both results are consistent with the existing literature and could be expected according to clinical experience [66,85–87,91].

In the 2-year period 2003–2004, having a university degree was associated with a decreased risk of comorbid SMI-SUD, whereas having a diagnosis of personality disorder was associated with an increased risk of comorbid SMI-SUD, but 10 years later we found educational level and diagnosis having no impact on comorbidity. As already described above, this may suggest possible changes in the pattern of SUD as far as problematic family issues are concerned; notwithstanding the fact that, in 2013–2014, educational level and diagnosis no longer represented risk factors, it would have been interesting to assess whether individuals with different cultural levels as assessed by schooling of with different diagnosis share the same pathways towards SUD and similar choices regarding type of substance and use. As far as educational level is concerned, in a recent study, we found that, although having a university degree was associated with a decreased risk of DD for males, it was associated with an increased risk of DD in females [65]. We hypothesized a different pattern of social functioning and performance in male and female SMI-SUD patients [44] and that males and females may access substances via different pathways and choose different types of substances as well [99–102], with a variable impact on their lives.

As far as diagnosis is concerned, the same study mentioned above, which assessed the period 2003–2012, found affective and "other" disorders associated with an increased risk of comorbid SUD, compared to personality disorders, which according to Baigent [94] would be more likely than Axis I disorders to be associated with chronic SUD. On the contrary, reports from the literature show mixed results about this issue, and recent studies suggest that the frequency of comorbid SUD is similar in schizophrenic psychoses and in personality disorders [37] and that primary mood and/or anxiety disorders are at high risk for comorbid SUD as well [96,97].

Last, in the 2-year period 2013–2014, we found that living in therapeutic rehabilitation centers was associated with a decreased risk (compared to living alone) of comorbidity with SUD. This result is encouraging and may support the effectiveness of such therapeutic settings in protecting patients from exposition and/or relapse into SUD.

5. Limitations

Some limitations should be underscored. The retrospective design and data gathering through clinical charts entail some limitations. Some information could not be retrieved, for example, detailed descriptions of type of self-harm or aggressive behavior. Psychiatric diagnoses were grouped into broad categories (affective disorders, schizophrenia and other psychosis, personality disorders, anxiety disorders, and others), and we did not discriminate between bipolar and unipolar affective disorders. We did not include data about laboratory tests objectively detecting drugs; nonetheless, it has been suggested that a urine drug screening can only identify a small additional rate (5%) of substance users [52]. Although it would have been interesting to assess details about reason for "acute" inpatient psychiatric admission, in this study, we focused specifically on a "snapshot" of comorbidity in a psychiatric ward over a 10-year period. Last, we cannot exclude that our results might have been influenced by broader systemic differences in the treatment of the DD population across time. Anyway, in our country, in the study period, there have neither been relevant changes in treatment options available for DD patients, not in the legal policies about drugs.

6. Conclusions

This study adds to the scant literature about this issue in our country, and the large sample size is a strength of this research. Both SMI and SUD are predictors of underachievement and failure in educational and occupational settings, difficulty facing family responsibilities, violent and abusing behaviors, poverty, legal problems, and scarce compliance to treatment [103]. Acute settings may be particularly appropriate for the development of targeted interventions [104], and the treatment of patients with comorbid psychiatric disorders and SUD should begin early during hospitalization [105].

Changes in the pathways leading to drug abuse and in the patterns of addiction should not be overlooked.

Author details

Carla Gramaglia[1], Ada Lombardi[1], Annalisa Rossi[1], Alessandro Feggi[1], Fabrizio Bert[2], Roberta Siliquini[3] and Patrizia Zeppegno[1,3*]

*Address all correspondence to: patrizia.zeppegno@med.uniupo.it

1 Psychiatry Institute, Department of Traslational Medicine, University of Eastern Piedmont, Novara, Italy

2 Psychiatry Institute, AOU Maggiore della Carità, Novara, Italy

3 Department of Public Health and Pediatrics, University of Turin, Turin, Italy

References

[1] Bierut LJ. Genetic vulnerability and susceptibility to substance dependence. Neuron. 2011;69(4):618–627. DOI: 10.1016/j.neuron.2011.02.015.

[2] Rhee SH, Hewitt JK, Young SE, Corley RP, Crowley TJ, Stallings MC. Genetic and environmental influences on substance initiation use and problem use in adolescents. Archives of Genetic Psychiatry. 2003;60(12):1256–1264.

[3] Furst Z, Riba P, Al-Khrasani M. New approach to the neurobiological mechanisms of addiction. Neuropsychopharmacologia Hungarica. 2013;15(4):189–205.

[4] Bierut LJ, Dinwiddie SH, Begleiter H, Crowe RR, Hesselborck V, Nurnberger JI Jr, Projesz B, Schuckit MA, Reich T. Familial transmission of substance dependence: alcohol, marijuana, cocaine and habitual smoking: a report from the collaborative study on genetics of alcoholism. Archives of Genetic Psychiatry. 1998;55(11):982–988.

[5] Heath AC, Bucholz KK, Madden PA, Dinwiddie SH, Slutske WS, Bierut LJ, Statham DJ, Dunne MP, Withfield JB, Martin NG. Genetic and environmental contributions to alcohol dependence risk in a national twin sample: consistency of findings in women and men. Psychological Medicine. 1997;27(6):1381–1396.

[6] Kendler KS, Karkowski LM, Corey LA, Prescott CA, Neale MC. Genetic and environmental risk factors in the aetiology of illicit drug initiation and subsequent misuse in women. The British Journal of Psychiatry. 1999;175:351–356.

[7] Kendler KS, Karkowski LM, Neale MC, Prescott CA. Illicit psychoactive substance use, heavy use, abuse, and dependence in US population based sample of male twins. Archives of Genetic Psychiatry. 2000;57(3):261–269.

[8] Kendler KS, Karlwoski L, Prescott CA. Hallucinogen, opiate, sedative and stimulated use and abuse in a population based sample of female twins. Acta Psychiatrica Scandinavia. 1999;99(5):368–376.

[9] Li MD, Cheng R, Ma JZ. A meta-analysis of estimated genetic and environmental effects on smoking behavior in male and female adult twins. Addiction. 2003;98(1):23–31.

[10] Tsuang MT, Lyons MJ, Eisen SA, Goldberg J, True W, Lin N, Meyer JM, Toomey R, Faraone SV, Eaves L. Genetic influences on DSM-III drug abuse and dependence: a study of 3.372 twin pairs. American Journal of Medical Genetics. 1996;67(5):473–477.

[11] Ducci F, Goldman D. The genetic basis of additive disorder. Psychiatric Clinics of North America Journal. 2012;35(2):495–519. DOI: 10.1016/j.psc.2012.03.010.

[12] Vink JM, Willemsen G, Boomsma DI. Heritability of smoking initiation and nicotine dependence. Behavior Genetics. 2005;35:397–406.

[13] Hosak L. Role of COMT gene val158Met polymorphism in mental disorders: a review. Science Direct. 2007;22:276–281.

[14] First M, Gladis MM. Diagnosis and differential diagnosis of psychiatric and substance use disorder. In: Solomon J, Zimberg S, Shollar E, editors, Dual Diagnosis: Evaluation and Treatment Training and Program Development. New York: Plenum Medical; 1993:23–38.

[15] Khantzian EJ. The self-medication hypothesis of substance use disorder: a reconsideration and recent applications. Harvard Review of Psychiatry. 1997;4(5):231–244.

[16] Kassel JD, Wardle M, Roberts JE. Adult attachment security and college student substance use. Addictive Behaviors. 2007;32(6):1164–1176.

[17] McKernan LC, Nash MR, Gottdiener WH, Anderson SE, Lambert WE, Carr ER. Further evidence of self medication: personality factors influencing drug choice in substance use disorder. Psychodynamic Psychiatry Journal. 2015;43(2):243–275. DOI: 10.1521/pdps.2015.43.2.243.

[18] Sagud M, Mihalijevic-Peles A, Muck-Seler D, Pivac N, Vuksan-Cusa B, Bratalijenovic T, Jakovlijevic M. Smoking and schizophrenia. Psychiatria Danubina. 2009;21(3):371–375.

[19] Sattler S, Schunck R. Associations between the big five personality traits and the non-medical use of prescription drugs for cognitive enhancement. Frontiers in Psychology. 2016;6:1971.

[20] Mueser KT, Yarnold PR, Bellack AS. Diagnostic and demographic correlates of substance abuse in schizophrenia and major affective disorder. Acta Psychiatrica Scandinavica. 1992;85:48–55.

[21] Mueser KT, Yarnold PR, Levinson DF, Singh H, Bellack AS, Kee K, Morrison RL, Yadalam KG. Prevalence of substance abuse in schizophrenia: demographic and clinical correlates. Schizophrenia Bulletin. 1990;16:31–56.

[22] Mueser KT, Yarnold PR, Rosenberg SD, Swet Jr C, Miles KM, Hill D. Substance use disorder in hospitalized severely mentally ill psychiatric patients: prevalence, correlates and subgroups. Schizophrenia Bullettin. 2000;26:179–192.

[23] Kavanagh DJ, Waghorn G, Jenner L, Chant DC, Carr V, Evans M, Herrman H, Jablensky A, McGrath JJ. Demographic and clinical correlates of comorbid substance use disorders in psychosis: multivariate analyses from an epidemiological sample. Schizophrenia Research. 2004;66:115–124.

[24] Rugani F, Bacciardi S, Rovai L, Pacini M, Maremmani AG, Deltito J, Dell'Osso L, Maremmani I. Symptomatology features of patients with and without ecstasy use during their first psychotic episode. International Journal of Environmental Research and Public Health. 2012;9(7):2283–2292. DOI: 10.3390/ijerph9072283.

[25] Torre E. Lezioni di Psichiatria e Psicologia Clinica. [Lessons of Psychiatry and Clinical Psychology]. Rome: Aracne Editrice; 2013

[26] Marquez-Arrico JE, Adan A. Dual diagnosis and personality traits: current situation and future research directions. Adicciones. 2013;25(3):195–202.

[27] Cloninger CR, Svrakic DM, Prybeck TR. A psychobiological model of temperament and character. Archives of General Psychiatry. 1993;50:975–990.

[28] Cloninger CR, Svrakic DM, Przybeck TR. Can personality assessment predict future depression? A twelve-month follow-up 631 subjects. Journal of Affective Disorders. 2006;92:35–44.

[29] Akiskal HS. The temperamental borders of affective disorder. Acta Psychiatrica Scandinavica Supplementum. 1994;379:32–37.

[30] Maina G, Rosso G, Salvi V, Bogetto F. Cyclothymic temperament and major depressive disorder: a study on Italian patients. Journal of Affective Disorder. 2010;121:199–203.

[31] Lukasiewicz M, Blecha L, Falissard B, Neveu X, Benyamina A, Reynaud M, Gasquet L. Dual diagnosis: prevalence, risk factors and relationship with suicide risk in a nation wide sample of French prisoners. Alcoholism: Clinical and Experimental Research. 2009;33:160–168.

[32] Latalova K, Prasko J, Kamaradova D, Sedlackova Z, Ociskova M. Comorbility bipolar disorder and personality disorder. Neuroendocrinology Letters. 2013;34:1–8.

[33] Fernandez-Mondragon S, Adan A. Personality in male patients with substance use disorder and/or severe mental illness. Psychiatry Research. 2015;228:448–494.

[34] Anthenelli RM. Focus on: comorbid mental health disorders. Alcohol Research and Health. 2010;33(1–2):109–117.

[35] Helzer J. Psychiatric diagnoses and substance abuse in the general population: the ECA data. NIDA Research Monograph. 1988;81:405–415.

[36] Torrens M, Gilchrist G, Domingo-Salvany A. Psychiatric comorbidity in illicit drug users: substance-induced versus independent disorders. Drug and Alcohol Dependence. 2011;113:147–156.

[37] Arias F, Szerman N, Vega P, Mesìas B, Basurte I, Morant C, Ochoa E, Poyo F, Babìn F. Estudio Madrid sobre prevalencia y caracterìsticas de los pacientes con patologìa dual en tratamiento en las redes de salud mental y de atencìon al drogo dependiente [Madrid study on the prevalence and characteristics of outpatients with dual pathology in community mental health and substance misuse services]. Addiciones. 2013;5:118–127.

[38] Bizzarri JV, Rucci P, Sbrana A, Gonnelli C, Massei GJ, Ravani L, Girelli M, Dell'Osso L, Cassano GB. Reasons for substance use and vulnerability factors in patients with substance use disorder and anxiety or mood disorders. Addictive Behaviors. 2007;32:384–391.

http://dx.doi.org/10.5772/63102

[39] Weiss RD, Kolodziej M, Griffin ML, Najavits LM, Jacobson LM, Greenfield SF. Substance use and perceived symptom improvement among patients with bipolar disorder and substance dependence. Journal of Affective Disorder. 2004;79:279–283.

[40] Regier DA, Farmer ME, Rae DS, Locke BZ, Keith SJ, Judd LL, Goodwin FK. Comorbidity of mental disorders with alcohol and other drug abuse. Results from Epidemiologic Catchment Area (ECA) Study. Journal of the American Medical Association. 1990;264:2511–2518.

[41] Goodwin RD, Stayner DA, Chinman MJ, Wu P, Tebes JK, Davidson L. The relationship between anxiety and substance use disorders among individuals with severe affective disorders. Comprehensive Psychiatry. 2002;43:245–252.

[42] Center for Behavioral Health Statistics and Quality. Behavioral health trends in the United States: Results from the 2014 National Survey on Drug Use and Health (HHS Publication No. SMA 15–4927, NSDUH Series H-50). Retrieved from http://www.samhsa.gov/ data/. 1 Choke Cherry Road, Rockville, MD 20857. 2015

[43] Rush B, Koegl C. Prevalence and profile of people with co-occurring mental and substance use disorders within a comprehensive mental health system. Canadian Journal of Psychiatry. 2008;53:810–821.

[44] Miguel L, Roncero C, Lopez-Ortiz C. Epidemiological and diagnostic axis I gender differences in dual diagnosis patients. Adicciones. 2011;23:165–172.

[45] Zhornitsky S, Rizkallah E, Pampoulova T, Chiasson JP, Lipp O, Stip E, Potvin S. Sensations-seeking, social anhedonia and impulsivity in substance use disorder patients with and without schizophrenia and in non-abusing schizophrenia patients. Psychiatric Research. 2012;200:237–241.

[46] Dragt S, Nieman DH, Schultze-Lutter F, Van der Meer F, Becker H, De Haan L, Dingemans PM, Birchwood M, Patterson P, Salokangas RK, Heinimaa M, Heinz A, Juckel G, Graf von Reventlow H, French P, Stevens H, Ruhrmann S, Klosterkotter J, Linszen DH. Cannabis use and age at onset of symptoms in subjects at clinical high risk for psychosis. Acta Psychiatrica Scandinavica. 2012;125:45–53.

[47] Morojele N, Saban A, Seedat S. Clinical presentations and diagnostic issues in dual diagnosis disorders. Current Opinion in Psychiatry. 2012;25:181–186.

[48] Benaiges I, Serra-Grabulosa JM, Prat G, Adan A. Executive functioning in individuals with schizophrenia and/or cocaine dependence. Human Psychopharmacology. 2013;28:29–39.

[49] Benaiges I, Prat G, Adan A. Health-related quality of life in patients with dual diagnosis: clinical correlates. Health and Quality of Life Outcomes. 2012;10:106.

[50] Szerman N, Vega P, Grau-Lopez L, Barral C, Basurte-Villamor I, Mesias B, Rodriguez-Cintas L, Martinez-Raga J, Casas M, Roncero C. Dual diagnosis resource needs in Spain: a national survey of professionals. Journal of Dual Diagnosis. 2014;10:84–90.

[51] Dervaux A, Laqueille X, Bourdel MC, Leborgne MH, Olié JP, Loo H, Krebs MO. Cannabis and schizophrenia: demographic and clinical correlates. Encephale. 2003;29:11–17.

[52] Latt N, Jurd S, Tennant C. Alcohol and substance use by patients with psychosis presenting to an emergency department: changing patterns. Australasian Psychiatry. 2011;9(4):354–359.

[53] Haddock G, Eisner E, Davies G, Coupe N, Barrowclough C. Psychotic symptoms, self-harm and violence in individuals with schizophrenia and substance misuse problems. Schizophrenia Research. 2013;151:215–220.

[54] Jiménez-Castro L, Raventòs-Vorst H, Escamilla M. Substance use disorder and schizophrenia: prevalence and sociodemographic characteristic in the Latin America population. Actas Espanolas de Psiquiatria. 2011;39:123–130.

[55] Schmidt LM, Hesse M, Lykke J. The impact of substance use disorders on the course of schizophrenia. A 15-years follow-up study: dual diagnosis over 15 years. Schizophrenia Research. 2011;130(1–3):228–233. DOI: 10.1016/j.schres2011.04.011.

[56] Maremmani AG, Rugani F, Bacciardi S, Rovai L, Pacini M, Dell'Osso L, Maremmani I. Does dual diagnosis affect violence and moderate-superficial self-harm in heroin addiction at treatment entry? Journal of Addiction Medicine. 2014;8:116–122.

[57] Fazel S, Lichtestein P, Grann M, Goodwin GM, Langstrom N. Bipolar disorder and violent crime: new evidence from population-based longitudinal studies and systematic review. Archives of General Psychiatry. 2010;67(9):931–938. DOI: 10.1001/archgenpsychiatry.2010.97.

[58] Drake RE, Wallach MA. Dual diagnosis: 15 years of progress. Psychiatric Services. 2000;51(9):1126–1129.

[59] Drake RE, Mueser KT, Clark RE, Wallach MA. The course, treatment and outcome of substance disorders in persons with severe mental illness. American Journal of Orthopsychiatry. 1996;66:42–51.

[60] Xie H, McHugo GJ, Fox MB, Drake RE. Substance abuse relapse in a ten year prospective follow-up of clients with mental and substance use disorder. Psychiatric Service. 2005;56:1282–1287.

[61] Buckley PF. Prevalence and consequences of the dual diagnosis of substance abuse and severe mental illness. Journal of Clinical Psychiatric. 2006;67(7):5–9.

[62] Deas D. Adolescent substance abuse and psychiatric comorbidities. Journal of Clinical Psychiatry. 2006;67(7):18–23.

[63] Vornik LA, Brown ES. Management of comorbid bipolar disorder and substance abuse. Journal of Clinical Psychiatry. 2006;67(7):24–30.

[64] Green AI. Treatment of schizophrenia and comorbid substance abuse: pharmacologic approaches. Journal of Clinical Psychiatry. 2006;67(7):31–35.

[65] Gramaglia C, Bert F, Lombardi A, Feggi A, Porro M, Siliquini R, Gualano MR, Torre E, Zeppegno P. Sex differences in first-admission psychiatric inpatients with and without a comorbid use disorder. Journal of Addiction Medicine. 2014;8(5):351–8. DOI: 10.1097/ADM.0000000000000062.

[66] Rodriguez-Jiménez R, Aragués M, Jiménez-Arriero MA, Ponce G, Munoz A, Bagney A, Hoenicka J, Palomo T. Dual diagnosis in psychiatric inpatients: prevalence and general characteristics. Investigacion Clinica. 2008;49(2):195–205.

[67] Ponizovsky AM, Rosca P, Haklai Z, Goldberger N. Trends in dual diagnosis of severe mental illness and substance use disorder, 1996–2010, Israel. Drug and Alcohol Dependence. 2015;148:203–208.

[68] Ritsner M, Ponizovsky A. Psychological distress through immigration: the two-phase temporal pattern? International Journal of Social Psychiatry. 1999;45:125–139.

[69] Ponizovsky AM, Radomiselensky I, Grinshpoon A. Psychological distress and its demographical associations in an immigrant population: findings from the Israeli National Health Survey. Australian & New Zealand Journal of Psychiatry. 2009;43:68–75.

[70] Margolese HC, Malchy L, Negrete JC, Tempier R, Gill K. Drug and alcohol use among patients with schizophrenia and related psychoses: level and consequences. Schizophrenia Research. 2004;67:157–166.

[71] Ziedonis DM. Integrated treatment of co-occurring mental illness and addiction: clinical intervention, program and system perspectives. CNS Spectrum. 2004;9:892–904, 925.

[72] Rassol GH. Dual Diagnosis: Substance Misuse and Psychiatric Disorders. Oxford: Blackwell Science; 2002.

[73] Carrà G, Clerici M. Dual diagnosis: policy and practice in Italy. The American Journal of Addictions. 2006;15:125–130.

[74] Pozzi G, Frustaci A, Janiri L. The challenge of psychiatric comorbidity to the public services for drug dependence in Italy: a national survey. Drug and Alcohol Dependence Journal. 2008;82:224–230.

[75] Canaway R, Merkes M. Barriers to comorbidity service delivery: the complexities of dual diagnosis and the need to agree on terminology and conceptual frameworks. Australian Health Review. 2010;34:262–268.

[76] Picci RL, Versino E, Oliva F. Does substance use disorder affect clinical expression in first-hospitalization patients with schizophrenia? Psychiatric Research. 2013;210(3):780–786.

[77] Preti A, Rucci P, Gigantesco A. Progress acute group. Patterns of care in patients discharged from acute psychiatric inpatients facilities: a national survey in Italy. Social Psychiatry and Psychiatric Epidemiology. 2009;44:767–776.

[78] Testa A, Giannuzzi R, Sollazzo F. Psychiatric emergencies (part II): psychiatric disorders coexisting with organic diseases. European Review for Medical and Pharmacological Sciences. 2013;17(1):65–85.

[79] Bizzarri JV, Rucci P, Sbrana A, Miniati M, Raimondi F, Ravani L, Massei GJ, Milani F, Massei G, Gonnelli C, Cassano GB. Substance use in severe mental illness: self-medication and vulnerability factors. Psychiatry Research. 2009;165:88–95.

[80] Maremmani AG, Dell'Osso L, Pacini M, Popovic D, Rovai L, Torrens M, Perugi G, Maremmani I. Dual diagnosis and chronology of illness in treatment-seeking Italian patients dependent on heroin. Journal of Addictive Disease. 2011;30:123–135.

[81] First MB, Spitzer RL, Gibbon M. SCID I Interviste Cliniche Strutturate per il DSM-IV. L'assessment secondo i criteri del DSM-IV [Structured Clinical Interview for DSM-IV. Assessment according to DSM-IV criteria]. Florence, Giunti O.S. Organizzazioni Speciali; 2000.

[82] First MB, Spitzer RL, Gibbon M. SCID II Interviste Cliniche Strutturate per il DSM-IV. L'assessment secondo i criteri del DSM-IV [Structured Clinical Interview for DSM-IV. Assessment according to DSM-IV criteria]. Florence, Giunti O.S. Organizzazioni Speciali; 2003.

[83] World Health Organization. International Classification of Disease. Roma: Istituto Poligrafico e Zecca dello Stato; 2002.

[84] Hosmer DW, Lemeshow S. Applied Logistic Regression. New York: Wiley & Sons; 1989.

[85] Katz G, Durst R, Shufman E. Substance abuse in hospitalized psychiatric patients. The Israel Medical Association Journal. 2008;10:672–675.

[86] Weich L, Pienaar W. Occurrence of comorbid substance use disorders among acute psychiatric inpatients at Stikland Hospital in the Western Cape, South Africa. African Journal of Psychiatry. 2009;12(3):213–217.

[87] Di Furia L, Pizza M, Cavarzeran F. Psychiatric co-morbidity in drug dependence. Bollettino per le Farmacodipendenze e l'Alcolismo [Drug Dependance and Alcoholism Bulletin]. 2005; Year XXVIII:1–2.

[88] Siliquini R, Piat SC, Zeppegno P, Ghico S, Torre E, Renga G. Psychoactive drug consumption and psychiatric disorders: a case control study. European Journal of Public Health. 2005;15:149.

[89] Zeppegno P, Airoldi P, Manzetti E, Panella M, Renna M, Torre E. Involuntary psychiatric admissions: a retrospective study of 460 cases. European Journal of Psychiatry. 2005;19:133–143.

[90] Zeppegno P, Probo M, Ferrante D, Lavatelli L, Airoldi P, Magnani C, Torre E. First admission for psychoses in Eastern Piedmont Italy. European Journal of Psychiatry. 2009;23:153–165.

[91] Relazione annuale al Parlamento sullo Stato delle Tossicodipendenze in Italia. 2015. Relazione annuale al Parlamento sullo Stato delle Tossicodipendenze in Italia. 2015. [Annual Report to Parliament on the State of Drug Addiction in Italy. 2015]. Available at: www.politicheantidroga.gov.it/attivita/pubblicazioni/relazioni-al-parlamento/relazioni-annuale-2005/presentazione.aspx [Accessed 08.01.2016].

[92] Hapangama A, Kuruppuarachchi KA, Pathmeswaran A. Substance use disorders among mentally ill patients in a general hospital in Sri Lanka: prevalence and correlates. Ceylon Medical Journal. 2013;58:111–115.

[93] Tosato S, Lasalvia A, Bonetto C, Mazzoncini R, Cristofalo D, De Santi K, Bertani M, Bissoli S, Lazzarotto L, Marrella G, Lamonaca D, Riolo R, Gardellin F, Urbani A, Tansella M, Ruggeri M. Psicos-Veneto Group. The impact of cannabis use on age of onset and clinical characteristics in first-episode psychotic patients. Journal of Psychiatric Research. 2013;47:438–444.

[94] Baigent M. Managing patients with dual diagnosis in psychiatric practice. Current Opinion in Psychiatry. 2012;25:201–205.

[95] Osuch E, Vinginilis E, Ross E, Forster C, Summerhurst C. Cannabis use, addiction risk and functional impairment in youth seeking treatment for primary mood or anxiety. International Journal of Adolescent Medicine and Health. 2013;25:309–314.

[96] Wu LT, Blazer DG, Gersing KR, Burchett B, Swarz MS, Mannelli P, NIDA AAPI Workgroup. Comorbid substance use disorders with other axis I and II mental disorders among treatment-seeking Asian Americans, Native Hawaiians/Pacific Islanders, and mixed-race people. Psychiatric Research. 2013;47:1940–1948.

[97] Torchalla I, Strehlau V, Li K, Aube Linden I, Noel F, Krausz M. Posttraumatic stress disorder and substance use disorder in comorbidity in homeless adults: prevalence, correlates and sex differences. Psychology of Addictive Behaviors. 2014;28(2):443–452.

[98] Zhuo Y, Bradizza CM, Maisto SA. The influence of treatment attendance on subsequent aggression among severely mentally ill substance abusers. Journal of Substance Abuse and Treatment. 2014;47(5):353–361. DOI: 10.1016/j.jsat.2014.06.010.

[99] Gearon JS, Nidecker M, Bellack A, Bennett M. Gender difference in drug use behavior in people with serious mental illness. The American Journal on Addiction. 2003;12:229–241.

[100] Maremmani I, Stefania C, Pacini M, Maremmani AG, Carlini M, Golia F, Deltito J, Dell'Osso L. Differential substance abuse patterns distribute according to gender in heroin addicts. Journal of Psychoactive Drugs. 2010;42:89–95.

[101] Chen KW, Banducci AN, Guller L, Mancatee RJ, Lavelle A, Daughters SB, Lejuez CW. An examination of psychiatric comorbidities as a function of gender type within an impatient substance use treatment program. Drug and Alcohol Dependence. 2011;118:92–99.

[102] Drapalski A, Bennet M, Bellack A. Gender differences in substance use, consequences, motivation to change and treatment seeking in people with serious mental illness. Substance Use and Misuse. 2011;46:808–818.

[103] Kessler RC, Nelson CB, McGonagle KA, Edlund MJ, Franck RG, Leaf PJ. The epidemiology of co-occurring addictive and mental disorders: implication for prevention and service utilization. American Journal of Orthopsychiatry. 1996;66:17–31.

[104] Carrà G, Johnson S. Variations in rates of comorbid substance use in psychosis between mental health settings and geographical areas in the UK. A systematic review. Social Psychiatry and Psychiatric Epidemiology. 2009;44:429–447.

[105] Bradizza CM, Stasiewicz PR. Integrating substance abuse treatment for the seriously mentally ill into inpatients psychiatric treatment. Journal of Substance Abuse Treatment. 1997;14:103–111.

Chapter 8

Review of Current Neuroimaging Studies of the Effects of Prenatal Drug Exposure: Brain Structure and Function

Jennifer Willford, Conner Smith, Tyler Kuhn,
Brady Weber and Gale Richardson

Additional information is available at the end of the chapter

http://dx.doi.org/10.5772/63389

Abstract

Neuroimaging tools have provided novel methods for understanding the impact of prenatal drug exposure on brain structure and function and its relation to development and behavior. Information gained from neuroimaging studies allows for the investigation of how prenatal drug exposure alters the typical developmental trajectory. The current prevalence and characteristics of prenatal drug exposure and its implications for vulnerable periods of brain development are reviewed. Structural and functional neuroimaging methods are introduced with examples of how study results from prenatal alcohol, cocaine, marijuana, and tobacco exposure further our understanding of the neurodevelopment impact of prenatal drug exposure. Prenatal drug neuroimaging studies have advanced our understanding of mechanisms and functional deficits associated with prenatal drug exposure. Studies have identified brain circuits associated with the default mode network, inhibitory control, and working memory that show differences in function as a result of prenatal drug exposure. The information gained from studies of prenatal drug exposure on brain structure and function can be used to make connections between animal models and human studies of prenatal drug exposure, identify biomarkers of documented effects of prenatal drug exposure on behavior, and inform prevention and intervention programs for young children.

Keywords: fMRI, prenatal substance exposure, alcohol, cocaine, marijuana, tobacco

1. Introduction

This chapter begins with a review of issues surrounding the assessment of the impact of prenatal drug exposure on developmental outcomes in children followed by a brief update of current trends in prenatal drug exposure including the prevalence, patterns, and characteristics of prenatal drug use, including alcohol, tobacco, marijuana, and other illicit drugs. Then, the impact of current neuroimaging methodology on our understanding of the effects of prenatal drug exposure is explored. The review considers examples of how neuroimaging tools have increased our understanding of the often subtle and complex impact of prenatal substance exposure on child brain development and behavior. The impact of prenatal drug exposure is challenging to assess due to characteristics of maternal drug use such as polydrug exposure and differences in the purity and legality of drugs. Developmental outcomes associated with prenatal drug exposure will also be affected by the timing, dose, and pattern of drug use during pregnancy, and the varying impact of other environmental factors such as maternal health and nutrition, access to prenatal care, and the home environment [1, 2]. For over 40 years, the impact of prenatal drug exposure has been studied in relation to growth, behavior, and cognitive outcomes using both longitudinal and cross-sectional designs, which have provided a depth of understanding. Overall, the most important outcome of decades of research has been that no safe levels of any type of prenatal drug use during pregnancy have been identified. Furthermore, the impact of prenatal drug exposure is often subtle and combined with other environmental risk factors, contributes to poor developmental outcomes for young children and adolescents.

2. Methodological Issues and Current Trends in Prevalence and Characteristics of Prenatal Drug Exposure

Prenatal drug exposure is a major public health concern for mothers and their children. In addition, society bears significant financial costs associated with social and child welfare services utilization [3, 4], neonatal intensive care unit costs, and longer hospital stays after delivery [3–8]. Children with prenatal drug exposure are also more likely to need intervention services to address medical, developmental, behavioral, academic, and socio-emotional issues [9]. Decades of research have documented the negative impact of prenatal drug exposure on child developmental outcomes including growth, emotion and behavior regulation, and cognitive function. The impact of prenatal drug exposure on the developing child has also been shown to interact with the quality of the child's environment. Given the complexities related to prenatal drug exposure and the influence of many potential external factors, the prevalence, characteristics, and effects on developmental outcomes can be difficult to assess. Difficulties arise from the dose, timing, and duration of prenatal drug exposure, the use of multiple drugs during pregnancy, methodology limitations in the ability to document prenatal drug exposure, differentiating between delayed and longer-term effects, genetic factors, and variability introduced by environmental experiences including the quality of relationships and the home environment [10]. In addition, methods used to measure prenatal drug exposure are varied, ranging from survey methods (e.g., national surveys) to prenatal interviewing (e.g., longitudinal cohort studies).

The main strategy for dealing with the complexities of research aimed at elucidating the impact and mechanisms of prenatal drug exposure on child development is to use longitudinal research designs that incorporate measurement of explanatory variables. Pregnant substance abusers are not studied based on whether they classify as "recreational" users or addicts. Rather, the timing (first, second, third trimester), dose, and pattern of drug use (continuous vs. binge exposure) are key variables. Among cohort studies, there are differences in sample characteristics that are important for the interpretation of any study results that suggest negative developmental outcomes associated with prenatal drug exposure. For example, some studies focus on "high- dose" exposure (e.g., Seattle Longitudinal Study of Fetal Alcohol Syndrome), whereas other studies focus on the full spectrum of exposures ranging from light-, moderate-, to high-dose exposure (e.g., Pittsburgh Maternal Health Practices and Child Development Project). Most studies have attempted to quantify the pattern of drug exposure as either continuous (e.g., average number of drinks/day) or binge (e.g., ≥4 drinks/occasion). Cross-sectional study designs are also used to study clinical populations, capturing the important characteristics of young children who have been referred for assessment and services.

Current trends suggest that while the prevalence of women using drugs during pregnancy is relatively low, maternal substance use has an impact on many children. Approximately 400,000–440,000 infants, 10–11% of all births, are prenatally exposed to alcohol, tobacco, or illicit drugs [11]. In addition, current trends in prenatal drug exposure suggest shifts in both the prevalence and patterns of maternal substance use that reflect both wide spread knowledge and perceptions of the impact of drugs of abuse in general, and prenatal drug exposure more specifically. Alcohol and tobacco are the most commonly used drugs during pregnancy, followed by marijuana, cocaine, and opioids [12]. For all types of prenatal drug exposure, the data show that reported use in pregnant women is lower compared to nonpregnant women in the same age category and that more pregnant women report use in the first trimester compared to second and third trimesters [12]. In general, a greater number of younger pregnant women (ages 18–25) report use compared to older women (ages 26–44) [12].

2.1. Current prevalence estimates of prenatal drug exposure

Recent estimates [12] show that the rates of prenatal alcohol use are approximately 9.4%, of which 2.3% of women report binge drinking and 0.4% report heavy drinking. Higher levels of drinking are reported in the first trimester compared to second and third trimesters. Patterns of alcohol use among pregnant women have changed over time. More recently, pregnant women are reported to drink more heavily and are more likely to develop an alcohol use disorder compared to earlier studies [13]. In addition, women of childbearing age have shown an increase in binge drinking, a trend that has decreased in males over time [14, 15]. Women who binge drink during pregnancy report, on average, 4.6 binge drinking episodes (nonpregnant women report 3.1 episodes) and the number of drinks consumed, while binge drinking does not differ from nonpregnant drinkers [2]. The Centers for Disease Control reports that medical record analysis shows a rate of 0.3 out of 1000 children ages 7–9 are diagnosed with fetal alcohol syndrome (FAS), while in-person assessments find higher rates (6–9 per 1000 children). Rates of fetal alcohol spectrum disorders are more difficult to ascertain, but community based studies in both the United State and Western Europe suggest that 24–48 per 1000 school children are affected by prenatal alcohol exposure [16, 17].

Reflecting national trends, the NSDUH [12] reports that cigarette use among women has been steadily decreasing from a rate of 30.7% in 2002–2003 to 24.0% in 2012–2013. However, during the same time period, the prevalence rate of cigarette use among pregnant women did not show a similar significant reduction. Eighteen percent of pregnant women reported cigarette use during pregnancy in 2002–2003 compared to 15.4% in 2012–2013. Other studies have shown that efforts to reduce smoking prevalence among female smokers before pregnancy have not been effective; however, efforts targeting pregnant women have met some success as rates have declined during pregnancy and after delivery [18,19].

The most commonly used illicit drug is marijuana, but illicit drug use also includes cocaine, opioids, and amphetamines. Among pregnant women, the rate of any illicit drug use is 5.4% and has not changed significantly since 2010–2011 [12]. Use remains higher in younger women (14.6%, ages 18–25) compared to older women (3.2%, ages 26–44). A high proportion of women are using marijuana illegally and fail to disclose their use to their providers. A recent study showed 81 percent of providers in urban outpatient clinics are asking their pregnant patients about illicit drug use and; of the women surveyed, 11% of women disclosed current use of marijuana, while 34% tested positive for one or more substances with marijuana being the most commonly detected (27%) [20]. Women who use methamphetamine during pregnancy show decreased prevalence and frequency of use from first to third trimester and women who decreased their use were more likely to seek prenatal care during pregnancy [21].

2.2. Maternal and environmental variables

There are a number of maternal and environmental characteristics that are associated with substance use during pregnancy [22]. Prenatal substance use is associated with younger maternal age [12] and socioeconomic factors such as lower level of education, unemployment, and higher levels of poverty [1]. Physical and mental health factors such as the utilization of health care during pregnancy [23, 24], fear of criminalization and/or stigma [25], higher rates of affective disorders including depression [1], and poly-substance exposure [1] are highly prevalent in pregnant substance users. Women using drugs during pregnancy are also more likely to have had either current and/or childhood exposure to violence and/or abuse [24]. Domestic violence is also associated with a higher proportion of substance use in women [24, 26].

The complex interactions of social, psychological, and physical variables that are at play in pregnant substance abusers also have an impact on the stability and quality of the child–parent relationship, a significant factor in healthy child development. The care that infants receive from their primary caretaker lays the foundation for the development of behavior and emotion regulation, social skills, and cognitive ability [18, 19, 27, 28], as well as physical and mental health [29, 30]. Substance abusing mothers show decreased responsivity to their infants. For example, opioid abusing mothers show a decreased ability to identify their infant's cues and to respond appropriately to them [31]. Addiction and mental illness, two factors associated with prenatal substance exposure are also associated with difficulty in forming healthy attachments [32]. The complex interactions of variables associated with prenatal substance exposure is important because the events that occur early in life, both in terms of the quality of relationships and environment, play a significant role in brain development. The important neural connections that support the brain circuitry that underlies emotional, social, and cognitive behavior are established early in life [33].

Prenatal drug exposures, the timing, and quality of other early experiences have a profound impact on child development because of their influence on early brain development. Early life experiences have an impact on the development of brain structure by influencing the timing and pattern of gene expression and the refinement of neural circuitry [34]. Neuroimaging methods that examine the structure and function of the brain have provided access to study the impact of prenatal drug exposure on the developing brain. Methods such as magnetic resonance imaging (MRI), diffusion tensor imaging (DTI), and functional magnetic resonance imaging (fMRI) are noninvasive allowing for their use in children. Neuroimaging tools have been used to better understand typical patterns of structural and functional development in the brain. This information can be used to examine how prenatal drug exposure affects normal brain development and how it relates to physical and behavioral outcomes.

3. Prenatal drug exposure and brain structure

3.1. Volume, symmetry, and cortical thickness

MRI uses the inherent magnetic properties of the body to create detailed images. Short radiofrequency pulses inside a strong magnetic field create patterns of excited molecules that can be used to create an image of the structure [35]. Offering detailed structural images of the brain, MRI is an essential tool for assessing structural characteristics including global and regional brain volumes, symmetry, and cortical thickness. Structural brain differences serve as biomarkers of the impact of the prenatal drug exposure and, eventually, may aid in identification and intervention. Overall, studies of prenatal drug exposure show consistent reductions in head circumference, overall and regional reductions in brain volumes, and differential reduction in gray and white matter volumes, results which are dependent on the accumulation of polydrug exposures [36].

Recent reports are consistent with previously documented widespread changes in brain structure in children and adolescents with moderate to heavy prenatal alcohol exposure [37]. Prenatal alcohol is associated with overall reductions in global [38, 39] and regional brain volume including the hippocampus, basal ganglia, cingulate cortex, and corpus callosum [37, 40–43]. Several studies indicate that reductions in brain volume linked to prenatal alcohol exposure were associated with deficits in cognitive function and facial dsymorphology. For example, prenatal alcohol exposed is linked to reductions in caudate volume which are also associated with deficits in cognitive control and verbal learning and memory [44] as well as palpebral fissure length [45]. Moreover, reductions in brain volume increase as a function of the amount of alcohol consumed during pregnancy and the severity of diagnosis [38, 46] and were reported from early childhood through young adulthood, suggesting long-term and persistent alterations in brain structure.

Prenatal alcohol exposure was also associated with increased asymmetry in the caudate nucleus, cingulate cortex, and corpus callosum. Specific to the caudate nucleus, moderate alcohol exposure was associated with increased volume in the left caudate compared to the right [43, 47]. Asymmetry in the cingulate cortex was due to reduced volume localized to the right caudal region of the cingulate [48], which may be related to differential loss of white matter compared to gray matter in this brain region [49].

Studies have evaluated the effects of prenatal alcohol on cortical morphology by examining cortical thickness. Several studies have reported increased cortical thickness in diffuse regions across the frontal, temporal, and parietal lobes [50–52] while another study reported cortical thinning [53]. Longitudinally, children with prenatal alcohol exposure show less developmentally appropriate cortical thinning across time compared to controls [54]. When cortical thickness is examined in contrast to surface area, prenatal alcohol exposure affects global surface area to a greater degree than cortical thickness especially in the right temporal gyrus [55].

Past neuroimaging studies show that prenatal cocaine exposure was also associated with long-term changes in brain structure. Recent studies confirm overall reductions in global brain volume as well as in the caudate, corpus callosum, and right cerebellum [56–58] differences in shape and volume characteristics of the striatum [45], and cortical thickness and volume of the right prefrontal cortex [59]. In adolescence, prenatal cocaine exposure was associated with specific reductions in gray matter volumes in frontal cortical and posterior regions [60]. In one study, the structural changes were correlated with impulsivity [59]. However, the prenatal cocaine exposure-related structural changes were subtle and may lose significance when covariates including other prenatal exposures are properly controlled [36].

Prenatal tobacco exposure was linked to overall reductions in intrauterine growth [61], which is also reflected in the brain. Prenatal tobacco exposure was associated with reductions in fetal head growth, reduced volume of the frontal lobes and cerebellum, and smaller width of the lateral ventricles [62, 63]. During childhood, prenatal tobacco exposure is associated with additional changes in brain structure including smaller total brain volume and smaller cortical gray matter volume [36, 64], cortical thinning in superior frontal and parietal cortices [64] and reduced gray matter volume in subcortical regions including the amygdala, thalamus, and pallidum [59, 65]. Increased volume in the frontal cortex with corresponding decreases in the anterior cingulate cortex was also observed [66]. Regional brain volume changes persisted into adolescence but may be explained by current adolescent tobacco use because children with prenatal tobacco exposure are at increased risk for early initiation and smoking behavior [67].

Fewer recent studies have been conducted on the impact of prenatal marijuana, methamphetamine, and opioid exposure on global and regional brain volume. But, some initial research indicates that prenatal exposure to these drugs is also associated with difference in brain structure. In contrast to other types of prenatal drug exposure, prenatal marijuana exposure was not related to reductions in global brain volume [36]. A small sample of children with prenatal opioid exposure showed reduced global brain volume as well as regional differences including reduced volume in the cerebral cortex, amygdala, nucleus accumbens, putamen, pallidum, brainstem, cerebellar cortex, cerebellar white matter, and inferior lateral ventricles [68]. Prenatal methamphetamine exposure was linked to regional volume reductions in both striatal and limbic structures including the caudate, anterior and posterior cingulate, inferior frontal gyrus, and ventral and lateral temporal lobes; regions that are vulnerable to the neurotoxic effects of methamphetamine in adult abusers [69]. Another study showed similar results, as well as sex-specific effects of prenatal methamphetamine exposure on brain structure, including increased volume in the striatum in males and increased cortical thickness in females [70].

3.2. Integrity of white matter tracts

DTI uses MRI to examine white matter microstructure by measuring the diffusion of water molecules in tissue and the integrity of water diffusion in one direction across a membrane. Unrestricted water molecules are capable of diffusing in any direction, however; in the presence of structural barriers such as cell membranes and myelin, water tends to diffuse in an increasingly directional manner. The degree to which water molecules are isotropic (directionally independent) versus anisotropic (directionally dependent) is determined using DTI. Anisotropy occurs in white matter tract fibers, particularly in myelinated axons [35, 71]. Functional anisotropy (FA) is used as a quantitative measure of diffusion and ranges in value from 0 (isotropic) to 1 (anisotropic) [72]. FA is highly sensitive to microstructural changes in white matter, but not to the type of change (radial or axial) [71]. Developmentally, FA undergoes the greatest amount of change during early childhood (through 5 years) [73, 74] and can be used to distinguish between stages of brain development [75]. In general, abnormal brain development or brain damage is associated with lower FA values in white matter [76]. Abnormalities in white matter that leads to decreases in FA may result from either increased radial (perpendicular and associated with changes in myelination) diffusivity and/or reduced axial (parallel and associated with axonal integrity) diffusivity [77]. Prenatal substance exposure is linked to lower FA and alterations in the structural integrity of myelin [78]. White matter microstructure, however, has been most widely studied in children with prenatal alcohol or cocaine exposure.

The impact of prenatal alcohol exposure on measures of white matter microstructure shows that effects can be detected at multiple stages of development, are associated with behavior, and fall on a continuum ranging from mild to severe Abnormalities in the corpus callosum are frequently reported, but also in anterior–posterior fiber bundles, corticospinal tracts, and the cerebellum [79–82]. Effects of prenatal alcohol exposure are linked to reduced white matter structural integrity in the cerebellum [83] and abnormalities in axial diffusivity [84] as early as infancy. In addition, subtle changes in FA have been associated with deficits in cognitive function including processing speed, math ability, executive function, and eye-blink conditioning [50, 81, 85–92] A recent study was also able to demonstrate that structural white matter changes are linked to disturbances in functional connectivity while at rest [83].

In contrast, DTI studies of the impact of prenatal cocaine or methamphetamine exposure on white matter integrity are mixed. Cocaine exposure has been associated with increased diffusion in left frontal callosal and right frontal fibers [93], but do not appear to remain significant after controlling for other prenatal drug exposures [36]. Another study that controlled carefully for other prenatal drug exposures showed that prenatal cocaine-related FA differences in fiber pathways including right cingulum, right arcuate fasciculus, left inferior longitudinal fasciculus, and splenium of the corpus callosum were associated with deficits in attention and response inhibition [94]. Only one study has reported a trend for higher FA associated with prenatal methamphetamine exposure [95]. These early studies and the lack of research on the impact of prenatal tobacco and marijuana exposure on white matter integrity indicate the need for additional research to better understand the impact of prenatal drug exposure on DTI measures.

4. Prenatal drug exposure and brain function

Neural circuits that control brain function have different patterns of activity that can be measured using fMRI. fMRI provides an indirect measure of brain function by quantifying the blood oxygen level-dependent (BOLD) response, which reflects changes in blood oxygen utilization throughout the brain. When neural circuits become active, MR signals will increase by a small amount, reflecting a signal change of approximately one percent. The ability to detect a change in MR signal depends on the different magnetic properties of oxygenated vs. deoxygenated blood and that blood flow to areas of the brain that are working are very sensitive. Different types of experimental designs are used in conjunction with fMRI methods to determine the location of brain activity. In the simplest type of experiment, patterns of brain activity are examined as a subject alternates between an experimental and control condition. The signal will increase and decrease as a function of the experimental conditions after adjusting for time. Functional neuroimaging studies produce group-averaged maps that show the level of brain activation that is associated with a specific task or in response to a specific stimulus. The group maps are then compared between conditions and/or between groups to examine the magnitude and extent of brain activation for a given response [96].

fMRI research has been used to determine if prenatal drug exposure has an impact on areas of the brain that receive more or less oxygenated blood in response to performing a cognitive task. The method has been used to demonstrate the effect of prenatal drug exposure on brain activation during a variety of cognitive behaviors. Recent work converges on three domains, the default mode network, inhibitory control, and working memory; all of which illustrate how fMRI methods can be used to better understand the impact of prenatal drug exposure on brain function. In addition, innovative functional connectivity studies have combined information from structural (MRI and DTI) with functional (fMRI) methods to understand the temporal relations between spatially distinct brain regions.

4.1. Default mode network

The default mode network (DMN) is comprised of a set of brain regions including ventral medial prefrontal cortex, posterior cingulate, inferior parietal lobe, lateral temporal cortex, dorsal medial prefrontal cortex, and the hippocampus (see **Figure 1**) [97]. This network is active when one appears to be at rest but is actually engaged in spontaneous and goal-directed mental

http://dx.doi.org/10.5772/63389

tasks such as free-thinking, remembering, and making future plans [98]. In contrast, the network is inhibited while performing tasks with high-cognitive demand and increased task difficulty [99, 100]. Behaviorally, both prenatal cocaine and alcohol exposure are associated with early and persistent deficits in arousal regulation and attention deficits [101–105] and an increased risk for a diagnosis of attention-deficit/hyperactivity disorder [106, 107]. One interpretation of the results of these studies is that the dysregulation of arousal and attention, in part, explains other observable deficits in higher-cognitive function.

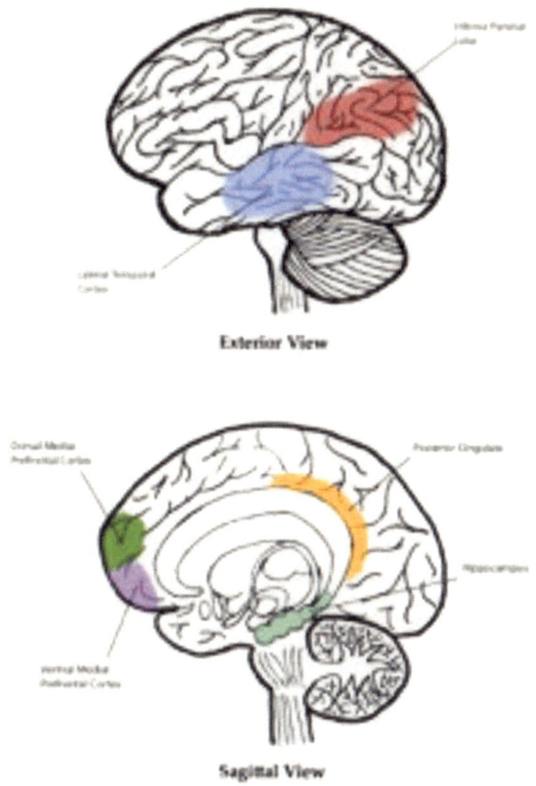

Figure 1. Key regions associated with the default mode brain network.

Current neuroimaging research suggests, however; that the underlying impact of prenatal cocaine or alcohol exposure on arousal and attention reflects changes in function of the DMN network. Results are summarized in **Table 1(A)**. Using resting-state fMRI, a recent large-scale study of neonates with prenatal cocaine exposure or polydrug exposure showed polydrug-related connectivity disruptions within frontal-amygdala, frontal-insula, and insula-sensori-motor circuits; and specific effects of prenatal cocaine exposure on the frontal-amygdala network [108]. Results showed that polydrug exposure was associated with negative connectivity within these networks. Negative connectivity is interpreted as a dysregulation in excitatory and inhibitory inputs [109–111], and in this case, a failure to inhibit the amygdala response from prefrontal cortex inputs.

A number of studies indicate that the effect of prenatal cocaine exposure on functional differences within the DMN persist into childhood and adolescence. Adolescents with prenatal cocaine exposure show overall reductions in regional cerebral blood flow at rest with compensatory, relative increases in anterior and superior brain regions [112]. Additionally, while in the resting state, adolescents with prenatal cocaine exposure show increased functional connectivity in the DMN compared to controls [113], and less deactivation of the network in the DMN, while performing a working memory task with emotional distracters.

Furthermore, the effects of prenatal cocaine and alcohol exposure on the DMN can be dissociated. Similar to prenatal cocaine exposure, prenatal alcohol exposure is associated with less deactivation in the DMN while performing a cognitive task [114]. In contrast to prenatal cocaine exposure, prenatal alcohol exposure is associated with decreased functional connectivity within the DMN at rest [114]. These results suggests that the underlying mechanism for prenatal cocaine or alcohol exposure effects on cognitive ability are due, in part, to changes in baseline levels of arousal and dysregulation of excitatory and inhibitory control of neural resources allocated to perform cognitive tasks.

4.2. Inhibitory control

The ability to engage in voluntary, goal-directed behavior requires activation of neural circuitry that supports cognitive control mechanisms. Response inhibition is considered to be a key component of cognitive control and refers to the ability to inhibit a response that is no longer needed or inappropriate given a change in either internal or external states [115]. The go/no-go task is a cognitive paradigm that can be used in conjunction with fMRI to evaluate response inhibition [115, 116]. In the go/no-go task, participants are required to respond or withhold a response depending on whether they are presented with a "go" stimulus or a "no-go" stimulus, respectively.

The go/no-go task has been used to determine independent effects of prenatal alcohol, cocaine, marijuana, and tobacco on response inhibition, allowing for a comparison across studies. Results are summarized in **Table 1(B)**. Children with prenatal tobacco [117] or marijuana [118] exposure were more likely to commit commission errors while performing the go/no-go task, but children with prenatal alcohol or cocaine exposure showed no behavioral differences in task performance. Prenatal alcohol exposure was associated with increased brain activation in prefrontal regions and less activation in the caudate compared to controls [119]. A similar pattern is demonstrated in adolescents with prenatal alcohol exposure suggesting long-term changes in brain function associated with response inhibition [120]. In contrast, prenatal cocaine exposed children showed increased activation in inferior frontal cortex and caudate and less activation in temporal and occipital regions [121]. Prenatal marijuana was associated with differential activation of frontal regions including and increased BOLD response in bilateral the prefrontal cortex and right premotor cortex, and a decreased response in the cerebellum [118]. Children with prenatal tobacco exposure showed increased activation in a more diverse set of brain regions including left frontal, right occipital, bilateral temporal, and parietal regions, and less activation in the cerebellum [117]. Young adults with prenatal tobacco exposure showed a similar pattern of results with increased activation inferior frontal, inferior parietal, basal ganglia, and cerebellum [122].

Results across multiple studies indicate that prenatal drug exposure leads to differential activation in frontal–striatal circuits, while performing the go/no-go task. In addition, across studies, prenatal drug-related increases in activation were reported in many brain regions, which indicates an increase in the demand for cognitive resources, while performing the response inhibition task. This pattern of results is indicative of an immature brain circuitry. Across development, the typical pattern observed in neuroimaging data is that for response inhibition, there is an increase in the magnitude of activation and a decrease in the extent of activation in frontal–striatal brain regions [123, 124]. Increased efficiency of neural processing is also associated with a peak in behavioral performance. Younger children show greater activation in similar brain regions as reported in the prenatal drug imaging studies [125, 126]. Although, the data collected in each of the studies were cross-sectional, the reported effects of prenatal drug exposure in childhood, adolescence, and adulthood indicate that the changes in brain circuitry underlying response inhibition may not be due to developmental delay, but instead due to long-term changes in the activation of the circuit.

4.3. Working memory

Working memory refers to the cognitive ability to hold and manipulate information for a short period of time. Brain imaging studies have shown a load-dependent role for the prefrontal cortex in working memory [127, 128]. Using fMRI methods, prenatal drug exposure is associated with differential brain activation within the prefrontal cortex, while performing working memory tasks. Results are summarized in **Table 1(C)**. For example, children prenatally exposed to tobacco experience more activation in the inferior parietal regions of the cortex, whereas children not exposed showed activation in the bilateral inferior frontal region of the cortex [129]. Prenatal marijuana is also associated with patterns of increased activation associated with working memory including the inferior and middle frontal gyri [130].

fMRI methods have also been used to demonstrate specific effects of prenatal drug exposure in both the visual–spatial and verbal working memory domains. Prenatal alcohol exposure leads to increased activation of the frontal–parietal–cerebellar network including the left dorsal frontal and left inferior parietal cortices, and bilateral posterior temporal regions during verbal working memory compared to controls [131]. The results showed that individuals prenatally exposed to alcohol recruit a larger, more extensive neural network than their peers. Across three studies, prenatal alcohol exposure was also associated with differential patterns of activation, while performing spatial working memory tasks [132–134]. In contrast, offspring with prenatal methamphetamine exposure had less activation than their unexposed counterparts in both the frontal and striatal regions; primarily in the left hemisphere of the brain on a spatial working memory task [135], but increased activation in bilateral temporal regions in response to performing a verbal working memory task [136].

(A) Default mode network			
Drug	**Effects on network**	**Behavioral effects**	**References**
Alcohol	Increased activity in DMN during cognitive tasks	Deficits in arousal regulation	[101–107, 114]
	Decreased activation of DMN at rest	Increased risk of ADHD diagnosis	
Cocaine	Increased activity in DMN during cognitive tasks	Deficits in arousal regulation	[101–107, 113, 114]
	Increased activation of DMN at rest	Increased risk of ADHD diagnosis	
(B) Inhibitory control			
Alcohol	Increased activity in prefrontal regions	Increased effort required for response inhibition	[119]
	Decreased activity in the caudate		
Tobacco	Increased activity in left frontal, right occipital, bilateral temporal, and parietal regions	Increased effort required for response inhibition	[117]
	Decreased activity in the cerebellum	More likely to commit commission errors	
Cocaine	Increased activity in inferior frontal cortex and caudate	Increased effort required for response inhibition	[121]
	Decreased activity in temporal and occipital regions		
(C) Working memory			
Alcohol	Increased activation in bilateral dorsal frontal, bilateral posterior temporal, and left inferior parietal regions	More effort required to maintain working memory	[131, 137, 138]
Tobacco	Activation of inferior parietal cortex as opposed to bilateral inferior frontal cortex	Different mechanisms are employed to maintain working memory	[129]
Methamphetamine	Decreased activation in frontal and striatal regions, particularly in left hemisphere	Decreased working memory performance	[135]

Table 1. Summary of prenatal drug exposure effects on (A) default mode network, (B) working memory, and (C) inhibitory control.

The impact of prenatal alcohol exposure can be dissociated from other potential explanatory variables. When examined in relation to family history of alcohol use disorders, prenatal alcohol exposure independently predicted increased activation in left middle and superior frontal brain regions [137]. In a direct comparison of adolescents with prenatal alcohol exposure or ADHD, behavioral profiles were similar but the two groups showed differences in how cortical brain regions were recruited for spatial working memory [138]. Overall, prenatal alcohol exposure was associated with an increased effort to compensate in relation to increasing task demands compared to the ADHD group.

Alterations in behavioral and brain function measures of working memory extend to prenatal cocaine exposure as well. The aforementioned deficits in arousal regulation associated with prenatal cocaine exposure appear to underlie brain and behavior-related working memory function. Li et al. [139] showed differential patterns of activation as a function of emotion–memory interactions. Increased demands on memory load diminished emotion-related activation in the amygdala in controls but not in the exposed group. In contrast, the exposed group failed to show an expected decrease in activation in the prefrontal cortex as memory load decreased in the presence of emotional stimuli. Results suggest that the impact of prenatal cocaine exposure on arousal regulation acts through both the dorsal cognitive and ventral emotional systems.

Overall, multiple studies demonstrate the complexities of prenatal drug-related effects on working memory. Patterns of brain activation associated with working memory are different by type of prenatal drug exposure, are present in the absence of behavioral differences, and show more extensive networks of activation compared to controls. Specific alterations in prefrontal cortex activation in response to working memory demand suggest that these regions are taxed to a greater degree as a result of prenatal drug exposure. Furthermore, changes in activation remained after controlling for other explanatory variables such as intelligence. Collectively, studies demonstrate that the effect of prenatal drug exposure on brain activation associated with working memory is less efficient and that increased levels of activation serve to compensate for any deficits in working memory function. Compensatory action, however, may not be sufficient in real-life situations characterized by increased demands on working memory function.

4.4. Novel applications of imaging methods and statistical techniques

Recently, a number of novel applications of functional neuroimaging and statistical methods have been employed to improve upon the limitations of current methods in detecting the subtle effects of prenatal drug exposure on brain function, develop connectivity maps, and aid in diagnosis. First, a variety of model-based or data-driven methods have been employed to analyze functional neuroimaging data. General linear modeling has been used most widely because it is effective, simple, and robust [140]. However, typical approaches to the statistical analysis of fMRI data are limited in that they are not able to detect activation in heterogeneous brain regions that have the potential to play diverse roles in multiple types of task performance [141]. A recent study successfully demonstrated the advantages of group-wise sparse representation of fMRI data and statistical coefficient mapping to evaluate the effect of prenatal alcohol exposure on functional activity. The advantages reported for this method included increased adaptability, more systematic in detecting diverse brain networks, and better able to identify commonalities and differences across subjects and groups [141].

fMRI data can also be analyzed to show how components of a neural system are working together when performing a specific task. The identification of associations between anatomically distinct time series is referred to as "functional connectivity" [140]. The ability to identify consistent, reproducible, and accurate regions of interest is the key to developing connectivity maps [142]. Using a new strategy to develop cortical landmarks (dense individualized and common connectivity-based cortical landmarks, DICCOLs), Li et al. [143] used functional connectomics signatures to identify 10 brain regions with structurally disrupted landmarks that could be used to distinctly identify prenatal cocaine exposed brains from that of controls.

Finally, a novel application of machine learning has been used to test whether brain images can be used to correctly identify prenatal cocaine-exposed young adults from socioeconomically matched controls [144]. Regional features were extracted from both structural and functional MR images, and the power of each to discriminate between prenatal cocaine exposed and control brains was accomplished through machine learning methods. The method accurately identified 91.8% of prenatally cocaine-exposed brains. The use of both structural and functional images was critical to improving the accuracy of the classification system compared to either type of image alone.

5. Conclusions

Prenatal drug exposure is a risk factor for increased vulnerability to difficulties in both behavior and cognition. Continued research to identify the structural and functional targets of prenatal drug-related neurotoxicity is important. Identifying biomarkers of prenatal drug-related changes in brain development and relating those changes to behavior, or in the case of alcohol to physical features, has the potential to inform diagnostic and treatment strategies. MRI, fMRI, and DTI neuroimaging methods provide powerful tools for visualizing the brain and, because they are noninvasive, are especially suited for research in young children. The impact of prenatal drug exposure on brain structure and function is subtle and often account for a small amount of variance that contributes to deficits in behavior regulation and cognition. These subtle effects can be explained by the complex interactions of the pattern of prenatal drug exposure both in terms of the timing and dose as well as the combination of multiple drugs, genetic, and environmental factors. Changes in brain structure and function in children and adolescents with prenatal drug exposure can be difficult to assess for a number of other reasons. To date, a neuropsychological profile for prenatal drug-related deficits in cognitive function has not been identified and there are diffuse individual differences in the expression of the impact of prenatal drug exposure on the brain and behavior. Furthermore, limitations in statistical approaches to the analysis of neuroimaging data can often lead to difficulty in detecting these subtle effects. Future studies will require large sample sizes and longitudinal research designs, and increasingly sophisticated neuroimaging and statistical

http://dx.doi.org/10.5772/63389

methods. A focus on connectivity measures will provide a better understanding of underlying mechanisms for the associations between brain structure and function, and behavior.

Author details

Jennifer Willford[1*], Conner Smith[1], Tyler Kuhn[1], Brady Weber[1] and Gale Richardson[2]

*Address all correspondence to: Jennifer.Willford@sru.edu

1 Slippery Rock University, Slippery Rock, PA, USA

2 University of Pittsburgh, Pittsburgh PA, USA

References

[1] Mark K, Desai A, Terplan M. Marijuana use and pregnancy: prevalence, associated characteristics, and birth outcomes. Arch Womens Ment Health. 2015;19(1):105–111. doi:10.1007/s00737-015-0529-9

[2] Tan C, Denny C, Cheal N, Sniezek J, Kanny D. Alcohol use and binge drinking among women of childbearing age—United States, 2011–2013. MMWR Morb Mortal Wkly Rep. 2015;64(37):1042–1046.

[3] Smith DK, Johnson AB, Pears KC, Fisher PA, DeGarmo DS. Child maltreatment and foster care: unpacking the effects of prenatal and postnatal parental substance use. Child Maltreat. 2007;12(2):150–160.

[4] Ryan JP, Marsh JC, Testa MF, Louderman R. Integrating substance abuse treatment and child welfare services: findings from the Illinois alcohol and other drug abuse waiver demonstration. Soc Work Res. 2006;30(2):95–107.

[5] Data & Statistics | FASD | NCBDDD | CDC [Internet]. Cdc.gov. 2016 [cited 9 May 2016]. Available from: http://www.cdc.gov/ncbddd/fasd/data.html.

[6] Czerkeys M, Blackstone J, Pulvino J. Buprenorphine versus methadone treatment for opiate addiction in pregnancy: an evaluation of neonatal outcomes. The American College of Obstetricians and Gynecologists: Papers on Current Clinical and Basic Investigation. 2010;4–10.

[7] Jones HE, Kaltenbach K, Heil SH, Stine SM, Coyle MG, Arria AM, O'Grady KE, Selby P, Martin PR, Fischer G. Neonatal abstinence syndrome after methadone or buprenorphine exposure. N Engl J Med. 2010;363(24):2320–2331.

[8] Popova S, Stade B, Bekmuradov D, Lange S, Rehm J. What do we know about the economic impact of fetal alcohol spectrum disorder? A systematic literature review. Alcohol Alcoholism. 2011;46(4):490–497.

[9] Huestis MA, Choo RE. Drug abuse's smallest victims: in utero drug exposure. Forensic Sci Int. 2002;128(1):20–30.

[10] Konijnenberg C, Methodological issues in assessing the impact of prenatal drug exposure. Subst Abuse. 2015;9(Suppl 2):39–44. doi:10.4137/SART.S23544

[11] Welfare N. NCSACW – Substance-Exposed Infants [Internet]. Ncsacw.samhsa.gov. 2016 [cited 9 May 2016]. Available from: https://ncsacw.samhsa.gov/resources/substance-exposed-infants.aspx.

[12] Substance Abuse and Mental Health Services Administration. Results from the 2013 National Survey on Drug Use and Health: Summary of National Findings. Rockville, MD: Substance Abuse and Mental Health Services Administration; 2014.

[13] Keyes K, Li G, Hasin D. Birth cohort effects and gender differences in alcohol epidemiology: a review and synthesis. Alcohol Clin Exp Res. 2011;35(12):2101–2112. doi: 10.1111/j.1530-0277.2011.01562.x

[14] Grucza RA, Norberg KE, Bierut LJ. Binge drinking among youths and young adults in the United States: 1979–2006. J Am Acad Child Adolesc Psychiatry. 2009;48(7):692–702. doi:10.1097/CHI.0b013e3181a2b32f

[15] Dawson DA, Goldstein RB, Saha TD, Grant BF. Changes in alcohol consumption: United States, 2001–2002 to 2012–2013. Drug Alcohol Depend. 2014;148:56–61. doi: 10.1016/j.drugalcdep.2014.12.016

[16] May P, Baete A, Russo J, Elliott A, Blankenship J, Kalberg W, et al. Prevalence and characteristics of fetal alcohol spectrum disorders. Pediatrics. 2014;134(5):855–866. doi:10.1016/j.drugalcdep.2014.10.017

[17] May P, Gossage J, Kalberg W, Robinson L, Buckley D, Manning M, et al. Prevalence and epidemiologic characteristics of FASD from various research methods with an emphasis on recent in-school studies. Dev Dis Res Rev. 2009;15(3):176–192. doi:10.1002/ddrr.68

[18] National Center for Health Statistics. Healthy People 2010 Final Review. Hyattsville: US Department of Health and Human Services; 2010.

[19] Tong VT, Dietz PM, Morrow B, D'Angelo DV, Farr SL, Rockhill KM, et al. Trends in smoking before, during, and after pregnancy–pregnancy risk assessment monitoring system, United States, 40 sites, 2000–2010. MMWR. 2013;62(SS06):1–19.

[20] Chang J, Holland C, Tarr J, Rubio D, Rodriguez K, Kraemer K, et al. Perinatal illicit drug and marijuana use: an observational study examining prevalence, screening, and disclosure. Am J Health Promot. In press. doi:10.4278/ajhp.141215-QUAL-625

[21] Della Grotta S, LaGasse LL, Arria AM, Derauf C, Grant P, Smith LM, Shah R, Huestis M, Liu J, Lester BM. Patterns of methamphetamine use during pregnancy: results from the Infant Development, Environment, and Lifestyle (IDEAL) Study. Matern Child Health J. 2010;14(4):519–527.

[22] Fentiman LC. Pursuing the perfect mother: why America's criminalization of maternal substance abuse is not the answer—a comparative legal analysis. MJGLAW. 2008;15:389.

[23] Roberts S, Nuru-Jeter A. Women's perspectives on screening for alcohol and drug use in prenatal care. Womens Health Issues. 2010;20(3):193–200. doi:10.1016/j.whi.2010.02.003

[24] Datner EM, Wiebe DJ, Brensinger CM, Nelson DB. Identifying pregnant women experiencing domestic violence in an urban emergency department. J Interpers Violence. 2007;22(1):124–135. doi:10.1177/0886260506295000

[25] Jessup MA, Humphreys JC, Brindis CD, Lee KA. Extrinsic barriers to substance abuse treatment among pregnant drug dependent women. J Drug Issues. 2003;33(2):285–304.

[26] Fals-Stewart W, Kennedy C. Addressing intimate partner violence in substance-abuse treatment. J Subst Abuse Treat. 2005;29(1):5–17. doi:10.1016/j.jsat.2005.03.001

[27] Morris A, Silk J, Steinberg L, Myers S, Robinson L. The role of the family context in the development of emotion regulation. Soc Dev. 2007;16(2):361–388. doi:10.1111/j.1467-9507.2007.00389.x

[28] Scaramella L, Leve L. Clarifying parent–child reciprocities during early childhood: the early childhood coercion model. Clin Child Fam Psychol Rev. 2004;7(2):89–107. doi:10.1023/B:CCFP.0000030287.13160.a3

[29] Schweinhart LJ, Montie J, Zongping X, Barnett WS, Belfield CR, Nores M. Lifetime effects: the High/Scope Perry Preschool study through age 40. Ypsilanti. 2005. Available at: http://works.bepress.com/william_barnett/3/

[30] Heckman J. The economics, technology, and neuroscience of human capability formation. Proc Natl Acad Sci USA. 2007;104(33):13250–13255. doi:10.1073/pnas.0701362104

[31] Hans S. Studies of prenatal exposure to drugs focusing on parental care of children. Neurotoxicol Teratol. 2002;24(3):329–337. doi:10.1016/S0892-0362(02)00195-2

[32] Barnard M, McKeganey N. The impact of parental problem drug use on children: what is the problem and what can be done to help? Addiction. 2004;99(5):552–559. doi:10.1111/j.1360-0443.2003.00664.x

[33] National Scientific Council on the Developing Child, National Forum on Early Childhood Policy and Programs. The foundations of lifelong health are built in early childhood. Center on the Developing Child at Harvard University; 2010.

[34] Fox S, Levitt P, Nelson III C. How the timing and quality of early experiences influence the development of brain architecture. Child Dev. 2010;81(1):28–40. doi:10.1111/j.1467-8624.2009.01380.x

[35] Horton M, Margolis A, Tang C, Wright R. Neuroimaging is a novel tool to understand the impact of environmental chemicals on neurodevelopment. Curr Opin Pediatr. 2014;26(2):230–236. doi:10.1097/MOP.0000000000000074

[36] Rivkin M, Davis P, Lemaster J, Cabral H, Warfield S, Mulkern R, et al. Volumetric MRI study of brain in children with intrauterine exposure to cocaine, alcohol, tobacco, and marijuana. Pediatrics. 2008;121(4):741–750. doi:10.1542/peds.2007-1399

[37] Lebel C, Roussotte F, Sowell E. Imaging the impact of prenatal alcohol exposure on the structure of the developing human brain. Neuropsychol Rev. 2011;21(2):102–118. doi:10.1007/s11065-011-9163-0

[38] Astley S, Aylward E, Olson H, Kerns K, Brooks A, Coggins T, et al. Functional magnetic resonance imaging outcomes from a comprehensive magnetic resonance study of children with fetal alcohol spectrum disorders. J Neurodev Disord. 2009;1(1):61–80. doi:10.1111/j.1530-0277.2009.01004.x

[39] Chen X, Coles C, Lynch M, Hu X. Understanding specific effects of prenatal alcohol exposure on brain structure in young adults. Hum Brain Mapp. 2011;33(7):1663–1676. doi:10.1002/hbm.21313

[40] Roussotte F, Rudie J, Smith L, O'Connor M, Bookheimer S, Narr K, et al. Frontostriatal connectivity in children during working memory and the effects of prenatal methamphetamine, alcohol, and polydrug exposure. Dev Neurosci. 2012;34(1):43–57. doi:10.1159/000336242

[41] Donald KA, Fouche JP, Roos A, Koen N, Howells FM, Riley EP, et al. Alcohol exposure in utero is associated with decreased gray matter volume in neonates. Metab Brain Dis. 2016;31(1):81–91. doi:10.1007/s11011-015-9771-0

[42] Willoughby KA, Sheard ED, Nash K, Rovet J. Effects of prenatal alcohol exposure on hippocampal volume, verbal learning, and verbal and spatial recall in late childhood. J Int Neuropsychol Soc. 2008;14(6):1022–1033. doi:10.10170S1355617708081368

[43] Yang Y, Phillips O, Kan E, Sulik K, Mattson S, Riley E, et al. Callosal thickness reductions relate to facial dysmorphology in fetal alcohol spectrum disorders. Alcohol Clin Exp Res. 2011;36(5):798–806. doi:10.1111/j.1530-0277.2011.01679.x

[44] Fryer S, Mattson S, Jernigan T, Archibald S, Jones K, Riley E. Caudate volume predicts neurocognitive performance in youth with heavy prenatal alcohol exposure. Alcohol Clin Exp Res. 2012;36(11):1932–1941. doi:10.1111/j.1530-0277.2012.01811.x

[45] Roussotte F, Sulik K, Mattson S, Riley E, Jones K, Adnams C, et al. Regional brain volume reductions relate to facial dysmorphology and neurocognitive function in fetal

alcohol spectrum disorders. Hum Brain Mapp. 2011;33(4):920–937. doi:10.1002/hbm.21260

[46] Eckstrand K, Ding Z, Dodge N, Cowan R, Jacobson J, Jacobson S, et al. Persistent dose-dependent changes in brain structure in young adults with low-to-moderate alcohol exposure in utero. Alcohol Clin Exp Res. 2012;36(11):1892–1902. doi:10.1111/j.1530-0277.2012.01819.x

[47] Willford J, Day R, Aizenstein H, Day N. Caudate asymmetry: a neurobiological marker of moderate prenatal alcohol exposure in young adults. Neurotoxicol Teratol. 2010;32(6):589–594. doi:10.1016/j.ntt.2010.06.012

[48] Migliorini R, Moore E, Glass L, Infante M, Tapert S, Jones K, et al. Anterior cingulate cortex surface area relates to behavioral inhibition in adolescents with and without heavy prenatal alcohol exposure. Behav Brain Res. 2015;292:26–35. doi:10.1016/j.bbr.2015.05.037

[49] Bjorkquist O, Fryer S, Reiss A, Mattson S, Riley E. Cingulate gyrus morphology in children and adolescents with fetal alcohol spectrum disorders. Psychiatry Res. 2010;181(2):101–107. doi:10.1016/j.pscychresns.2009.10.004

[50] Sowell E, Johnson A, Kan E, Lu L, Van Horn J, Toga A, et al. Mapping white matter integrity and neurobehavioral correlates in children with fetal alcohol spectrum disorders. J Neurosci. 2008;28(6):1313–1319. doi:10.1523/JNEUROSCI.5067-07.2008

[51] Fernández-Jaén A, Fernández-Mayoralas DM, Tapia DQ, Calleja-Pérez B, García-Segura JM, Arribas SL, et al. Cortical thickness in fetal alcohol syndrome and attention deficit disorder. Pediatr Neurol. 2011;45(6):387–391. doi:10.1016/j.pediatrneurol.2011.09.004

[52] Yang Y, Roussotte F, Kan E, Sulik K, Mattson S, Riley E, et al. Abnormal cortical thickness alterations in fetal alcohol spectrum disorders and their relationships with facial dysmorphology. Cereb Cortex. 2011;22(5):1170–1179. doi:10.1093/cercor/bhr193

[53] Zhou D, Lebel C, Lepage C, Rasmussen C, Evans A, Wyper K, et al. Developmental cortical thinning in fetal alcohol spectrum disorders. Neuroimage. 2011;58(1):16–25. doi:10.1016/j.neuroimage.2011.06.026

[54] Treit S, Zhou D, Lebel C, Rasmussen C, Andrew G, Beaulieu C. Longitudinal MRI reveals impaired cortical thinning in children and adolescents prenatally exposed to alcohol. Hum Brain Mapp. 2014;35(9):4892–4903. doi:10.1002/hbm.22520

[55] Rajaprakash M, Chakravarty M, Lerch J, Rovet J. Cortical morphology in children with alcohol-related neurodevelopmental disorder. Brain Behav. 2013;4(1):41–50. doi:10.1002/brb3.191

[56] Akyuz N, Kekatpure M, Liu J, Sheinkopf S, Quinn B, Lala M, et al. Structural brain imaging in children and adolescents following prenatal cocaine exposure: preliminary longitudinal findings. Dev Neurosci. 2014;36(3–4):316–328. doi:10.1159/000362685

[57] Avants B, Hurt H, Giannetta J, Epstein C, Shera D, Rao H, et al. Effects of heavy in utero cocaine exposure on adolescent caudate morphology. Pediatr Neurol. 2007;37(4):275–279. doi:10.1016/j.pediatrneurol.2007.06.012

[58] Grewen K, Burchinal M, Vachet C, Gouttard S, Gilmore J, Lin W, et al. Prenatal cocaine effects on brain structure in early infancy. Neuroimage. 2014;101:114–123. doi:10.1016/j.neuroimage.2014.06.070

[59] Liu J, Lester B, Neyzi N, Sheinkopf S, Gracia L, Kekatpure M, et al. Regional brain morphometry and impulsivity in adolescents following prenatal exposure to cocaine and tobacco. JAMA Pediatr. 2013;167(4):348. doi:10.1001/jamapediatrics.2013.550.

[60] Rando K, Chaplin T, Potenza M, Mayes L, Sinha R. Prenatal cocaine exposure and gray matter volume in adolescent boys and girls: relationship to substance use initiation. Biol Psychiatry. 2013;74(7):482–489. doi:10.1016/j.biopsych.2013.04.030

[61] Abbott L, Winzer-Serhan U. Smoking during pregnancy: lessons learned from epidemiological studies and experimental studies using animal models. Crit Rev Toxicol. 2012;42(4):279–303. doi:10.3109/10408444.2012.658506

[62] Ekblad M, Korkeila J, Parkkola R, Lapinleimu H, Haataja L, Lehtonen L. Maternal smoking during pregnancy and regional brain volumes in preterm infants. J Pediatr. 2010;156(2):185–190. doi:10.1016/j.jpeds.2009.07.061

[63] Roza S, Verburg B, Jaddoe V, Hofman A, Mackenbach J, Steegers E, et al. Effects of maternal smoking in pregnancy on prenatal brain development. The Generation R Study. Eur J Neuroscience. 2007;25(3):611–617. doi:10.1111/j.1460-9568.2007.05393.x

[64] El Marroun H, Schmidt M, Franken I, Jaddoe V, Hofman A, van der Lugt A, et al. Prenatal tobacco exposure and brain morphology: a prospective study in young children. Neuropsychopharmacology. 2013;39(4):792–800. doi:10.1038/npp.2013.273

[65] Haghighi A, Schwartz D, Abrahamowicz M, Leonard G, Perron M, Richer L, et al. Prenatal exposure to maternal cigarette smoking, amygdala volume, and fat intake in adolescence. JAMA Psychiatry. 2013;70(1):98. doi:10.1001/archgenpsychiatry.2012.1101.

[66] Derauf C, Lester B, Neyzi N, Kekatpure M, Gracia L, Davis J, et al. Subcortical and cortical structural central nervous system changes and attention processing deficits in preschool-aged children with prenatal methamphetamine and tobacco exposure. Dev Neurosci. 2012;34(4):327–341. doi:10.1159/000341119

[67] Cornelius MD, Leech SL, Goldschmidt L, Day NL. Prenatal tobacco exposure: is it a risk factor for early tobacco experimentation? Nicotine Tob Res. 2000;2(1):45–52. doi:10.1080/14622200050011295

[68] Walhovd K, Moe V, Slinning K, Due-Tonnessen P, Bjornerud A, Dale A, et al. Volumetric cerebral characteristics of children exposed to opiates and other substances in utero. Neuroimage. 2007;36(4):1331–1344. doi:10.1016/j.neuroimage.2007.03.070

[69] Sowell E, Leow AD, Bookheimer SY, Smith LM, O'Connor MJ, Kan E, Rosso C, Houston S, Dinov ID, Thompson PM. Differentiating prenatal exposure to methamphetamine and alcohol versus alcohol and not methamphetamine using tensor-based brain morphometry and discriminant analysis. J Neurosci. 2010;17;30(11):3876–85. doi: 10.1523/JNEUROSCI.4967-09.2010

[70] Roos A, Jones G, Howells F, Stein D, Donald K. Structural brain changes in prenatal methamphetamine-exposed children. Metab Brain Dis. 2014;29(2):341–349. doi: 10.1007/s11011-014-9500-0

[71] Alexander A, Lee J, Lazar M, Field A. Diffusion tensor imaging of the brain. Neurotherapeutics. 2007;4(3):316–329. doi:10.1016/j.nurt.2007.05.011

[72] Uluğ AM, van Zijl PC. Orientation-independent diffusion imaging without tensor diagonalization: anisotropy definitions based on physical attributes of the diffusion ellipsoid. J Magn Reson Imaging. 1999;9(6):804–13. doi:10.1002/(SICI)1522-2586(199906)9:6<804::AID-JMRI7>3.0.CO;2-B

[73] Ben Bashat D, Sira L, Graif M, Pianka P, Hendler T, Cohen Y, et al. Normal white matter development from infancy to adulthood: comparing diffusion tensor and high b value diffusion weighted MR images. J Magn Reson Imaging. 2005;21(5):503–511. doi: 10.1002/jmri.20281

[74] Ben Bashat D, Kronfeld-Duenias V, Zachor D, Ekstein P, Hendler T, Tarrasch R, et al. Accelerated maturation of white matter in young children with autism: a high b value DWI study. Neuroimage. 2007;37(1):40–47. doi:10.1016/j.neuroimage.2007.04.060

[75] Eluvathingal T, Hasan K, Kramer L, Fletcher J, Ewing-Cobbs L. Quantitative diffusion tensor tractography of association and projection fibers in normally developing children and adolescents. Cereb Cortex. 2007;17(12):2760–2768. doi:10.1093/cercor/bhm003

[76] Neil J, Miller J, Mukherjee P, Huppi P. Diffusion tensor imaging of normal and injured developing human brain—a technical review. NMR Biomed. 2002;15(7–8):543–552. doi:10.1002/nbm.784

[77] Alexander A, Hurley S, Samsonov A, Adluru N, Hosseinbor A, Mossahebi P, et al. Characterization of cerebral white matter properties using quantitative magnetic resonance imaging stains. Brain Connect. 2011;1(6):423–446. doi:10.1089/brain.2011.0071

[78] Walhovd K, Westlye L, Moe V, Slinning K, Due-Tonnessen P, Bjornerud A, et al. White matter characteristics and cognition in prenatally opiate- and polysubstance-exposed children: a diffusion tensor imaging study. AJNR Am J Neuroradiol. 2010;31(5):894–900. doi:10.3174/ajnr.A1957

[79] Ma X, Coles C, Lynch M, LaConte S, Zurkiya O, Wang D, et al. Evaluation of corpus callosum anisotropy in young adults with fetal alcohol syndrome according to

diffusion tensor imaging. Alcohol Clin Exp Res. 2005;29(7):1214–1222. doi: 10.1097/01.ALC.0000171934.22755.6D

[80] Donald KA, Eastman E, Howells FM, Adnams C, Riley EP, Woods RP, Narr KL, Stein DJ. Neuroimaging effects of prenatal alcohol exposure on the developing human brain: a magnetic resonance imaging review. Acta Neuropsychiatr. 201;27(5):251–269. doi: 10.1017/neu.2015.12

[81] Wozniak J, Muetzel R, Mueller B, McGee C, Freerks M, Ward E, et al. Microstructural corpus callosum anomalies in children with prenatal alcohol exposure: an extension of previous diffusion tensor imaging findings. Alcohol Clin Exp Res. 2009;33(10):1825–1835. doi:10.1111/j.1530-0277.2009.01021.x

[82] Wozniak J, Muetzel R. What does diffusion tensor imaging reveal about the brain and cognition in fetal alcohol spectrum disorders? Neuropsychol Rev. 2011;21(2):133–147. doi:10.1007/s11065-011-9162-1

[83] Donald K, Roos A, Fouche J, Koen N, Howells F, Woods R, et al. A study of the effects of prenatal alcohol exposure on white matter microstructural integrity at birth. Acta Neuropsychiatrica. 2015;27(04):197–205. doi:10.1017/neu.2015.35

[84] Taylor P, Jacobson S, van der Kouwe A, Molteno C, Chen G, Wintermark P, et al. A DTI-based tractography study of effects on brain structure associated with prenatal alcohol exposure in newborns. Hum Brain Mapp. 2014;36(1):170–186. doi:10.1002/hbm.22620

[85] Fan J, Meintjes E, Molteno C, Spottiswoode B, Dodge N, Alhamud A, et al. White matter integrity of the cerebellar peduncles as a mediator of effects of prenatal alcohol exposure on eyeblink conditioning. Hum Brain Mapp. 2015;36(7):2470–2482. doi: 10.1002/hbm.22785

[86] Fryer S, Frank L, Spadoni A, Theilmann R, Nagel B, Schweinsburg A, et al. Microstructural integrity of the corpus callosum linked with neuropsychological performance in adolescents. Brain Cogn. 2008;67(2):225–233. doi:10.1016/j.bandc.2008.01.009

[87] Fryer S, Schweinsburg B, Bjorkquist O, Frank L, Mattson S, Spadoni A, et al. Characterization of white matter microstructure in fetal alcohol spectrum disorders. Alcohol Clin Exp Res. 2009;33(3):514–521. doi:10.1111/j.1530-0277.2008.00864.x

[88] Lebel C, Rasmussen C, Wyper K, Walker L, Andrew G, Yager J, Beaulieu C. Brain diffusion abnormalities in children with fetal alcohol spectrum disorder. Alcohol Clin Exp Res. 2008;32(10):1732–1740. doi:10.1111/j.1530-0277.2008.00750.x

[89] Lebel C, Rasmussen C, Wyper K, Andrew G, Beaulieu C. Brain microstructure is related to math ability in children with fetal alcohol spectrum disorder. Alcohol Clin Exp Res. 2010;34(2):354–363. doi:10.1111/j.1530-0277.2009.01097.x

[90] Li L, Coles C, Lynch M, Hu X. Voxelwise and skeleton-based region of interest analysis of fetal alcohol syndrome and fetal alcohol spectrum disorders in young adults. Neuroimage. 2009;47:S47. doi:10.1002/hbm.20747

[91] Ma X, Coles C, Lynch M, LaConte S, Zurkiya O, Wang D, et al. Evaluation of corpus callosum anisotropy in young adults with fetal alcohol syndrome according to diffusion tensor imaging. Alcohol Clin Exp Res. 2005;29(7):1214–1222. doi:10.1097/01.ALC.0000171934.22755.6D

[92] Wozniak J, Mueller B, Muetzel R, Bell C, Hoecker H, Nelson M, et al. Inter-hemispheric functional connectivity disruption in children with prenatal alcohol exposure. Alcohol Clin Exp Res. 2011;35(5):849–861.

[93] Warner T, Behnke M, Eyler F, Padgett K, Leonard C, Hou W, et al. Diffusion tensor imaging of frontal white matter and executive functioning in cocaine-exposed children. Pediatrics. 2006;118(5):2014–2024. doi:10.1111/j.1530-0277.2010.01415.x

[94] Lebel C, Warner T, Colby J, Soderberg L, Roussotte F, Behnke M, et al. White matter microstructure abnormalities and executive function in adolescents with prenatal cocaine exposure. Psychiatry Res. 2013;213(2):161–168. doi:10.1016/j.pscychresns.2013.04.002

[95] Cloak C, Ernst T, Fuji L, Hedemark B, Chang L. Lower diffusion in white matter of children with prenatal methamphetamine exposure. Neurology. 2009;72(24):2068–2075. doi:10.1212/01.wnl.0000346516.49126.20

[96] Rogers B, Morgan V, Newton A, Gore J. Assessing functional connectivity in the human brain by fMRI. J Magn Reson Imaging. 2007;25(10):1347–1357. doi:10.1016/j.mri.2007.03.007

[97] Buckner RL, Andrews-Hanna JR, Schacter DL. The brain's default network: anatomy, function, and relevance to disease. Ann N Y Acad Sci. 2008;1124:1–38. doi:10.1196/annals.1440.011

[98] Andrews-Hanna JR. The brain's default network and its adaptive role in internal mentation. The Neuroscientist. 2012 Jun 1;18(3):251–70. doi :10.1177/1073858411403316

[99] McKiernan KA, D'Angelo BR, Kaufman JN, Binder JR. Interrupting the "stream of consciousness": an fMRI investigation. Neuroimage. 2006;29:1185–1191. doi:10.1016/j.neuroimage.2005.09.030

[100] Singh K, Fawcett I. Transient and linearly graded deactivation of the human default-mode network by a visual detection task. Neuroimage. 2008;41(1):100–112. doi:10.1016/j.neuroimage.2008.01.051

[101] Accornero VH, Amado AJ, Morrow CE, Xue L, Anthony JC, Bandstra ES. Impact of prenatal cocaine exposure on attention and response inhibition as assessed by continuous performance tests. J Dev Behav Pediatr. 2007;28(3):195–205. doi:10.1097/01.DBP.0000268560.72580.f9

[102] Beeghly M, Rose-Jacobs R, Martin B, Cabral H, Heeren T, Frank D. Level of intrauterine cocaine exposure and neuropsychological test scores in preadolescence: subtle effects on auditory attention and narrative memory. Neurotoxicol Teratol. 2014;45:1–17. doi:10.1016/j.ntt.2014.06.007

[103] Carmody DP, Bennett DS, Lewis M. The effects of prenatal cocaine exposure and gender on inhibitory control and attention. Neurotoxicol Teratol. 2011;33(1):61–68. doi:10.1016/j.ntt.2010.07.004

[104] Chiriboga CA, Starr D, Kuhn L, Wasserman GA. Prenatal cocaine exposure and prolonged focus attention. Poor infant information processing ability or precocious maturation of attentional systems? Dev Neurosci. 2009;31(1–2):149–158. doi:10.1159/000207502

[105] Underbjerg M, Kesmodel US, Landrø NI, Bakketeig L, Grove J, Wimberley T, Kilburn TR, Særke C, Thorsen P, Mortensen EL. The effects of low to moderate alcohol consumption and binge drinking in early pregnancy on selective and sustained attention in 5-year-old children. BJOG. 2012;119(10):1211–1221. doi:10.1111/j.1471-0528.2012.03396.x

[106] Han JY, Kwon HJ, Ha M, Paik KC, Lim MH, Gyu Lee S, Yoo SJ, Kim EJ. The effects of prenatal exposure to alcohol and environmental tobacco smoke on risk for ADHD: a large population-based study. Psychiatry Res. 2015;225(1–2):164–168. doi:10.1016/j.psychres.2014.11.009

[107] Yolton K, Cornelius M, Ornoy A, McGough J, Makris S, Schantz S. Exposure to neurotoxicants and the development of attention deficit hyperactivity disorder and its related behaviors in childhood. Neurotoxicol Teratol. 2014;44:30–45. doi:10.1016/j.ntt.2014.05.003

[108] Salzwedel A, Grewen K, Vachet C, Gerig G, Lin W, Gao W. Prenatal drug exposure affects neonatal brain functional connectivity. J Neurosci. 2015;35(14):5860–5869. doi:10.1523/JNEUROSCI.4333-14.2015

[109] Fox M, Snyder A, Vincent J, Corbetta M, Van Essen D, Raichle M. From The cover: the human brain is intrinsically organized into dynamic, anticorrelated functional networks. Proc Natl Acad Sci USA. 2005;102(27):9673–9678. doi:10.1073/pnas.0504136102

[110] Kelly A, Uddin L, Biswal B, Castellanos F, Milham M. Competition between functional brain networks mediates behavioral variability. Neuroimage. 2008;39(1):527–537. doi:10.1016/j.neuroimage.2007.08.008

[111] Gao W, Lin W. Frontal parietal control network regulates the anti-correlated default and dorsal attention networks. Hum Brain Mapp. 2011;33(1):192–202. doi:10.1002/hbm.21204

[112] Rao H, Wang J, Giannetta J, Korczykowski M, Shera D, Avants B, et al. Altered resting cerebral blood flow in adolescents with in utero cocaine exposure revealed by perfusion functional MRI. Pediatrics. 2007;120(5):e1245–e1254. doi:10.1542/peds.2006-2596

[113] Li Z, Santhanam P, Coles C, Lynch M, Hamann S, Peltier S, et al. Increased "default mode" activity in adolescents prenatally exposed to cocaine. Hum Brain Mapp. 2011;32(5):759–770. doi:10.1002/hbm.21059

[114] Santhanam P, Coles C, Li Z, Li L, Lynch M, Hu X. Default mode network dysfunction in adults with prenatal alcohol exposure. Psychiatry Res. 2011;194(3):354–362. doi: 10.1016/j.pscychresns.2011.05.004

[115] Verbruggen F, Logan G. Response inhibition in the stop-signal paradigm. Trends Cogn Sci. 2008;12(11):418–424. doi:10.1016/j.tics.2008.07.005

[116] Verbruggen F, Logan G. Models of response inhibition in the stop-signal and stop-change paradigms. Neurosci Biobehav Rev. 2009;33(5):647–661. doi:10.1016/j.neubiorev.2008.08.014

[117] Bennett D, Mohamed F, Carmody D, Bendersky M, Patel S, Khorrami M, et al. Response inhibition among early adolescents prenatally exposed to tobacco: an fMRI study. Neurotoxicol Teratol. 2009;31(5):283–290. doi:10.1016/j.ntt.2009.03.003

[118] Smith A, Fried P, Hogan M, Cameron I. Effects of prenatal marijuana on response inhibition: an fMRI study of young adults. Neurotoxicol Teratol. 2004;26(4):533–542. doi:10.1016/j.ntt.2004.04.004

[119] Fryer S, Tapert S, Mattson S, Paulus M, Spadoni A, Riley E. Prenatal alcohol exposure affects frontal-striatal BOLD response during inhibitory control. Alcohol Clin Exp Res. 2007;31(8):1415–1424. doi:10.1111/j.1530-0277.2007.00443.x

[120] Ware A, Infante M, O'Brien J, Tapert S, Jones K, Riley E, et al. An fMRI study of behavioral response inhibition in adolescents with and without histories of heavy prenatal alcohol exposure. Behav Brain Res. 2015;278:137–146. doi:10.1016/j.bbr.2014.09.037

[121] Sheinkopf S, Lester B, Sanes J, Eliassen J, Hutchison E, Seifer R, et al. Functional MRI and response inhibition in children exposed to cocaine in utero. Dev Neurosci. 2009;31(1–2):159–166. doi:10.1159/000207503

[122] Longo C, Fried P, Cameron I, Smith A. The long-term effects of prenatal nicotine exposure on response inhibition: an fMRI study of young adults. Neurotoxicol Teratol. 2013;39:9–18. doi:10.1016/j.ntt.2013.05.007

[123] Rubia K. Neuro-anatomic evidence for the maturational delay hypothesis of ADHD. Proc Natl Acad Sci USA. 2007;104(50):19663–19664. doi:10.1073/pnas.0710329105

[124] Bunge S, Dudukovic N, Thomason M, Vaidya C, Gabrieli J. Immature frontal lobe contributions to cognitive control in children. Neuron. 2002;33(2):301–311. doi:10.1016/S0896-6273(01)00583-9

[125] Casey B, Trainor R, Orendi J, Schubert A, Nystrom L, Giedd J, et al. A developmental functional MRI study of prefrontal activation during performance of a go-no-go task. J Cogn Neurosci. 1997;9(6):835–847. doi:10.1162/jocn.1997.9.6.835

[126] Tamm L, Menon V, Reiss A. Maturation of brain function associated with response inhibition. J Am Acad Child Adolesc Psychiatry. 2002;41(10):1231–1238. doi:10.1097/00004583-200210000-00013

[127] Braver T, Cohen J, Nystrom L, Jonides J, Smith E, Noll D. A parametric study of prefrontal cortex involvement in human working memory. Neuroimage. 1997;5(1):49–62. doi:10.1006/nimg.1996.0247

[128] Rypma B, Prabhakaran V, Desmond J, Glover G, Gabrieli J. Load-dependent roles of frontal brain regions in the maintenance of working memory. Neuroimage. 1999;9(2):216–226. doi:10.1006/nimg.1998.0404

[129] Bennett D, Mohamed F, Carmody D, Malik M, Faro S, Lewis M. Prenatal tobacco exposure predicts differential brain function during working memory in early adolescence: a preliminary investigation. Brain Imaging Behav. 2012;7(1):49–59. doi:10.1007/s11682-012-9192-1

[130] Smith A, Longo C, Fried P, Hogan M, Cameron I. Effects of marijuana on visuospatial working memory: an fMRI study in young adults. Psychopharmacology. 2010;210(3):429–438. doi:10.1016/j.ntt.2005.12.008

[131] O'Hare E, Lu L, Houston S, Bookheimer S, Mattson S, O'Connor M, et al. Altered frontal-parietal functioning during verbal working memory in children and adolescents with heavy prenatal alcohol exposure. Hum Brain Mapp. 2009;30(10):3200–3208. doi:10.1002/hbm.20741

[132] Malisza K, Allman A, Shiloff D, Jakobson L, Longstaffe S, Chudley A. Evaluation of spatial working memory function in children and adults with fetal alcohol spectrum disorders: a functional magnetic resonance imaging study. Pediatr Res. 2005;58(6):1150–1157. doi:10.1203/01.pdr.0000185479.92484.a1

[133] Spadoni A, Bazinet A, Fryer S, Tapert S, Mattson S, Riley E. BOLD response during spatial working memory in youth with heavy prenatal alcohol exposure. Alcohol Clin Exp Res. 2009;33(12):2067–2076. doi:10.111.j.1530-0277.2009.01046.x

[134] Astley S, Aylward E, Olson H, Kerns K, Brooks A, Coggins T, et al. Magnetic resonance imaging outcomes from a comprehensive magnetic resonance study of children with fetal alcohol spectrum disorders. Alcohol Clin Exp Res. 2009;33(10):1671–1689. doi:10.1111.j.1530-0277.2009.01004.x

[135] Roussotte F, Bramen J, Nunez S, Quandt L, Smith L, O'Connor M, et al. Abnormal brain activation during working memory in children with prenatal exposure to drugs of

abuse: the effects of methamphetamine, alcohol, and polydrug exposure. NeuroImage. 2011;54(4):3067–3075. doi:10.1016.j.neuroimage.2010.10.072

[136] Lu L, Johnson A, O'Hare E, Bookheimer S, Smith L, O'Connor M, et al. Effects of prenatal methamphetamine exposure on verbal memory revealed with functional magnetic resonance imaging. J Dev Behav Pediatr. 2009;30(3):185–192. doi:10.1097.DBP.0b013e3181a7ee6b

[137] Norman A, O'Brien J, Spadoni A, Tapert S, Jones K, Riley E, et al. A functional magnetic resonance imaging study of spatial working memory in children with prenatal alcohol exposure: contribution of familial history of alcohol use disorders. Alcohol Clin Exp Res. 2012;37(1):132–140. doi:10.1111/j.1530-0277.2012.01880.x

[138] Malisza K, Buss J, Bolster R, de Gervai P, Woods-Frohlich L, Summers R, et al. Comparison of spatial working memory in children with prenatal alcohol exposure and those diagnosed with ADHD: a functional magnetic resonance imaging study. J Neurodev Disord. 2012;4(1):12. doi:10.1186/1866-1955-4-12

[139] Li Z, Coles C, Lynch M, Hamann S, Peltier S, LaConte S, et al. Prenatal cocaine exposure alters emotional arousal regulation and its effects on working memory. Neurotoxicol Teratol. 2009;31(6):342–348. doi:10.1016/j.ntt.2009.08.005

[140] Friston K, Jezzard P, Turner R. Analysis of functional MRI time-series. Hum Brain Mapp. 1994;1(2):153–171. doi:10.1002/hbm.460010207

[141] Lv J, Jiang X, Li X, Zhu D, Zhao S, Zhang T, et al. Assessing effects of prenatal alcohol exposure using group-wise sparse representation of fMRI data. Psychiatry Res. 2015;233(2):254–268. doi:10.1016/j.pscychresns.2015.07.012

[142] Liu T. A few thoughts on brain ROIs. Brain Imaging Behav. 2011;5(3):189–202. doi:10.1007/s11682-011-9123-6

[143] Li Z, Santhanam P, Coles C, Ellen Lynch M, Hamann S, Peltier S, et al. Prenatal cocaine exposure alters functional activation in the ventral prefrontal cortex and its structural connectivity with the amygdala. Psychiatry Res. 2013;213(1):47–55. doi:10.1016/j.pscychresns.2012.12.005

[144] Fan Y, Rao H, Hurt H, Giannetta J, Korczykowski M, Shera D, Avants BB, Gee JC, Wang J, Shen D. Multivariate examination of brain abnormality using both structural and functional MRI. NeuroImage. 2007 Jul 15;36(4):1189–99. doi:10.1016/j.neuroimage.2007.04.009